Cancer, Communication and Aging

HEALTH COMMUNICATION
Gary L. Kreps, *series editor*

Communication in Recovery: Perspectives on Twelve-Step Groups
Lynette S. Eastland, Sandra L. Herndon, & Jeanine R. Barr (eds.)

Communicating in the Clinic: Negotiating Frontstage and Backstage Teamwork
Laura L. Ellingson

Media-Mediated Aids
Linda K. Fuller (ed.)

Cancer-Related Information Seeking
J. David Johnson

Changing the Culture of College Drinking: A Socially Situated Health Communication Campaign
Linda C. Lederman & Lea P. Stewart

Handbook of Communication and Cancer Care
Dan O'Hair, Gary L. Kreps, & Lisa Sparks, (eds.)

Crisis Communication and the Public Health
Matthew Seeger and *Timothy Sellnow (eds.)*

Cancer, Communication and Aging
Lisa Sparks, Dan O'Hair, & Gary L. Kreps (eds.)

Cancer and Death: A Love Story in two Voices
Leah Vande Berg & Nick Trujillo

forthcoming

A Natural History of Family Cancer
Wayne Beach

E-Health: The Advent of Online Cancer Information Systems
Pamela Whitten, Gary L. Kreps, and Matthew S. Eastin (eds.)

Communicating Spirituality in Health Care
Maggie Wills (ed.)

Cancer, Communication and Aging

edited by

Lisa Sparks
Chapman University

H. Dan O'Hair
University of Oklahoma

Gary L. Kreps
George Mason University

HAMPTON PRESS, INC.
CRESSKILL, NJ 07626

Printed in the United States of America

Library of Congress Cataloging-in-Publication Data

Cancer, communication and aging / edited by Lisa Sparks, H. Dan O'Hair, Gary L. Kreps

p. cm. -- (Health communication)

Includes bibliographic references and indexes.

ISBN 978-1-57273-754-9 (hardbound) -- ISBN 978-1-57273-755-6 (paperbound)

1. Geriatric oncology. 2. Communication in medicine. 3. Older people--communication. I. Sparks, Lisa. II. O'Hair, Dan. III. Kreps, Gary L. IV. Series: Health communication (Cresskill, N.J.)

[DNLM: 1. Neoplasms-psychology. 2. Aged. 3. Communication. 4. Interpersonal Relations. 5. Neoplasms--nursing. 6. Patients--psychology.
QZ 200 C2151228 2008]

RC281.A34C363 2008

618.97'6994--dc22

2008017231

Hampton Press, Inc.
23 Broadway
Cresskill, NJ 07626

Contents

1

Conceptualizing Cancer, Communication and Aging

New Directions for Research

Lisa Sparks

Chapman University

H. Dan O'Hair

University of Oklahoma

Gary L. Kreps

George Mason University

Cancer is one of the most significant health challenges facing society, being the second leading cause of death in the United States (American Cancer Society, 2006). According to the Centers for Disease Control and Prevention (CDC, 2006) cancer is largely controllable through prevention, early detection, and treatment. Reducing the nation's cancer burden requires reducing the prevalence of the behavioral and environmental factors that increase cancer risk. Cancer screening services and high-quality treatment must be continually available and accessible, particularly to medically underserved populations (CDC, 2006). The CDC's Center for Healthy Aging Community Outreach and Demonstration Project identifies the following 10 keys to healthy aging, by addressing the following 10 conditions that are considered essential for maintaining health in older adults:

1. Prevent bone loss and muscle weakness.
2. Control blood pressure.
3. Increase physical activity.
4. Regulate blood sugar.
5. Stop smoking.
6. Maintain social contact.
7. Participate in cancer screening.
8. Get regular immunizations.
9. Lower cholesterol.
10. Combat depression.

Many of these conditions are linked to cancer. Health-damaging behaviors, particularly tobacco use, lack of physical activity, and poor eating habits, are major contributors to the nation's leading chronic diseases including cancer (CDC, 2006a). Clearly, promoting and communicating healthy behavior choices, effective communication, education, community policies and practices, is vital to reducing the cancer burden—especially for the older adult population.

Cancer is an older adult disease (Wallace, 2001). According to the American Cancer Society (2006) more than 1 million people get cancer each year and a majority of those diagnosed are older adults. Approximately one out of every two American men and one out of every three American women will be diagnosed with cancer at some point during their lifetime. Anyone can get cancer at any age; however, about 77% of all cancers are diagnosed in people aged 55 and older. More than 25% of all deaths in the United States are attributable to cancer (Wallace, 2001) and only cardiovascular disease accounts for more deaths in adults aged 65 and older. Of all deaths, 25% are attributable to cancer for adults between the ages of 65 and 74. Furthermore, about 20% of all deaths are caused by cancer for those aged between 74 and 84. After the age of 85, the percentage of adults dying of cancer decreases to about 12% (Solomon, 1999). Males over the age of 65 are most likely to contract to cancers of the lung, prostate, colon, rectum, urinary system, and bladder. Females of the same age cohort are most susceptible to cancers of the breast, colon, rectum, lung, and pancreas (Solomon, 1999).

Old age has generally been associated with lower competence, independence, health, and vitality, but more benevolence and wisdom (Harwood et al., 1996, Harwood et al., 2001; Nelson, 2002, 2005). That said, the distinctive aging characteristics older adults bring to the cancer context has remained relatively unexplored. Notwithstanding the significant attention afforded the study of physician–patient communication (e.g., Cegala, 1997; Cegala & Broz, 2003; Dutta-Bergman, 2005; Thompson & Parrott, 2002), relatively recent research has emerged germane to salient and more specific issues of cancer communication (O'Hair, Kreps, & Sparks, 2007), although relatively few studies have centered on cancer communication and aging (see Sparks, 2003), particularly from such perspectives grounded in communication and aging research such as intergroup and/or social identity (see, however, Harwood & Sparks, 2003). Such research addressing the unique issues of cancer communication and aging has certainly flourished since 2001. Biomedical scientists, physician–researchers, other medical personnel, and social scientists have made great progress in cancer care research over the last few decades and patients and families are the beneficiaries of such research. The foundation of cancer communication helps to prevent cancer incidents via health prevention campaigns to change health behaviors, by promotion of early detection through health campaigns, through diagnoses and treatment in communicating with health care providers, and to survivors and their family members in helping them to communicate more effectively about their illness as it alters their activities of daily living, and for many, their ways of dealing with the delicate issues surrounding death and dying. Furthermore, the CDC and research at the National Cancer Institute (NCI) claim that more than 9.8 million people in the United States are cancer survivors (CDC, 2004) with the greatest proportion of cancer diagnoses existing with the older adult population.

Cancer is a disease of older adults and their family members. By affecting the diagnosed, the diagnoser, the health system, and the family system, it changes the ways in which we communicate and process relevant and important health information to make informed decisions. Cancer impacts our organizations, businesses, schools, and our nation. It is vitally important that we understand how communicating about cancer with older adults and their family members in appropriate and effective ways can reduce incidence and mortality, understand complicated diagnoses, enhance treatment and survivorship, and can even reduce malpractice. In fact, according to Kaplan (2004) malpractice is best reduced by communicating clear evidence that the health care provider has fully informed the patient about the risks and benefits of intervention, and offered the patient the opportunity to make an informed choice. Health care providers are negatively evaluated when providers fail to disclose risks and when medicine promises more than can be delivered. Thus, cancer communication is a crucial component of healthcare delivery.

As O'Hair, Kreps, and Sparks (2007) stated in the *Handbook of Communication and Cancer Care*, perhaps the one aspect of cancer care that has received little research attention until recently is communication. Compelling, empirically based research in cancer communication did not emerge until the 1990s when funding for communication research began to find its way into the hands of communication scholars and research-practitioners. A major movement for this funding was the development of the

Health Communication and Informatics Research Branch of the NCI, and the development of cancer communications research as a significant area of investment (Kreps, 2005). Through various programs and funding mechanisms, cancer communication research has been dramatically increasing (Kreps, 2003b).

Given that a cancer diagnosis is one of the most significant events in an individual's life (Sorenson, Rossel, & Holm, 2004) and treatment has high personal relevance (Fallowfield, Ford, & Lewis, 1994) for the patient as well as those caring for the patient, it is not surprising that effective and appropriate communication is a crucial component of cancer care. Being diagnosed with cancer is often frightening for all involved and treatments can often be quite complex and uncomfortable. Some types of cancer are more easily managed than others. For example, although breast, colon, and skin cancers are still quite dangerous, especially when diagnosed at advanced stages of development, many patients who are able to detect these diseases in the early stages are living full lives for many years. The critical issue we stress is that although being diagnosed with cancer is not necessarily a path to a life cut short, it also is a disease that must be continually and carefully managed. It is a health problem that demands attention, examination, and decision making. An extraordinary number of issues must be considered in the conduct of cancer care, not the least of which are critical communication factors, including gathering and interpreting relevant health information, eliciting coordination among interdependent patients, providers, and family members, and/or caregivers, and providing social support and promoting psychosocial adjustment (O'Hair et al., 2003). The contributors to this volume make convincing cases that communication is an intrinsic element of cancer care, and holds unique communicative challenges for older adults. Although we understand communication processes much better than we did even 10 years ago, there is still much work to do before we arrive at levels of excellence in cancer communication, particularly for the aged. It is important that we gain a deeper understanding of the complexities involved in effective and appropriate communication with patients who have cancer across the continuum of cancer care from diagnosis to survivorship. Effective health communication is the crucial link that can provide and encourage cancer prevention, inform cancer detection and diagnosis, guide cancer treatment, support successful cancer survivorship, and finally promote the best end-of-life care in unique ways (Kreps, 2003a). To influence entrenched health behaviors, communicative messages of all types need to be relevant and compelling, with appropriate and pertinent health information that provides direction and rationale for making the best health-related decisions and adopting health-preserving behaviors. By gaining this knowledge, researchers and health care providers can give better cancer care to patients, and partners and family members can more easily acquire health information that will help them to help themselves in more productive and efficient ways.

The sections of the volume are arranged into the following three parts: Communicating About Cancer Information and Aging: Issues of Prevention, Diagnosis, Treatment, and Identity; Communicating About Cancer Survivorship and Aging: Issues of Comfort, Healing, and Social Support; Communicating About Cancer Contexts and Aging: Issues of Cultural Values, Spirituality, and End of Life.

COMMUNICATING ABOUT CANCER INFORMATION AND AGING: ISSUES OF PREVENTION, DIAGNOSIS, TREATMENT, AND IDENTITY

Cancer is a dreadful disease in terms of how it impacts an individual's life. Just days earlier, the patient was living life with all of the normal annoyances, joys, and pains and then life as it has been known is suddenly turned emotionally and physically upside-down. Life is never the same after a cancer occurrence. Life with cancer brings about unfathomable psychological and emotional turmoil as patients face the fact that they now have cancer and many of their same-age friends and family members have not received a cancer diagnosis in their lifetime. Cancer often results in new ways of living and unknown paths toward preparing for dying.

The first part of this book begins with a selection of chapters that focus on some aspect of how older adults deal with issues of prevention, diagnosis, treatment, and how their unique identities play a role. In Chapter 2, Sparks and Turner review previous research on message processing and health information germane to the older adult population as they navigate the cancer experience.

Sparks and Turner analyze the ways by which cancer communication messages can be designed and delivered to match the specific communication skills, needs, and pre-dispositions of the older adult population. The authors offer suggestions for specificity in designing messages and interventions focused on encouraging aging patients to be active participants in health communication environments, particularly when it comes to cancer care by focusing on effective and appropriately tailored message strategies. Sparks and Turner take a perspective grounded in life-span development by focusing on complexities of particular age-related communication barriers that may hinder or help in caring for the aging patient by providing an application of the Selection, Optimization, and Compensation Model. The authors offer a summary of ways of understanding the various elements of older adult cognitive and emotional processing of difficult messages and the impact of other age-related communication barriers so that providers of all types can begin to construct interpersonal and mediated messages in systematic and understandable ways. The authors offer a summary of the ways in which tailored research-based messages will have a greater likelihood of reaching the aging patient diagnosed with cancer.

Chapter 3 by Parrott, Krieger, Silk, and Egbert explores findings related to indirect relationships between age and education for Internet use to search for health information. The authors examine situations in which an information-rich resource exists that may motivate aging adults to participate in treatments including clinical trials, extend their life spans, and enhance the quality of their lives, but may be largely inaccessible because of the characteristics of the technology. Aging adults and online cancer information comprise such a dilemma. The authors discuss how this potential problem represents a "digital divide" of sorts that is not so much related to the accessibility of computers and related technology, but to the usability and accuracy of Internet materials.

In Chapter 4 by Nussbaum, Fisher, Baringer, and Kundrat, the authors explain interesting ways of connecting health, communication, and aging by examining the unique aspects inherent in communicating about cancer with older adults. The authors posit how the diagnosis of cancer not only greatly impacts the patient, but also impacts the formal and informal relationship support networks of the individual who must now cope with the disease. The authors highlight the significant interpersonal communication and relationship issues that affect the overall quality of life for an older individual who has been diagnosed with cancer. The discussion concludes that not only is the diagnosis of cancer life changing for the patient, but it also changes the dynamics of each relationship between the older adult who has cancer and those who will help to care for the patient both in a formal institutional setting and at home.

Particularly germane to health communication and aging issues, the focus of Sparks' and Harwood's Chapter 5 centers on issues of social identity and health from an intergroup perspective. The chapter builds on research from an earlier article (Harwood & Sparks, 2003), where the authors argued for the general applicability of Social Identity Theory (SIT; Tajfel & Turner, 1986; see also Harwood & Giles, 2005) to the health communication literature, and most specifically to issues surrounding cancer diagnosis, treatment, and recovery. Sparks and Harwood further explain that SIT is a broad sociopsychologically grounded theory of intergroup relations, which focuses particularly on the importance people ascribe to their identities, the ways in which they protect them, and the ways in which they respond when their identities are threatened. It deals primarily with identification with large social groups (age, culture, sexuality, etc.), but can also be applied to smaller and more specialized groups (an alma mater, a family, a victim of a particular disease). Building on Harwood and Sparks (2003), the authors introduce an intriguing and potentially useful social identity model of cancer communication. The model aims to elaborate on the role of social identity processes in determining prevention, preparation and response strategies to cancer.

COMMUNICATING ABOUT CANCER SURVIVORSHIP AND AGING: ISSUES OF COMFORT, HEALING, AND SOCIAL SUPPORT

The second section shifts attention to some of the more salient survivorship issues inherent in cancer communication research. This part opens with a particularly compelling chapter by du Pré and Ray, who argue that the evolving meanings that arise from queries during the cancer experience such as those centering around the "why cancer?" and "why me?" are personal, social, and cultural. The authors state that the true answers lie more in the realm of social interaction (communication) than biomedicine. The stories presented in this chapter show the reader lessons about the power of faith and emotional strength. The authors explain that such stories are important in the communication exchange, both for the teller and the listener. Finally, du Pré and Ray argue that if there is one overall lesson to be learned, it is that no experience is entirely good or bad but instead there is possibility within the miracles that emerge within the most heart-wrenching moments as well as unexpected moments of serenity that sometimes arise from the painful experiences.

Taking a slightly different but complementary perspective, Anderson and Geist-Martin (Chapter 7) explore one family's story of cancer survivorship by examining the role narratives play in their lives. The authors specifically examine the narratives of the cancer survivor and her family members as they struggle to cope with their situation, provide support for one another, and consider their changing personal identities. The study first advocates the need for learning about the composition of survivor identities over the course of a life-threatening illness. The authors then reveal how this study attempts to understand how illness survivors and their family members use narratives as a method of communicating their changing identities. Finally, the authors provide a discussion about the ways in which communicating illness is often perceived as "taboo," however they argue that the study sets the stage to encourage others to be a part of the participants' stories and learn more about why those stories are often concealed.

In Chapter 8, Wilmoth, Davis, and Sanders describe key issues for health care educators and health care workers (HCW) to consider when working with African-American women diagnosed with breast cancer, focusing specifically on the ways Black women communicate about the diagnostic process and the subsequent impact of breast cancer on their lives. The authors accomplish this goal by linking intercultural and interethnic communication and patient-to-HCW communication, and by identifying African-American women's ways of speaking in focus groups about their breast cancer experience. The authors provide analysis and insights to HCWs who have been educated in the mainstream medical model and how this impacts communication and health care in such intercultural and interethnic interactions.

In their chapter, Robinson, Turner, and Thompson focus on social support issues germane to the older adult population. They first provide a comprehensive review of the social support literature and then more specifically examine the various ways patients with cancer need assistance as they battle the disease and how technology plays an increasingly supportive role in their lives. The authors first describe and define social support by stating that it tends to refer to those situations where one person provides help or services to others. They then explain the ways in which social support and supportive communicative relationships have been shown to play an important role in our mental and physical health. Finally, the authors provide an intriguing and relevant discussion of "optimal matching" and computer use of older adults as well as how via the selection, optimization, and compensation processes, older adults can more easily maintain satisfying, successful and efficacious lives by selecting behaviors that will help them fulfill their needs at a reasonable cost.

In Query and Wright's complementary Chapter 10, the potential of online support groups for older adults with cancer and their lay caregivers is explored in terms of potential health benefits. The chapter begins by reviewing literature on computer-mediated support groups for older adults, individuals with cancer, and caregivers. The authors then present a model of online support-group participation based on communication competence, social support, and coping theory, social network theory, and theories of computer-mediated communication. Finally, the authors provide a discussion of the implications of this model for individuals with cancer and their lay caregivers.

In the final contribution of this section, Harzold and Sparks (Chapter 11) provide an interesting study of the impact of such communicative processes that adult children go through during the parent's cancer experience. This study stems from the first author's thesis where a life-span developmental communicative approach was used to examine the relationships between communication competency, humor orientation, and relational satisfaction in the older adult parent–adult child dyad when the parent has been diagnosed with cancer. The authors found that communication competency is associated with humor orientation and relational satisfaction while humor itself may operate in more complex ways within the family cancer context. Communication competency had a significantly positive correlation with both humor orientation and relational satisfaction, whereas humor orientation was not significantly correlated with relational satisfaction. Finally, the authors provide content analysis of open-ended data, which showed that discussing diagnosis and treatment procedures with children most often resulted in a satisfying conversation, whereas withholding information had an adverse affect, and humor was often used as a coping or relief function for discussing side effects of cancer treatment.

COMMUNICATING ABOUT CANCER CONTEXTS AND AGING: ISSUES OF CULTURAL VALUES, SPIRITUALITY, AND END OF LIFE

This section raises a number of issues that seek to identify issues of cultural values, spirituality, and end of life to help patients cope with their internal strife. In Chapter 12, Pecchioni, Krieger, Sparks, Pitts, and Ota provide an exceptionally compelling examination of the ways in which culture influences the social context of cancer among older adults. The authors open the chapter with a discussion of the role of culture in social life. They then investigate intersections of communication and aging with a focus on Eastern and Western cultural perspectives. Finally, the authors use the intriguing context of cancer clinical trials as an example to illustrate how culture shapes the experience of aging and cancer.

Also taking a cultural perspective, Chapter 13 by Villagran and Hoffman focuses more specifically on issues germane to the Latino/a population. The authors describe that minority patients with cancer who enter into the health care system often must overcome unique organizational barriers that arise based on cultural and linguistic differences between themselves and their providers. The authors introduce some of the relevant programs that have emerged in recent years in an effort to provide organizational socialization of new cancer patients into health organizations and how they call for the inclusion of specific accommodations to make services more accessible to minority and limited English proficiency (LEP) patients (Hablamos Juntos, 2005).

The authors provide a brief review of literature related to Latino cultural issues and values specific to cancer care, and then propose a culturally appropriate model of organizational communication to improve Latino patient socialization in the cancer context. Villagran and Hoffman provide a compelling case encouraging health organizations seeking to reduce health disparities among Latinos to consider the role of cultural values in patients' information management and decision making. They end with a discussion of how such values can then be used to create culture-specific strategies to increase support for intended health outcomes.

In Chapter 14, Egbert, Sparks, Kreps, and du Pré expand our thinking about the role spirituality plays for older adults diagnosed with cancer. These authors take up a little studied cancer phenomenon, but one that is highly salient for many patients with cancer by exploring spirituality and cancer. As the stories in this chapter illustrate, the authors argue that a key component of coping with cancer is managing uncertainties and identifying meaning within the experience. In this respect, older adults may have an advantage over younger adults. The authors provide a discussion of the role communication plays in facilitating coping with cancer through spirituality, a person's search for meaning in life's experiences. The authors then conceptualize "spirituality" and how this concept connects with related terms such as *religion* and *religiosity*. In their effort to present a broad overview of spiritual coping mechanisms for people living with cancer, the authors chose to focus on the concept of spirituality, as opposed to religiosity, arguing that spirituality is the more inclusive term. The authors then provide an analysis by examining individuals' search for meaning within cancer experiences. They conclude the chapter by arguing that despite cultural assumptions that often suggest that cancer is a dreadful diagnosis that leads to death, closer observation and analysis reveals that, along with the fear and uncertainty of cancer often comes unprecedented understanding, awareness, and appreciation for life. Finally, the authors point out that as our understanding of spirituality, meaning, and health grows, our ideas about what constitutes comforting communication may change.

In Chapter 15, Lannamann, Harris, Bakos, and Baker argue that providers and their dying patients are often caught in a dysfunctional interpersonal logic that has emerged within the hospital context. Their impasse delays the palliative care that can relieve physical and emotional suffering, dramatically impacting their quality of life. In an effort to alleviate these potential problems, the authors then propose a dialogic intervention: An ongoing conversation in which patients and their families bring life to their personal meanings for post-diagnosis caregiving decisions and caregiving tasks. Based on multiple theoretical models as well as therapeutic and organizational experience, the authors offer several suggestions for breaking the end-of-life communication impasse. They argue that giving patients and their families the opportunity to self-organize around caregiving will end the end-of-life impasse and suggest that family-centered post-diagnosis care planning conversations with patients and their loved ones will better prepare them to accept hospice earlier than they do today. The authors conclude by proposing that patients and their significant others who engage in repeated family-centered care planning scenarios will overcome the impasse that exists in the current decision-making process.

PROLOGUE TO THE VOLUME

The goal of this chapter was to introduce the major communication approaches to cancer, communication and aging that are covered in the chapters that follow. It is our hope that the chapters in this book will encourage concerted investigation into the important functions and strategies for effective communication with older adults confronting cancer care. Researchers have the potential to conduct important studies that will inform health communication practice, providing health care consumers and providers with evidence-based strategies for using communication to build meaningful collaborative relationships that can help reduce cancer risks, incidence, morbidity, and mortality, while enhancing quality of life across the continuum of cancer care. Health communication scholars have an overabundance of theoretical, methodological, and pragmatic communication-based approaches that can greatly contribute to enhancing our understanding of the many complex yet unique communicative contexts of cancer care (O'Hair, 2003; Sparks, 2003). Health communication scholars must engage the health care community in cancer care research and actively translate research findings into strategies for effective cancer care. It is our sincere hope that the chapters in this book will begin this important process of applying communication research and theory to enhancing cancer care.

ACKNOWLEDGMENTS

Many of the ideas within these chapters were initially derived from the first symposium on Cancer, Communication and Aging held at George Mason University in 2002. This volume is a dramatic extension of those underdeveloped ideas, which have now materialized into incredible scholarly contributions to the germane issues that arise in the cancer communication and aging area. The editors extend deep appreciation to the contributors who shared their scholarship and experiences in each of the chapters contained here. We are also deeply grateful to Barbara Bernstein, Publisher of Hampton Press, for having the faith and diligence in seeing this important project come to fruition. Finally, we thank our families who gave us the time to bring this book together, Daniele, Elena, Arianna, Marcia, Grant, John O., Mary John, Erica, Jonathan, Stephanie, Becky, David. We also deeply appreciate the inspiration from our many friends and family members whom have confronted cancer. This book is dedicated to you and to all of the cancer patients, providers and their families.

This book is dedicated to dear friend Steve Mandell who is the ultimate ultramarathoner of friendship and life. Steve-o we love you!

Proceeds from this volume are being dedicated to the Association for Cancer Online Resources which provides a very important and powerful communication forum for tens of thousands of cancer survivors and their loved ones.

REFERENCES

American Cancer Society. (2006). *Cancer statistics.* Retrieved June 19, 2006 from http://www.cancer.org/docroot/CRI/content/CRI_2_4_1x_Who_gets_cancer.asp?sitearea=

Centers for Disease Control and Prevention. (2004). Cancer Survivorship—United States, 1971—2001. *Morbidity and Mortality Weekly Report, 53*(24), 526-529.

Centers for Disease Control and Prevention. (2006a). Center for Healthy Aging Community Outreach and Demonstration Project. http://www.cdc.gov/prc/research-projects/core-projects/center-healthy-aging-community-outreach.htm

Centers for Disease Control and Prevention. (2006b). Health information for older adults. http://www.cdc.gov/aging/info.htm

Cegala, D. J. (1997). A study of doctors' and patients' patterns of information exchange and relational communication during a primary care consultation: Implications for communication skills training. *Journal of Health Communication,* 2, 169-194.

Cegala, D. J., & Broz, S. L. (2003). Provider and patient communication skills training. In T. L. Thompson, A. M. Dorsey, K. I. Miller, & R. Parrot (Eds.), *Handbook of health communication* (pp. 95-120). Mahwah, NJ: Erlbaum.

Dutta-Bergman, M. (2005). The relation between health-orientation, provider-patient communication, and satisfaction: An individual-difference approach. *Health Communication, 18,* 291-303.

Fallowfield, L., Ford, S., & Lewis, S. (1994). Information preferences of patients with cancer. *Lancet, 344,* 1576.

Hablamos Juntos (2005). A program of the Robert Wood Johnson Foundation. Retrieved August 9, 2005, from http://www.hablamosjuntos.org/default.asp

Harwood, J., & Giles, H. (2005). *Intergroup communication: Multiple perspectives.* New York: Peter Lang.

Harwood, J., Giles, H., McCann, R.M., Cai, D., Somera, L., Ng, S-H., Gallois, C., & Noels, K.A. (2001). Older adults' trait ratings of three age groups around the Pacific Rim. *Journal of Cross-Cultural Gerontology, 16*, 157-171.

Harwood, J., Giles, H., Ota, H., Pierson, H.D., Gallois, C., Ng, S.H., Lim, T-S., & Somera, L. (1996). College students' trait ratings of three age groups around the Pacific Rim. *Journal of Cross-Cultural Gerontology, 11*, 307-317.

Harwood, J., & Sparks, L. (2003). Social identity and health: An intergroup communication approach to cancer. *Health Communication, 15*, 145-159.

Kaplan, R. M. (2004). Shared medical decision making: A new tool for preventative medicine. *American Journal of Preventative Medicine, 26*(1), 81-83.

Kreps, G.L. (2003a). The impact of communication on cancer risk, incidence, morbidity, mortality, and quality of life. *Health Communication, 15*(2), 163-171.

Kreps, G. L. (2003b). Opportunities for health communication scholarship to shape public health policy and practice: Examples from the National Cancer Institute. In T. Thompson, R. Parrott, K. Miller, and A. Dorsey, (Eds.), *The handbook of health communication* (pp. 609-624), Hillsdale, NJ: Erlbaum.

Kreps, G. L. (2005). Cancer communication research at the National Cancer Institute. In M. Haider (Ed.), *Public health communications utility, values, and challenges*. Sudbury, MA: Jones & Bartlett.

Nelson, T. D. (Ed.). (2002). *Ageism: Stereotyping and prejudice against older persons*. Cambridge, MA: MIT Press.

Nelson, T. D. (Ed.). (2005). Ageism [special issue]. *Journal of Social Issues, 61(2).*

O'Hair, D. (2003). Research traditions in provider–consumer interaction: Implications for cancer care. *Patient Education and Counseling, 50*, 5-8.

O'Hair, D., Villagran, M., Wittenberg, E., Brown, K., Hall, T., Ferguson, M., & Doty, T. (2003). Cancer survivorship and agency model (CSAM): Implications for patient choice, decision making, and influence. *Health Communication, 15*, 193-202.

O'Hair, H. D., Kreps, G. L., & Sparks, L. (Eds.). (2007). *Handbook of communication and cancer care*. Cresskill, NJ: Hampton Press.

O'Hair, H. D., Kreps, G. L., & Sparks, L. (2007). Conceptualizing cancer care and communication. In H. D. O'Hair, L. Sparks, & G. L. Kreps (Eds.), *Handbook of communication and cancer care* (pp. 1-10). Cresskill, NJ: Hampton Press.

Solomon, D. H. (1999). The role of aging processes in aging-dependent diseases. In V. L. Bengsten & K. W. Schaie (Eds.), *Handbook of theories of aging* (pp. 133-150). New York: Springer.

Sorenson, J. B., Rossel, P., & Holm, S. (2004). Patient-physician communication concerning participation in cancer chemotherapy trials. *British Journal of Cancer, 90*, 328-322.

Sparks, L. (Ed.). (2003a). Cancer communication and aging [special Issue]. *Health Communication, 15*(2).

Sparks, L. (2003b). An introduction to cancer communication and aging: Theoretical and research insights. *Health Communication, 15*, 123-132.

Tajfel, H., & Turner, J. C. (1986). The social identity theory of intergroup behavior. In S. Worschel & W. G. Austin (Eds.), *The social psychology of intergroup relations* (2nd ed., pp. 7-24). Chicago: Nelson-Hall.

Thompson, T. L., & Parrott, R. (2002). Interpersonal communication and health care. In M. L. Knapp & J. A. Daly (Eds.), *Handbook of interpersonal communication* (3rd ed., pp. 680-725). Thousand Oaks, CA: Sage.

Wallace, R. B. (2001). Prevention of cancer in the elderly. In E. Swanson, T. Tripp-Reimer, & K. Buckwalter (Eds.), *Health promotion and disease prevention in the older adult: Interventions and recommendations* (pp. 146–155). Springer: New York.

PART I

COMMUNICATING ABOUT CANCER INFORMATION AND AGING

Issues of Prevention, Diagnosis, Treatment, and Identity

2

The Impact of Cognitive and Emotive Communication Barriers on Older Adult Message Processing of Cancer-Related Health Information

New Directions for Research

Lisa Sparks
Chapman University

Monique Mitchell Turner
University of Maryland

For the aging patient, the new cultural world of cancer is frequently burdened with a new technical and medical-oriented language along with a new set of unknown relationships. The focus of this chapter is to highlight the significant potential contributions to our understanding of cancer communication that can be made by integrating scholarship from the communication, aging, and health arenas combined with relevant literature drawn from persuasion and message-processing literature. We must begin to pay attention to the subtle complexities of age-related communication barriers, how older adults use strategies of selection and optimization with compensation to deal with such barriers, and how cognitive barriers can potentially affect message processing and information seeking of cancer information. In order to provide the best care for aging patients, we must first understand such complexities that many older adults face and how cognitive and emotive barriers impact older adult preferences for, and ability to, process messages potentially influencing health outcomes.

OLDER ADULTS AND CANCER

Recent estimates indicate that nearly 9 million Americans have a history of cancer. Cancer was second only to heart disease as the leading cause of death in the United States for those aged 65 and over (NCHS, 2000). Older adults account for 61% of all new cancer cases and 70% of all cancer deaths, and it is estimated that those aged 65 and over have 11 times the cancer risk of those under the age of 65 years (Lewis et al., 2003). Moreover, the number is expected to increase as the U.S. population ages even with increased improvements in early detection and treatment of cancer (Edwards et al., 1997). Cancer survivors aged 65 and older are already estimated to be 16% and rising. Increasingly, older adults are diagnosed with cancer more than any other segment of the population (see Hewitt, Rowland, & Yancik, 2003; Sparks, 2003). What's more is that older adults diagnosed with cancer are the population group over and above any other who are at increased risk for poor communication with health professionals (Adelman & Greene, 2000; Greene & Adelman, 2001, 2002). It is crucial that we begin to understand how to communicate with aging cancer patients across the continuum of cancer care from diagnosis to survivorship. Thus, the study of communication practices during cancer care for the aging patient is critical for improving geriatric care as well as for considering the lives of those affected by the disease. Consequently, the unique aspects of cancer care for the aging patient will become increasingly important.

Research involving the communication of cancer care for the aging patient includes such topics as social identity (Harwood & Sparks, 2003), successful adaptation across the life span (Nussbaum, Baringer, & Kundrat, 2003), narratives (Anderson & Geist-Martin, 2003), palliative care (Ragan, Wittenberg, & Hall, 2003), social support (Robinson & Turner, 2003), communicative competence online (Query & Wright, 2003), decision-making processes (O'Hair et al., 2003), and communicating about cancer risk (Rowan, Sparks, Pecchioni, & Villagran, 2003). Furthermore, Kreps (2003) stated that the study and application of health communication has the greatest potential to help reduce cancer risks, incidence, morbidity, and mortality, while enhancing quality of life across the continuum of cancer care (prevention, detection, diagnosis, treatment, survivorship, and end-of-life care).

In order to implement more sound communicative practices during cancer care, it is crucial that we first begin to understand that just as not all cancer diagnoses are alike, not all patients are alike. Most importantly, not all older adult patients are alike. Younger older adults ranging from 50 to 64 years of age have very different message-processing and information-seeking strategies than their older counterparts (i.e., ages 65-74, 75-99, and 100+!). Also note that individuals of similar chronological age often undergo very different life experiences. These different experiences can influence communication in relationships. One life experience that can differ between individuals of the same chronological age is the presence or absence of a cancer diagnosis. Health care providers of various specialties beyond oncology are often the first to discover the cancer and have to cope with communicating the bad news to the fearful and/or angry patient (Ong et al., 1998).

OLDER ADULTS AND CANCER COMMUNICATION

The impact of such a diagnosis, and subsequent interactions related to it, can be remarkably overwhelming for older adults as well as for those caring for them. Although many older adults have known others who have been diagnosed with cancer, more often than not these individuals have little to no experience with the cancer culture and any norms associated with this unknown world (Sparks, 2003). The communication surrounding each diagnosis for older adult patients must begin to be tailored to account for such complexities and barriers impacting message processing of the older adults including young-old, middle-old, old-old, as well as those reaching 100 years of age and older.

Recognizing the complexities of effective cancer communication with the aging patient must no longer be ignored. Cancer messages must be designed and delivered to match the communication skills, needs, and predispositions of specific audiences such as the older adult population. To influence entrenched health behaviors, messages need to be relevant and compelling, with health information that provides direction and rationale for making the best health-related decisions and adopting health-preserving behaviors (Maibach, Kreps, & Bonaguro, 1996).

Cancer poses a series of significant health threats that demand effective health communication (Kreps & Chapelsky-Massimilla, in press). Effective health communication can encourage cancer prevention, inform cancer detection and diagnosis, guide cancer treatment, support successful cancer survivorship, and finally, promote the best end-of-life care. Implications of this analysis are drawn for directing informed cancer communication research and practice. This chapter sheds light on the powerful potential to strategically use health communication to reduce cancer risks, incidence, morbidity, and mortality, while enhancing quality of life across the continuum of cancer care germane to the aging patient (prevention, detection, diagnosis, treatment, survivorship, and end-of-life care; Byock, 2000; Hiatt & Rimer, 1999). This chapter reviews the unique physical, cognitive, language, and interactive-relationship characteristics of caring for the aging patient as well as the family members connected to the patient in the complex, confusing, and overwhelming cancer-related health environment. It should be evident that age-related physiological changes, cognitive changes, and life experiences of older individuals tend to complicate the ways health care providers and family members care for the aging patient who has been diagnosed with cancer. From a perspective grounded in life-span developmental communication, the notion of understanding the impact of potential cognitive, emotional, and other conversational barriers that are unique to caring for the aging patient is first put forth followed by an explanation of the selection and optimization with compensation model that aids older adults in adjusting to their communicative, psychological, affective, and behavioral environment. Once such conversational barriers are addressed and better understood in terms of older adult adaptation to such deficits across the life span, researchers, practitioners, and family members involved in caring for aging patients will have more clearly defined ways of constructing messages that aging patients will likely comprehend and process, which may contribute to better health outcomes. Cancer messages must be designed specifically for the different segments of the older adult population (e.g., ages 50-64, 65-74, 75-99, 100+). Insight into the unique difficulties of cognitive, emotive, and related communication barriers that get in the way of older adult message-processing and information-seeking strategies is pertinent and long overdue. This chapter attempts to answer that call so that more effective and relevant health campaigns can ultimately be launched to reach this specific, albeit complex and interesting aging population. Persuasion and health communication scholars alike must focus on designing messages and interventions focused on encouraging patients of all ages to be active participants in health communication environments, particularly within the complex cancer environment.

COGNITIVE PROCESSING OF CANCER-RELATED MESSAGES

Developing the most effective communication to encourage cancer detection and prevention assumes that the patient will engage in message-relevant thinking. That is, health practitioners and scholars develop effective messages hoping that the message will gain the attention of the audience, the audience will read and/or listen to the message, and the audience will ultimately engage in thoughtful message processing. Early research on thoughtful processing of persuasive messages focused on issues such as the time and attention allocated to the message, the comprehension of the message content, and the acceptance of the message conclusions (Hovland, Janis, & Kelley, 1953;

Todorov, Chaiken, & Henderson, 2002). Yet, we know that although people can carefully process health messages they do not always do so.

According to the Heuristic Systematic Model (Chaiken, 1980) and the theoretically similar Elaboration Likelihood Model (ELM) people will process messages via systematic processing, heuristic processing, or both. When people process a health message heuristically, they consider few message cues, and instead form their judgment based on simple decision making. For instance, the patient may read a Web site encouraging meditation as a therapy for cancer. The Web site is written, ostensibly, by a medical doctor. Thus, the patient thinks "medical doctors can be trusted" and believes the Web site instead of critically thinking about (and cross-checking) the message. Other simple cues may be "longer messages are better," "older people are more trustworthy," "all my friends are doing it," or "physically attractive people are more likeable." People processing in this mode do not differentiate between weak and strong health messages, but rather are persuaded by variables irrelevant to message processing (Chaiken, 1980; Petty & Cacioppo, 1986; Petty, Cacioppo, & Goldman, 1981). This kind of processing can be dangerous in the realm of cancer communication where misinformation can lead to poor prevention practices, or an inability to detect cancer.

People who process messages systematically will think carefully about the message and engage in thinking that is relevant to the message content. Human beings, however, are economical and will invest only the necessary cognitive effort to complete the task at hand. And, in order to engage in systematic processing, people must be sufficiently motivated, and have sufficient cognitive resources. Motivation is affected by how personally relevant the message is (Chaiken, 1980), the reader's need for cognition (Cacioppo, Petty, Kao, & Rodriguez, 1986), exposure to unexpected message contents (Maheswaran & Chaiken, 1991), and, in many cases, the number of messages received. Cognitive resources, or ability to process a message, are affected by distraction (Festinger & Maccoby, 1964; Petty, Wells, & Brock, 1976), message repetition (Cacioppo & Petty, 1979), time pressure (Moore, Hauskneckt, & Thamodaran, 1986), communication modality (Eagly & Chaiken, 1993), and knowledge and expertise (Alba & Marmorstein, 1987).

Attitude change that occurs because of systematic processing is more durable, and indicative of future behavior change. This is because such attitudes were formed by careful evaluation of the merits of the arguments and thus reflect the content of the thoughts that were generated during reading to (or listening to) the message. If these arguments are perceived to be high quality, the message receiver should generate positive thoughts. But, if the message is reviewed to be low quality the thoughts generated by the message will be negative, leading to less persuasion. In this way, systematic processing is the "holy grail" of cognitive-processing scholars. It is believed that if we can motivate careful processing, message receivers will engage in message elaboration and convince themselves to engage in the recommended actions. Furthermore, they will be more likely to engage in long-term change. For cancer scholars, this may be the difference between detecting cancer and living, or failing to detect cancer and dying.

Systematic processing manifests itself in various ways. Cognitive processes refer to such information-processing activities as perceiving, abstracting, judging, elaborating, rehearsing, and recalling from memory. The most common means of examining cognitive responses in research is to ask participants to list or report all of their thoughts after having read (or heard) a message. These messages can be mass-mediated or interpersonal in nature. Categorically, these thoughts can be counterarguments, favorable thoughts, or irrelevant thoughts. And, it should be noted that these thoughts can regard the message, the source, the audience of the message, or the channel in which the message was transmitted (Cacioppo, Harkins, & Petty, 1981).

Positive thoughts reflect relative agreement with the message. If such thoughts occur after having read a message carefully, these positive cognitions will be predictive of long-term change. That is, when positive thoughts occur because people have carefully considered the merits of an appeal, have cross-checked that message, and/or have researched the issue themselves, then the likelihood that they will actually engage in the actions recommended in the message is high. Yet, people can have positive thoughts after having hardly attended to a message, or after having heuristically processed a message. Therefore, it is important to also look at where the positive thoughts were directed. Positive thoughts about the source (the source is a likeable person, the source is an expert) may reveal a lack of careful thinking.

Counterarguments are negative thoughts regarding the persuasive message where the message receiver counters an argument in the message. The more counterarguments people generate after having received a message, the less likely they are to be motivated to engage in the actions recommended in the message. Thus, when developing cancer prevention and detection messages, message designers must be aware of the potential arguments against their stance. Several factors are known to increase counterarguing. If a person is motivated to form an unfavorable opinion (e.g., if he or she is cynical about colorectal cancer exams), careful thought can take the form of arguing against the message (Petty et al., 1976). Also, if a person has an unbalanced amount of information about the message topic, he or she may be more biased when processing the message (Petty & Wegener, 1999). Counterarguing is decreased as the message arguments increase in quality. Thus, the more well throughout the arguments, the more the source of the message understands the arguments against the recommendations (e.g., the side effects of treatment), the more statistical and narrative evidence that can be provided, the less likely the patient will counterargue. It must be noted, however, that counterarguing is also decreased when people are distracted (Buller, 1986) or when people are in a good mood (Janis, Kaye, & Kirschner, 1965), indicating that decreased counterarguing is not always a good thing. Instead, scholars must recognize why people have reduced counterargumentation.

Message receivers can also have irrelevant thoughts when receiving a health message. In such cases, the message receiver thinks about entirely different issues when receiving a message. Irrelevant thoughts can take the form of "I was thinking about grocery shopping while my doctor was talking to me" or "I am afraid of dying so I turned my thoughts to something more positive." Especially in cancer communication where the topic is likely to conjure up thoughts of death, fear, or even recollections of a loss of a loved one, message designers must take into consideration how to keep thoughts on task (Sparks, 2003).

Importantly, persuasion researchers have acknowledged the importance of designing persuasive messages to induce motivation in receivers to increase the likelihood of systematic processing. Yet, older adults have unique barriers that will affect their likelihood of processing. Importantly, message-processing scholars have not paid attention to the growing population of older adults. Therefore, although we know that this group has unique barriers to processing (as discussed subsequently), the exact impact of these barriers is unclear at best. We must tackle these unknowns in order to develop better, clearer, more effective cancer communication.

COMPLEXITIES OF AGE-RELATED COMMUNICATION BARRIERS

Throughout this chapter it is suggested that a significant relationship exists between communication messages and the satisfaction that people obtain from such messages whether such exchanges stem from interpersonal, small group, organizational, public, or mass-mediated contexts. We also argue that the motivation and ability to process messages is integral to thinking carefully about cancer messages (and that the message must stimulate such ability and motivation). The next reasonable argument then would be that an individual's ability to create and maintain satisfaction with interactions and message exchanges ultimately affects his or her health. Epidemiological researchers Berkman and Syme (1979) suggested that individuals without close interpersonal interactions and relationships are twice as likely to die as those with strong interpersonal ties. Thus, further understanding of how the communicative interactions of older adults play out in the construction and processing of such messages across the communication continuum (e.g., interpersonal, small group, organizational, public, mass) is another element that may contribute greatly to increased health outcomes for aging patients.

The importance of understanding the complexities underlying communicating with the aging patient diagnosed with cancer works in another important way. Communication not only plays a crucial role in assessing a patient's mental and physical health, but, additionally, after the individual is diagnosed with an illness such as cancer, his or her communicative relationships seem to influence how he or she will get well (Nussbaum, Pecchioni, Robinson, & Thompson, 2000; Pecchioni, Ota, & Sparks, 2004). Because of the complexities of the health care provider–older adult patient relationship, barriers that older adults and their partners and caregivers face in conversation and some implications of such barriers must be better understood, as well as the connection to the ways in which older adults adapt to deficits acquired across the life span. As Cohen (1994) stated, the nature and management of cancer for older adults depends on not only biological processes, but psychological and social processes as well. The barriers that we present affect the patient in a multitude of ways, not only their health, but their ultimate ability to process messages.

Barrier 1: Aging Characteristics. Before diving into communication and relational barriers, one must understand Busse's (1969) discussion of primary and secondary characteristics of aging. A gerontological theorist, Busse first recognized that many of the declining characteristics associated with aging were not a function of growing old, but most often were tied to other elements of the individual's life. The primary characteristics of aging include developmental changes that result solely from the process of aging (i.e., wrinkles), whereas secondary characteristics are changes that occur due to events that take place during the life span (e.g., poor diet). Eisdorfer and Cohen's (1980) research suggests that much of the cognitive decline associated with aging is not due to the aging process, but is the result of high blood pressure, which can occur at any age. Thus, it is important to first understand that communication barriers in cancer care for the aging patient can be caused by both primary and secondary characteristics of aging (Nussbaum et al., 2000).

Barrier 2: Aging and Presbyopia. Presbyopia is a thickening of the crystalline lenses of the eye, along with a decrease in elasticity of the lenses of the eye (Corso, 1971; Kline & Scialfa, 1996; McFarland, 1968), and begins around the age of 40. At this point, many individuals begin to hold printed material farther away from their eyes than before. At age 50, most individuals have trouble seeing small objects and details with an increased need for glasses when reading (Botwinick, 1978). By the age of 70, less than 30% have retained 20/20 eyesight and most do not have normal vision even with correction (Botwinick, 1978). Thus, older adults increasingly have to adjust to problems related to seeing objects both near and far. Certain losses resulting from aging also begin to affect everyday activities (Kline & Scialfa, 1996). Such increased difficulties include spatial acuity, depth perception, motion perception, and being able to see in shadowed areas. Older individuals diagnosed with cancer need to have access to relevant cancer-related health information. Thus, health messages need to not only pay attention to issues of message framing, but also to elements of messages including font sizes and multiple media outlets for delivering messages (e.g., aural and visual, etc.).

Barrier 3: Aging and Presbycusis. Not surprisingly, the aging process also impacts the ability to process aural information. *Presbycusis* is the term used to describe the hearing loss associated with aging. Characteristics of presbycusis include a decrease in ability to distinguish between consonants and among adjacent frequencies as well as a reduced sensitivity to higher frequency sounds (Botwinick, 1977, 1978; Corso, 1971; Willeford, 1971). Hearing problems increase considerably after the age of 45, although deafness in older adult is rare, with only 15% of individuals over the age of 75 considered to be deaf (Darbyshire, 1984; Verbrugge, 1984). Still, 20% of older adults over the age of 75 suffer from mild hearing loss. Often, the declining ability to hear mixed with a decline in confidence about hearing result in more requests for repetition of information from the interactant or an avoidance of conversations (Nussbaum et al., 2000). Elderly individuals experiencing hearing loss will try to overcompensate via a number of strategies including an attempt to fill in the semantic and syntactic gaps whenever possible (Villaume, Brown, & Darling, 1994). Of course, as with any conversational snafu, inappropriate fillers can create an uncomfortable conversation. When conversations do not follow conventional norms, the wrong words bring about unintended difficulties. Even the slightest impairments in both sight and hearing are often worse when combined than a more significant impairment in either sight or hearing. Such sensory difficulties contribute to decreases in confidence with one's conversational abilities, which in turn may contribute to problems in other areas such as message processing or particular information-seeking strategies for older adults.

Hearing problems have been linked to difficulties in the production of speech sounds for older adults (Hutchinson & Beasley, 1981). Message exchange and understanding is likely to be impacted by such declines acquired across one's life span. Another problem in the message exchange is the increase in time it takes for older adults to encode and decode messages (Nussbaum et al., 2000). The increase in such coding processes is attributed to physiological changes in the brain and a decrease in the information-processing efficiency of the central nervous system (CNS; Birren, Woods, & Williams, 1980; MacKay & Abrams, 1996; Smith, Thompson, &

Michalewski, 1980; Takeda & Matsuzawa, 1985). Although encoding and decoding process problems are likely to be minor, delays during conversation are often awkward and seem to be longer than usual, which can be attributed to negative personality characteristics of the older adult. Again, health messages must be constructed in ways that are sensitive to older adult cognitive and emotional barriers to processing as well as age-related message-processing problems that are likely to arise.

Barrier 4: Aging and Messages. Word retrieval, name recall, and planning what to say during a conversation can also present problems along with delays in processing (Cohen, 1994; MacKay & Abrams, 1996), all of which can impact the typical conversational flow. Such difficulties lead interactants to begin to question the older speaker's competence. Thus, memory difficulties are just some of the problems associated with message transmission and exchange.

Information-seeking with aging patients, however, does have added barriers. Although a number of cancer interventions and campaigns are currently launched, it is unknown the extent to which older adults pay attention to, or even seek out this information. In fact, Pecchioni and Sparks' (2007) data reveal that the only source of health information that older adults use consistently is their doctor. After doctors, the most important information sources were (in order): family members, nurses, friends, the Internet, other medical personnel, and other patients. Yet, the source of information that patients were most satisfied with is their friends and family. The source of information they are least satisfied with was listed as their doctor. These data indicate a serious discrepancy between information sought, and information persons are satisfied with (see also Sparks, Pecchioni, & Mittapalli, 2003, 2004). For aging patients in particular, it is important to understand the extent by which satisfaction with information is correlated with message effectiveness. If this is indeed the case, then it is reasonable to assume that older adults will be most persuaded by information provided by friends and family. This is a critical issue for health practitioners because friends' and family information may lack up-to-date research, clarity, or even accuracy. Thus, it is imperative that we examine the complexities of age-related communication barriers by understanding how aging patients process cognitive, affective, and behavioral information in unique ways, how older adults are persuaded to seek out information, and thus be active participants in their cancer-related health care.

Barrier 5: Aging and Cognitive Function. A simplistic relationship between aging and decline in cognitive ability does not exist, however, some dimensions of intelligence slightly decrease as we age, particularly for those over the age of 70 (see e.g., Jarvik & Bank, 1983; Schaie, 1983, 1996).

Moreover, research indicates that some of the cognitive decline related to aging can be overcompensated for with mental and physical activity (see e.g., Botwinick, 1977; Schaie, 1996). Recent research in cognitive aging indicates that for normal cognitive aging, older adults will maintain the relative strengths and weaknesses acquired and practiced earlier in their lives (Anstey, Hofer, & Luszcz, 2003). In other words, these new and contrasting findings suggest that even the very old are able to retain their unique patterns of cognitive strengths and weaknesses. Prior research suggests that explanations for cognitive deficits across the life span are primarily due to genetic factors, neurochemical factors, CNS efficiency and integrity (Anstey, Lord, & Williams, 1997; Anstey & Smith, 1999; Li, 2002; Li & Lindenberger, 1999). Another theme in the cognitive aging literature that is worth noting is the importance of distinguishing between chronological age as an index of time and the physiological and contextual processes that may be a better indicator of adult development that is more informative for explaining cognitive change (Birren & Cunningham, 1985; Wohlwill, 1970). Individuals of the same chronological age are not automatically in the same physical or mental state of mind (Rubin & Rubin, 1986). Contextual age is "a transactional view of aging that incorporates physiological, psychological, social, and communication influences on life-position" (Rubin & Rubin, 1986, p. 30). It is the state affected by physical health, interpersonal interactions, mobility, life satisfaction, social activity, and economic security (Rubin & Rubin, 1986). Despite differences in chronological age, contextual age allows individuals to identify with one another in ways that are sometimes invisible (Kundrat & Nussbaum, 2003).

Evidence related to drastic declines in cognition processes for older adults does not strongly support a negative relationship and has been overstated. However, significant declines in cognitive ability have been found to occur in older adults about 5 years before death (Kleemeier, 1962). The decline is likely to be related to distance from death more than being related to age (Berg, 1996). Cohen's (1979) research suggests that when older adults are able to understand a spoken message in the same manner as a younger adult, they are often not able to use the information. Older adults frequently have a more difficult time in making inferences from information obtained from an interaction than younger adults, which leads conversants to believe that the older adult is not getting the point of the conversation.

Everyday problem solving can also be a problem for older adults simply because the strategies employed differ from those used by younger adults (Willis, 1996). Nussbaum et al., (2000) stated that such differences are shown on declarative (i.e., searching for the information) and procedural (i.e., using prior experiential knowledge) levels. On the declarative level, older adults can sift through vast amounts of information and pull out the relevant pieces of information necessary for choosing the best option available. Younger adults tend to act more like novices by searching for extensive information. If successful decision making is established by the amount of information gathered, then older adults show a poorer performance than their younger counterparts. On the procedural level of problem solving, older adults rely on well-established procedural strategies for obtaining solutions to the problem. Poor problem solving may emerge when old skills are applied to newer problems (Nussbaum et al., 2000).

Schaie's (1975) research has suggested that the intellectual abilities and skills of reasonably healthy older adults have not diminished but have instead become obsolete. Older adults simply need retraining to adjust to contemporary society. Some dimensions of intelligence decrease with age and are typically divided into two categories, crystallized and fluid. As Nussbaum et al. (2000) described, crystallized intelligence includes verbal skills, comprehension skills, and vocabulary typically acquired via education and personal experience and remain relatively stable until the age of 70 (Botwinick, 1977). Fluid intelligence is typically unrelated to experience or education, but rather refers to mainly nonverbal skills such as abstract reasoning, response time, and mathematics. Fluid intelligence tends to decline after the age of 35. The decline is usually due to a decreased functioning of the CNS (Horn & Donaldson, 1980). One way to greatly slow down the decreases in fluid intelligence is through interaction with others (Nussbaum et al., 2000). Research into the influence of fluid intelligence on conversation is untouched and desperately needed. Cancer-related health messages for older adults should take into account the older adult changes in fluid intelligence. Thus, health messages including an interpersonal-based component will be much more likely to reach the older adult population. We must begin to consider constructing health messages across the continuum of communication ranging from interpersonal to mediated.

Barrier 6: Aging and Memory. Similar to the research on aging and cognitive abilities, research studying the influence of aging on memory indicates memory to be a multidimensional construct (Nussbaum et al., 2000). In short, the relationship between age and memory is incredibly complex. Three types of memory tend to dominate the aging and memory literature: sensory, short-term, and long-term, and all are differentially impacted by the aging process. *Sensory memory* is defined as one's ability to remember an image or memory of stimuli within a fraction of a second after exposure (see e.g., Baltes, Reese, & Lipsitt, 1980). The authors further stated that sensory memory does not appear to diminish with age if sensory limitations fail to get in the way of the reception of stimuli. *Short-term memory* is defined as the ability to remember an image or memory of stimuli within seconds or minutes after exposure and tends to slowly decline with age (see e.g., Baltes et al., 1980). Decline in short-term memory processes varies with each individual because of aspects such as cognitive style (Monge, 1969), complexity of material (Botwinick & Storandt, 1974), amount of emotional threat in terms of stress the older adult receives, rapid pace of presentation, amount or complexity of organizing needed to encode vast amounts of information (Arenberg & Robertson-Tchabo, 1977; Craik & Rabinowitz, 1985), fear of failure (Okun, 1976), and recognizable recall material (Chase & Simon, 1973; Hanley-Dunn & McIntosh, 1984). Conversational difficulties tend to arise for older adults because of problems with simultaneously processing and storing information (Smith, 1996). In terms of short-term memory recall of information, younger adults have an advantage over older adults. Although such declines in short-term memory associated with aging make conversations slightly more difficult for older adults, research indicates that such difficulties can be reduced and increases in affect can be achieved simply by conversing in a relaxed and nonevaluative style (Nussbaum, Robinson, & Grew, 1983, 1985). *Long-term memory* is comprised of specific experiences or episodic memory, knowledge or semantic memory, and procedural memory (Smith, 1996). Declines in age-related long-term memory tend to be more drastic in some components than those for short-term memory (Craik, 1977). Such dramatic declines are primarily due to encoding or organizational difficulties, or the procedural component of memory (see e.g., Arenberg & Robertson-Tchabo, 1977; Craik & Rabinowitz, 1985; Smith, 1996). A number of other factors contribute to declines in long-term memory. It takes more time for older adults to retrieve information from memory (Craik, 1977). Other factors impacting long-term recall include recognition of the material being recalled (see e.g., Chase & Simon, 1973; Hanley-Dunn & McIntosh, 1984), as well as one's learning style (Monge, 1969), salience of information, number of items to remember, type of task and task structure (Botwinick, 1973), and motivation level (Elias & Elias, 1977). However, older adults have been found to have better narrative recall and tend to remember stories in more accurate detail than their younger counterparts. Furthermore, older adults have a more complex and developed scripted knowledge of daily activities and tend to be more efficient at identifying problems and finding reasonable solutions (Blanchard-Fields & Abeles, 1996). Older adults and younger adults have different problem-solving strategies and social-knowledge scripts because they do not share the same schema (Nussbaum et al., 2000). Understanding such differences is the first step toward reducing misunderstandings and miscommunication of health messages, particularly when it comes to serious diagnoses such as cancer.

Barrier 7: Aging, Emotion, and Relationships. Nussbaum et al. (2003) stated that an understanding of successful adaptation and effective management of cancer by older adults cannot be accomplished without the study of the interpersonal communication of older adults. First, the nature and management of cancer for older adults depends on not only biological processes, but psychological and social processes as well (Cohen, 1994).

Socioemotional Selectivity Theory, advanced by Carstensen (1992), proposes that older adults reduce their overall social interactions while maintaining those relationships that provide the most emotional support. This can enlighten our understanding of where a diagnosis of cancer will be most disruptive in an older adult's relational world. Understanding how family and friend relationships function in old age can help us to predict and explain the process of an older individual's successful adaptation to living with cancer (Nussbaum et al., 2003).

Cancer information is often highly emotionally charged because of the serious, often life-threatening, nature of many forms of cancer. Receiving a diagnosis of cancer can be a major shock to most people. It is important that cancer communications programs are strategically designed to address the important psychological and socioemotional issues surrounding different individuals' experiences with cancer (Kreps, 2003). Care must be taken to coordinate content and relational aspects of communication to both inform people about cancer and cancer treatment, without confusing or upsetting them (Buckman, 1996; Gillotti, Thompson, & McNeilis, 2002). To increase the likelihood that health messages will be understood and processed, it is critical that we create cancer-related health messages by sending similar messages in a variety of ways (i.e., provide the information in a pamphlet to take home; provide the same information in various interpersonal conversations from physicians involved, different members of the family, and friends; provide the same information via a video to take home, as well as an Internet website).

SELECTIVE OPTIMIZATION WITH COMPENSATION MODEL

Underlying the notion that older adult cancer patients adapt to their illness through communication is a meta-model of adaptation developed by Baltes and Baltes (selective optimization with compensation [SOC] model; 1990). Baltes and Baltes viewed aging as a life-long adaptive process by suggesting that as one grows older, adaptation to the losses associated with aging can be best explained by examining the relationships among the processes of selective optimization based on compensation. Based on social exchange theory, it is believed that people make determinations about the behaviors they will enact based on the goals they have selected, the resources and opportunities available to them, and their perceptions of their ability to enact behaviors that will help them attain those goals. Although the individual may not be able to perform particular task as well as they once did, through the selective optimization with compensation process older adults are able to maintain satisfying, successful, efficacious, and arguably healthier lives.

The SOC model can be explained succinctly by defining three terms. Selection is viewed as adaptation through limiting the number of goals the individual may pursue. Optimization is a positioning of skills and resources within a limited goal or life domain to remain effective. Compensation is used to describe the individual's response to a loss in behavioral capacity. Because our skills often exceed requirements of the task, a slight loss in a skill or ability as a consequence of aging may not present much of a problem because the losses tend to occur in those skill or ability areas that are not typically used.

DESIGNING HEALTH MESSAGES FOR OLDER ADULTS

Health communication scholars must also make special considerations regarding designing messages and interventions that encourage older adults to be active participants in cancer communication. We need to focus on message strategies that will prove effective with the unique complexities and barriers facing the elderly population. That said, such a goal must be pursued by focusing on an understanding of older adult cognitive and emotional processes followed by particular message framing that will more likely reach this unique population. As has been laid out, older adults have unique barriers that mandate careful thought prior to message design. We must create messages that can be seen, recalled, and systematically processed. Here we present several design options that can be taken into consideration when developing messages for older adults. Of course, there is a dearth of information on message effectiveness geared toward older adults, therefore, these message recommendations are viewed by us as potential research programs—not as solutions with clear results.

Message Framing

Seeking out cancer information is a risky endeavor. That is, knowledge gained from such information-seeking strategies will not cure cancer, but rather it may help one find out if one is at risk for cancer. Health communication and persuasion scholars, as well as health practitioners have utilized the framing postulate of Prospect Theory as a way to understand the communication involved in risky decisions (see e.g., Kahneman & Tversky, 1979). The theory suggests that individuals will act differentially to information presented as gains or losses. The framing postulate further hypothesizes that individuals avoid risks when considering gains but prefer risks when considering losses. Older adult patients may differentially face decisions about cancer treatments relative to their unique characteristics and life circumstances (e.g., chemotherapy regimens, etc.) in considering gains and losses germane to the aging population.

Negatively framed messages are referred to in terms of losses whereas positively framed messages are typically referred to in terms of gains. The message-framing postulate of Prospect Theory has been utilized in the health domain fairly extensively, particularly given that the outcome of disease detection is an uncertain and often risky behavior (see e.g., Banks, Zimmerman, Ishak, & Harter, 1995; Meyerowitz & Chaiken, 1987; Rothman, Salovey, Antone, Keough, & Martin, 1993). For instance, research by Meyerowitz and Chaiken (1987) suggests that female participants were more convinced to conduct breast self-examinations after being exposed to negatively framed messages than to positively framed messages. Negatively framed messages have also been found to be more effective in persuading persons in terms of detection behaviors such as seeking health information or discovering a lump or mole (see Rothman et al., 1993). One way in which health messages differ is whether they recommend preventing a health risk or hazard (e.g., wearing seatbelts) or recommend detecting a health risk or hazard (e.g., breast self examinations). Information-seeking is often considered a detection behavior (see e.g., Mitchell, 2000). Detecting a health problem is viewed as more risky because in the process of gathering health information about particular symptoms, individuals may find out they have a serious health problem, such as cancer. Presumably, not knowing about a disease is less risky than knowing that you have a disease. Prevention is less risky because you are taking measures to ensure not becoming sick or hurt. That said, negatively framed messages are more likely to smooth the progress of detection behaviors, largely because risky options are preferred when individuals are considering losses (Rothman et al., 1993). In fact, research has indicated that individuals who are exposed to negatively framed messages are more likely to change their behavioral intentions toward health detection behaviors.

In such a discussion of message framing, it is interesting to point out that positively and negatively framed information are equal numerically speaking—but it is the tone of the information that leads individuals to perceive it differently. And, therefore, individuals may cognitively process messages differentially based on framing, particularly older adults. Researchers have long recognized the magnitude of examining cognitive processing as mediating the link between messages and subsequent behavior. For instance, Mitchell (2000) and Mitchell Brown, Villagran, and Villagran. (2001) examined the role of cognitive processing in understanding the emotion by message quality interaction. By experimentally varying emotion, involvement, and message quality, the researchers investigated the impact that emotion and message quality jointly have on cognitive processes in terms of thought valence, counterarguing, and message recall. Results indicated that overall, message quality is the best predictor of attitude change, and that cognitive processing is a key mediator of that relationship. Furthermore, Lapinski and Levine (2000) found similar results with this finding across cultural groups. Both studies also showed a strong linear correlation between counterarguments and attitude change such that, as participants' ability to counterargue increases, their attitude change decreases. This line of research suggests that communication scholars need to begin addressing the unique ways by which older adults process and receive messages, as well as the ways the older adult population begins to adapt to difficult health diagnoses such as cancer in different ways than their younger counterparts.

Emotional Appeals

By far, the most common message design tactic used in public health is the emotional appeal—particularly fear appeals. In fact, some estimate that 26% of all public service announcements make use of fear appeals.

Fear appeals, or threat appeals, can be defined in terms of their content, or by the reaction they engender from the audience. Fear appeals may contain gory pictures, vivid language, or personalistic language. Theoretically, the most common account for why fear tactics work (and why they can fail) is through the Extended Parallel Processing Model (EPPM; Witte, 1992, 1994).

The EPPM makes the argument that an effective fear appeal has two basic components: threat and efficacy. Specifically, threat is composed of both perceptions of severity (can has severe outcomes) and susceptibility (cancer can affect me). Efficacy is also broken into two parts: self-efficacy (I can do the recommended behavior) and response efficacy (the recommended behavior will work). The EPPM predicts that high levels of perceived risk, especially in combination with low perceptions of self (self-efficacy) and/or low evaluations of the recommended response (response efficacy), often lead to rejection of recommendations and may result in negative, maladaptive responses (Witte, 1992). For example, people who have extreme anxiety about lung cancer but doubt their ability to alter smoking habits (low self-efficacy) may justify smoking by rationalizing that they may die tomorrow in a car accident. Alternatively, people who have extreme anxiety about heart disease but believe heredity, not smoking, determines risks (low response efficacy) may continue smoking a pack of cigarettes per day, rationalizing that poor health is genetically predetermined.

Persuasive health interventions, therefore, should be designed to include all four components. Messages must stimulate a high level of threat while simultaneously communicating an effective answer, and empowering individuals to adopt that answer. Meta-analytic data suggests that strong fear appeals are those that produce high levels of perceived severity and susceptibility, and are more persuasive than low or weak fear appeals (Witte & Allen, 2000). Witte and Allen's data also indicate that fear appeals motivate adaptive danger control actions such as message acceptance and maladaptive fear control actions such as defensive avoidance or reactance. It appears that strong fear appeals and high-efficacy messages produce the greatest behavior change, whereas strong fear appeals with low-efficacy messages produce the greatest levels of defensive responses.

Despite the fact that individuals experienced "fear" derived from the long-term knowledge of harmful effects of smoking, the literature seems to be relatively pessimistic about the long-term effectiveness of fear appeals (Bandura, 1977; Mittelmark, 1978). For instance, Pee and Hammond (1997) argued that such fear appeals have long-term detrimental effects based on the concept of escape-avoidance behavior. It is perceived that with exposure to such fear appeal campaigns, individuals would rather not risk the knowledge of having contracted certain diseases. One example is the decreased adherence to breast screening guidelines due to intensified distress of contracting breast cancer.

Although most emotional appeals are fear appeals, other emotions have the ability to motivate people—most notably, guilt and anger. We turn our attention briefly to both emotions.

Guilt, which is aroused when people's behavior is incongruent with their perception of appropriate conduct (Baumeister, Stillwell, & Heatherton, 1994), is a powerful motivator. The study of guilt as antecedent to behavior change is not new. As early as 1966, Darlington and Macker as well as Wallace and Sadalla experimentally induced participants to feel guilty, and subsequently measured their likelihood of engaging in altruistic acts. The data from research teams revealed that those who experienced guilt were more likely to engage in altruistic behavior.

Given the robust effects that guilt has on compliance, it may also be true that health interventions that elicit guilt will change individuals' behaviors via the attitude–intention–behavior link (Ajzen & Fishbein, 1969, 1970, 1973; Fishbein, 1967; Howard & Sheth, 1969). Nonetheless, examining guilt as elicited by a persuasive message has a much shorter history than studying guilt from a compliance paradigm; especially in health interventions. Those studies that have examined guilt appeals have done so from a marketing perspective—that is, they used guilt appeals to persuade people to buy products. Although research in advertising does indicate that advertisements that induce guilt in persons may be more likely to have increased purchase intentions (Edomondson, 1986), guilt studies have not focused on health communication in a breast cancer context.

Pinto and Priest (1991) examined the impact of low, moderate, and high guilt on purchase intentions. They posited a curvilinear effect of guilt on the amount of guilt people will actually experience. They rationalized that, as with fear appeals (Janis & Feshbach, 1953), as the intensity of guilt messages increase, felt guilt decreases and felt anger increases; their data was consistent with this hypothesis. Similarly, Pinto and Worobetz (1992) aroused guilt through food product advertisements. Pinto et al. aroused guilt in working mothers by showing dental floss and bread advertisements eliciting low, moderate, and high levels of guilt. Their data indicated that moderate appeals of guilt are more effective than high or low appeals of guilt and that anger mediates levels of guilt, such that as guilt increases, so does anger and ultimately, attitude change decreases.

Coulter and Pinto (1995) also induced guilt via food advertisements. Again, these scholars found a curvilinear effect of guilt on purchase intentions, and their data was consistent with a linear effect of guilt appeal on felt anger. Together, these data indicate that high guilt appeals are ineffective, and that this is due to participants feeling angry about receiving the message, and feeling manipulated by it. In fact, Coulter and Pinto examined participants' corporate attributions after receiving the guilt appeals. The high guilt appeals led to feelings that the corporation was manipulative and desired to make money.

In an extension of this research program, Alden and Crowley's (1995) research on sex guilt (SG) found that after participants viewed booklets of condom advertisements, they reported that SG impacted the cognitive processing of ads. Their data indicated that high SG females had fewer relevant thoughts regarding the message. This also illuminates the rationale behind the failure of high-guilt messages. Perhaps persons who receive a high-guilt appeal become angry, feel manipulated, and therefore focus on alternative issues as a means to resolve negative affect (vs. focusing on the appeal). This is consistent with the theoretical underpinnings of the negative state relief model (NSR; Bauman, Cialdini, & Kendrick, 1981). Baumann et al. explained that a negative mood is accompanied by an intrinsic drive to alleviate the bad feelings. Because people do not enjoy negative moods, they work toward moving back to their baseline mood (Mitchell, 2000). Moreover, individuals are motivated to distract themselves from unpleasant thoughts and engage in other activities, such helping others, that divert their attention from the unpleasant affect (Isen & Simmonds, 1978). Additionally, participants may be likely to ignore any stimulus that prolongs the negative affect.

Statistical Versus Narrative Appeals

Another issue with regard to designing messages is how to present the evidence. Controversy continues with respect to the relative persuasiveness of narrative versus statistical appeals. Although some data is consistent with narrative appeals being more persuasive than statistical ones (Harte, 1976;

Koballa, 1986), others have indicated the exact opposite (Baesler & Burgoon, 1994; Dickson, 1982; Wells & Harvey, 1977).

Attempting to resolve the above debate, Allen and Preiss (1997) undertook a meta-analysis comparing the relative persuasiveness of narrative versus statistical appeals. Although the meta-analysis revealed that statistical evidence was more persuasive than narrative evidence, the effect size between message type and persuasiveness was rather meager.

Kopfman, Smith, Ah Yun, and Hodges (1998) studied differences between narrative and statistical appeals with respect to organ donation. In their study, they were interested in affective versus cognitive reactions to narrative and statistical appeals. Their data indicated, overall, that statistical appeals impact cognitive responses (such as recall) and narrative appeals are more likely to impact emotional responses. Therefore, perhaps message designers must consider the responses they desire before concluding how the evidence should be written. Moreover, most messages have the capability of including both kinds of evidence.

These message recommendations are hardly exhaustive. There are multitudes of theories suggesting ways to develop persuasive health interventions—many of which are not mentioned here. Ultimately, the job of the message designer is to develop a message that takes into consideration the unique qualities of the disease, the modality, and most certainly the audience.

CONCLUSION

This chapter reviewed the unique physical, cognitive, affective, language, and interactive-relationship characteristics likely to be involved when caring for the aging patient as well as the family members connected to the patient in the complex, confusing, and overwhelming cancer-related health environment. Age-related physiological, cognitive, emotive, and life changes and experiences often complicate the ways care is provided for an older adult diagnosed with cancer. By better understanding such conversational barriers, researchers, practitioners, and family members involved in caring for aging patients will be able to deliver relevant and compelling messages that aging patients can better understand and process, and better health outcomes will be achieved. Designing and delivering cancer communication messages to match the specific communication skills, needs, and predispositions of the older adult population is a crucial component of health care delivery. This chapter has provided concrete suggestions for a focus on message design and framing for health interventions tailored to the older adult population. Such systematic, communication research-based campaigns can aid older adults in becoming active participants in health communication environments. By focusing on such complexities of particular age-related communication barriers that may hinder or help in caring for the aging patient, researchers, family members and health practitioners can provide much better cancer care. It is vitally important that health messages can be understood and processed. Thus, it is time that we begin paying closer attention to creating cancer-related health messages by repeating messages through multiple communication channels (e.g., pamphlets, interpersonal conversations from physicians, family, and friends, video, and the Internet).

Furthermore, the SOC model (Baltes & Baltes, 1990) is important as it explains how adaptation occurs in a general sense and provides a framework for understanding the middle range theories employed above to generate specific hypotheses. SOC also provides a rationale for what constitutes an optimal match in terms of a good or desirable message. From the social exchange perspective, which underlies the SOC model, a good message is one where the rewards of listening to and absorbing the message exceed the costs—relative to the available message alternatives. Thus, the SOC model and designing of relevant and compelling messages for aging patients can aid in pushing through the age-related barriers older adults face to achieve increased health outcomes. By gaining this knowledge, researchers and health care providers can give better care to aging patients and aging patients as well as partners and family members can more easily acquire health information that will help them to help themselves in more productive and efficient ways!

Health communication scholars must do a better job of translating relevant communication theories and literature into the lives of aging patients, caregivers, and health care provider teams. Communication theories from interpersonal relationship development and processes to persuasion and mass-mediated provide sound building blocks for those interested in using reliable research-based empirical evidence to aid in explaining the critical features of a successful older adult who has received the news of a cancer diagnosis. Thus, further understanding of how older adults' communicative interactions play out in the construction and processing of such messages across the communication continuum (e.g., interpersonal, small group, organizational, public, mass) is an essential step that is greatly needed for increased health outcomes for aging patients. Recognizing the complexities of effective cancer care communication with the aging patient must no longer be ignored. Cancer communication messages must be designed and delivered to match the communication skills, needs, and predispositions of such specific audiences. To influence entrenched health behaviors, messages (from interpersonal to mediated) need to be relevant and compelling, with health information that provides direction and rationale for making the best health-related decisions and adopting health-preserving behaviors. Effective health communication can encourage cancer prevention, inform cancer detection and diagnosis, guide cancer treatment, support successful cancer survivorship, and finally, promote the best end-of-life care in unique ways. This goal of this chapter was to highlight the powerful potential to strategically construct health communication messages to reduce cancer risks, incidence, morbidity, and mortality, while enhancing quality of life across the continuum of cancer care germane to the aging patient (prevention, detection, diagnosis, treatment, survivorship, and end-of-life care). It is argued that by first understanding such unique age-related communication barriers, researchers, practitioners, and family members can then begin to construct interpersonal and mediated messages in a systematic, understandable way. Such tailored research-based messages will have a greater likelihood of reaching and impacting the aging patient diagnosed with cancer. Health communication scholars have a plethora of theoretical, methodological, and pragmatic communication-based approaches to greatly contribute to the complex yet unique communicative contexts of cancer care for the aging patient. There is no better way to inform the health care and research community than to engage in care and get involved in interdisciplinary research teams and to translate such research efforts into practice.

REFERENCES

Adelman R., & Greene M. (2000). Communication between older patients and their physicians. *Clinics in Geriatric Medicine 16*(1), 1-24.

Ajzen, I., & Fishbein, M. (1969). The prediction of behavioral intentions in a choice situation. *Journal of Experimental Social Psychology, 5,* 400-416.

Ajzen, I., & Fishbein, M. (1970). The prediction of behaviour from attitudinal and normative beliefs. *Journal of Personality and Social Psychology*, *6*, 466-487.

Ajzen, I., & Fishbein, M. (1973). Attitudinal and normative variables as predictors of specific behaviours. *Journal of Personality and Social Psychology*, *27*, 41-27.

Alba, J. W., & Marmorstein, H. (1987). The effects of frequency knowledge on consumer decision making. *Journal of Consumer Research, 14,* 14-25.

Alden, D. L., & Crowley, A. E. (1995). Sex guilt and receptivity to condom advertising. *Journal of Applied Social Psychology, 25,* 1446-1463.

Anderson, J., & Geist-Martin, P. (2003). Narratives and healing: Exploring one family's stories of cancer survivorship. *Health Communication, 15*(2), 133-144.

Anstey, K. J., Hofer, S. M., & Luszcz, M. A. (2003). Cross-sectional and longitudinal patterns of dedifferentiation in late-life cognitive and sensory function: The effects of age, ability, attrition, and occasion of measurement. *Journal of Experimental Psychology: General, 32*(3), 470-487.

Anstey, K. J., Lord, S. R., & Williams, P. (1997). Strength in the lower limbs, visual contrast sensitivity, and simple reaction time predict cognition in older women. *Psychology and Aging, 12,* 137-144.

Anstey, K. J., & Smith, G. A. (1999). Interrelationships among biological markers of aging, health, activity, acculturation, and cognitive performance in older adults. *Psychology and Aging, 14,* 615-618.

Arenberg, D., & Robertson-Tchabo, E. (1977). Learning and aging. In J. Birren & K. Schaie (Eds.), *Handbook of the psychology of aging* (pp. 721-749). New York: Van Nostrand Reinhold.

Baesler, E. J., & Burgoon, J. K. (1994). The temporal effects of story and statistical evidence on belief change. *Communication Research, 21,* 582-602.

Baltes, P. B., & Baltes, M. M. (1990). Psychological perspectives on successful aging: The model of selective optimization with compensation. In P. B. Baltes & M. M. Baltes (Eds.), *Successful aging: Perspectives from the behavioral sciences.* New York: Cambridge University Press.

Baltes, P. B., Reese, H., & Lipsitt, L. (1980). Life-span developmental psychology. In M. Rosenzweig & L. Porter (Eds.), *Annual review of psychology* (pp. 65-110). Palo Alto, CA: Annual Reviews.

Bandura, A. (1977). *Social learning theory.* Englewood Cliffs, NJ: Prentice Hall.

Banks, A.T., Zimmerman, H.J., Ishak, K.G., & Harter, J.G. (1995). Diclofenac-associated hepatotoxicity: Analysis of 180 cases reported to the Food and Drug Administration as adverse reactions. *Hepatology,* 22, 820-827.

Bauman, D. J., Cialdini, R. B., & Kendrick, D. T. (1981). Altruism as hedonism: Helping and self-gratification as equivalent responses. *Journal of Personality and Social Psychology, 40,* 1039-1046.

Baumeister, R. F., Stillwell, A. M., & Heatherton, T. F. (1994). Guilt: An interpersonal approach. *Psychological Bulletin, 115,* 243-267.

Berg, S. (1996). Aging, behavior, and terminal decline. In J. E. Birren & K. W. Schaie (Eds.), *Handbook of the psychology of aging* (4th ed., pp. 323-337). San Diego, CA: Academic Press.

Berkman, L., & Syme, S. (1979). Social networks, host resistance, and mortality. *American Journal of Epidemiology, 109,* 186-204.

Birren, J. E., & Cunningham, W. (1985). Research on the psychology of aging: Principles, concepts, and theory. In J. E. Birren & W. Schaie (Eds.), *Handbook of the psychology of aging* (2nd ed., pp. 3-34). New York: Van Nostrand Reinhold.

Birren, J. E., Woods, A., & Williams, M. (1980). Behavioral slowing with age: Causes, organization, and consequences. In L. Poon (Ed.), *Aging in the 1980s* (pp. 293-308). Washington, DC: American Psychological Association.

Blanchard-Fields, F., & Abeles, R. (1996). Social cognition and aging. In J. E. Birren & K. W. Schaie (Eds.), *Handbook of the psychology of aging* (4th ed., pp. 150-161). San Diego, CA: Academic Press.

Botwinick, J. (1973). *Aging and behavior.* New York: Springer.

Botwinick, J. (1977). Intellectual abilities. In J. Birren & K. Schaie (Eds.), *Handbook of the psychology of aging* (pp. 580-605). New York: Van Nostrand Reinhold.

Botwinick, J. (1978). *Aging and behavior* (2nd ed.). New York: Springer.

Botwinick, J., & Storandt, M. (1974). *Memory related functions and age.* Springfield, IL: Thomas.

Buckman, R. (1996). Talking to patients about cancer. *British Medical Journal, 31,* 699-700.

Buller, D. B. (1986). Distraction during persuasive communication: A meta-analytic review. *Communication Monographs, 53*, 91-114.

Busse, E. (1969). Theories of aging. In E. Busse & E. Pfeiffer (Eds.), *Behavior and adaptation in later life* (pp. 11-32). Boston: Little, Brown.

Byock, I. (2000). Completing the continuum of cancer care: Integrating life-prolongation and palliation. *CA: A Cancer Journal for Clinicians, 50,* 123-132.

Cacioppo, J.T., Harkins, S.G., Petty, R.E. (1981). The nature of attitudes and cognitive responses and their relationships to behavior, In R. E. Petty, T. M. Ostrom, & T. C. Brock (Eds.), *Cognitive responses in persuasion* (pp. 31-54). Hillsdale, NJ: Erlbaum.

Cacioppo, J. T., & Petty, R. E. (1979). Effects of message repetition and position on cognitive response, recall, and persuasion. *Journal of Personality and Social Psychology*, 37, 97-109.

Cacioppo, J. T., Petty, R. E., Kao, C. F., & Rodriguez, R. (1986). Central and peripheral routes to persuasion: An individual difference perspective. *Journal of Personality and Social Psychology, 51*, 1032-1043.

Carstensen, L.L. (1992). Social and emotional patterns in adulthood: Support for socioemotional selectivity theory. *Psychology and Aging, 7*, 331-338.

Chaiken, S. (1980). Heuristic versus systematic information processing and the use of source versus message cues in persuasion. *Journal of Personality and Social Psychology, 39,* 752-766.

Chase, W., & Simon, H. (1973). The mind's eye in chess. In W. G. Chase (Ed.), *Visual information processing* (pp. 215-281). New York: Academic Press.

Cohen, G. (1979). Language comprehension in old age. *Cognitive Psychology, 11,* 423-429.

Cohen, G. (1994). Age-related problems in the use of proper names in communication. In M. L. Hummert, J. M. Wiemann, & J. F. Nussbaum (Eds.), *Interpersonal communication in older adulthood: Interdisciplinary theory and research* (pp. 40- 57). Thousand Oaks, CA: Sage.

Corso, J. (1971). Sensory processes and age effects in normal adults. *Journal of Gerontology, 26,* 90-105.

Craik, F. (1977). Age differences in human memory. In J. Birren & K. W. Schaie (Eds.), *Handbook of the psychology of aging* (pp. 384-420). New York: Van Nostrand Reinhold.

Craik, F., & Rabinowitz, J. (1985). The effects of presentation rate and encoding task on age-related memory deficits. *Journal of Gerontology, 40,* 309-315.

Darbyshire, J. (1984). The hearing loss epidemic: A challenge to gerontology. *Research on Aging, 6,* 384-394.

Dickson, P. R. (1982). The impact of enriching case and statistical information on consumer judgments. *Journal of Consumer Research, 8,* 398-406.

Eagly, A.H., & Chaiken, S. (1993). *The psychology of attitudes*. Fort Worth, TX: Harcourt Brace Jovanovich.

Edwards B.K., Howe H.L., Ries L.A.G., Thun M.J., Rosenberg H.M., Yancik R., Wingo, P.A., Jemal A., & Feigal, E.G. (2002). Annual report to the nation on the status of cancer, 1973-1999, featuring implications of age and aging on the US cancer burden. *Cancer, 94*(10), 2766-2792.

Eisdorfer, C., & Cohen, D. (1980). The issue of biological and psychological deficits. In E. Borgatta & N. McCluskey (Eds.), *Aging and society: Current research and policy perspectives* (pp. 49-70). Beverly Hills, CA: Sage.

Elias, M. F., & Elias, P. K. (1977). Motivation and activity. In J. Birren & K. W. Schaie (Eds.), *Handbook of the psychology of aging* (pp. 357-383). New York: Van Nostrand Reinhold.

Festinger, L., & Maccoby, N. (1964). On resistance to persuasive communications. *Journal of Abnormal and Social Psychology, 68*, 359-366

Fishbein, M (1967). Attitude and the prediction of behaviour. In M. Fishbein (Ed.), *Readings in attitude theory and measurement*. New York: Wiley.

Gillotti, C., Thompson, T., & McNeilis, K. (2002). Communicative competence in the delivery of bad news. *Social Science and Medicine, 54,* 1011-1023.

Greene, M. G., & Adelman, R. D. (2001). Building the physician-older patient relationship. In M. L. Hummert & J. F. Nussbaum (Eds.), *Aging, communication, and health: Linking research and practice for successful aging* (pp. 101-120). Mahwah, NJ: Erlbaum.

Greene, M., & Adelman, R. (2002, January). Physician–older adult patient communication about cancer. In G. L. Kreps (Chair), *Consumer-Provider Communication Symposium*, Bethesda, MD.

Hanley-Dunn, P., & McIntosh, J. (1984). Meaningfulness and recall of names by young and old adults. *Journal of Gerontology, 39,* 583-585.

Harwood, J., & Sparks, L. (2003). Social identity and health: An intergroup communication approach to cancer. *Health Communication, 15*(2), 145-170.

Harte, Y. (1976). The effects of evidence in persuasive communication. *Central States Speech Journal, 27,* 42-46.

Hewitt, M., Rowland, J., & Yancik, R. (2003). Cancer survivors in the United States: Age, health, and disability. *The Journals of Gerontology, Series A, 58(1)*, 82-92.

Hiatt, R. A., & Rimer, B. K. (1999). A new strategy for cancer control research. *Cancer Epidemiology, Biomarkers, & Prevention, 8,* 957-964.

Horn, J. L., & Donaldson, G. (1980). Cognitive development in adulthood. In O. G. Brim, Jr. & J. Kagen (Eds.), *Constancy and change in human development* (pp. 445-529). Cambridge, MA: Harvard University Press.

Howard, J. A., & Sheth, J. N. (1969). *The theory of buyer behavior.* New York: Wiley.

Hovland, C., Janis, I., & Kelley, H. (1953). *Communication and persuasion*. New Haven, CT: Yale University Press.

Hutchinson, J., & Beasley, D. (1981). Speech and language functioning among the aging. In H. Oyer & E. Oyer (Eds.), *Aging and communication* (pp. 155-174). Baltimore: University Park Press.

Isen, A., & Simmonds, S. (1978). The effect of feeling good on a helping task that is incompatible with good mood. *Social Psychology, 41*, 346-349.

Janis, I.L., Kaye, D., & Kirshner, P. (1965). Facilitating effects of eating while reading on responsiveness to persuasive communications. *Journal of Personality and Social Psychology, 1*, 181-186.

Jarvik, L., & Bank, L. (1983). Aging twins: Longitudinal psychometric data. In K. Schaie (Ed.), *Longitudinal studies of adult psychological development* (pp. 40-63). New York: Guilford.

Kahneman, D., & Tversky, A. (1979). "Prospect theory": An analysis of decision under risk. *Econometrica*, 47, 263-291.

Kleemeier, R. (1962). Intellectual changes in the senium. *Proceedings of the Social Statistics Section of the American Statistics Association, 1,* 290-295.

Kline, D.W., & Scialfa, C.T. (1996). Visual and auditory aging. In J.E. Birren & K.W. Schaie (Eds.), *Handbook of the psychology of aging* (4th ed., pp. 181-203). San Diego, CA: Academic Press.

Koballa, T. R., Jr. (1986). Persuading teachers to reexamine the innovative elementary science programs of yesterday: The effect of anecdotal versus data-summary communications. *Journal of Research in Science Teaching, 23,* 437-449.

Kopfman, J.E., Smith, S.W., Ah Yun, J.K., & Hodges, A. (1998). Affective and cognitive reactions to narrative versus statistical evidence organ donation messages. *Journal of Applied Communication Research, 26,* 279-300.

Kreps, G.L. (1988). Relational communication in health care. *Southern Speech Communication Journal, 53*, 344-359.

Kreps, G.L. (2003). Impact of communication on cancer risk, incidence, morbidity, and quality of life [special issue]. *Health Communication, 15*(2), 163-170.

Kreps, G.L., & Chapelsky-Massimilla, D. (in press). Cancer communications research and health outcomes: Review and challenge. *Communication Studies.*

Kundrat, A., & Nussbaum, J.F. (2003). The impact of invisible illness on identity and contextual age across the life span. *Health Communication, 15*(3).

Lapinski, M.K., & Levine, T.R. (2000). Culture and manipulation theory: The effects of self-construal and locus of benefit on information manipulation. *Communication Studies, 51*(1), 55-73.

Lewis, J., Ng, K., Hung, K.E., Bilker, W.B., Berlin, J.A., Brensinger, C., & Rustgi, A.K. (2003). Detection of proximal adenomatous polyps with screening sigmoidoscopy: A systematic review and meta-analysis of screening colonoscopy. *Archives of Internal Medicine, 163*(4), 413-421.

Li, S.-C. (2002). Connecting the many levels and facets of cognitive aging. *Trends in Cognitive Neuroscience, 11,* 38-43.

Li, S.-C., & Lindenberger, U. (1999). Cross-level unification: A computational exploration of the link between deterioration of neurotransmitter systems and dedifferentiation of cognitive abilities in old age. In L.-G. Nilsson & H. Markowitsch (Eds.), *Cognitive neuroscience and memory* (pp. 103-146). Toronto, Ontario, Canada: Hogrefe & Huber.

MacKay, D.G., & Abrams, L. (1996). Language, memory, and aging: Distributed deficits and the structure of new-versus-old connections. In J. E. Birren & K. W. Schaie (Eds.), *Handbook of the psychology of aging* (4th ed., pp. 251-265). San Diego, CA: Academic Press.

Maibach, E. W., Kreps, G.L., & Bonaguro, E.W. (1996). Developing strategic communication campaigns for HIV/AIDS prevention. In S. Ratzan (Ed.), *AIDS: Effective communication for the 90s* (pp. 15-35). Washington, DC: Taylor & Francis.

Maheswaran, D., & Chaiken, S. (1991), Promoting systematic processing in low-motivation settings: Effect of incongruent information on processing and judgment. *Journal of Personality and Social Psychology, 61,* 13-25.

McFarland, R. (1968). The sensory and perceptual processes in aging. In K. Schaie (Ed.), *Theory and methods in research on aging* (pp. 9-52). Morgantown: West Virginia University Press.

Meyerowitz, B.E., & Chaiken, S. (1987). The effect of message framing on breast self-examination attitudes, intentions, and behaviors. *Journal of Personality and Social Psychology, 52*(3), 500-511.

Mitchell, M. M. (2000) Motivated, but not able? The effects of positive and negative mood on persuasive message processing. *Communication Monographs, 67,* 215-225.

Mitchell, M. M., Brown, K. M., Villagran, M., & Villagran, P. D. (2001). The effects of anger, sadness and happiness on persuasive message processing: A test of the negative state relief model. *Communication Monographs, 68,* 347-359.

Mittlemark, M.B. (1978). *Information on imminent versus long term health consequences: Impact on children's smoking behaviour, intentions and knowledge.* Unpublished doctoral dissertation, University of Houston, Houston, TX.

Monge, R. (1969). Learning in adult years set or rigidity. *Human Development, 12,* 131-140.

Moore, D. L., Hausknecht, D. L., & Thamodaran, K. (1986). Time compression, response opportunity, and persuasion. *Journal of Consumer Research, 13,* 85-99.

National Center for Health Statistics. (2000). *Health, United States, 2000.* Hyattsville, MD: U.S. Department of Health and Human Services.

Nussbaum, J. F., Baringer, D., & Kundrat, A. (2003). Health, communication, and aging: Cancer and the older adult [special issue]. *Health Communication, 15*(2), 185-194.

Nussbaum, J. F., Pecchioni, L., Robinson, J. D., & Thompson, T. (2000). *Communication and aging* (2nd ed.). Mahwah, NJ: Erlbaum.

Nussbaum, J. F., Robinson, J. D., & Grew, D. (1983, May). *Nursing staff-resident communication within the long-term health care facility.* Paper presented at the International Communication Association, Dallas, TX.

Nussbaum, J. F., Robinson, J. D., & Grew, D. (1985). Communicative behavior of the long-term health care employee: Implications for the elderly resident. *Communication Research Reports, 2,* 16-22.

O'Hair, H.D., Villagran, M. M., Wittenberg, E., Brown, K., Ferguson, M., Hall, H. T., & Doty, T. (2003). Cancer survivorship and agency model (CSAM): Implications for patient choice, decision-making, and influence [special issue]. *Health Communication,15*(2), 195-202.

Okun, M. (1976). Adult age and cautiousness in decision. *Human Development, 19,* 220-233.

Ong, L., Visser, M., Kruyver, I., Bensing, J. M., Brink-Muinen, A., Stouthard, J., Lammes, F., & de Haes, J. (1998). The Roter Interaction Analysis System (RIAS) in oncological consultations: Psychometric properties. *Psycho-oncology, 7,* 387-401.

Pecchioni, L., Ota, H., & Sparks, L. (2004). Cultural issues in communication and aging. In J. F. Nussbaum & J. Coupland (Eds.), *Handbook of communication and aging research* (pp. 167-207). Mahwah, NJ: Erlbaum.

Pecchioni, L., & Sparks, L. (2007). Health information sources of individuals with cancer and their family members. *Health Communication.*

Pee, B., & Hammond, S. (1997). Sensitive issues in health education practice: Cancer prevention and adolescents. *Health Education, 97,* 233-243.

Petty, R. E., & Cacioppo, J. T. (1986). *Communication and persuasion: Central and peripheral routes to attitude change.* New York: Springer.

Petty, R. E., Cacioppo, J. T., & Goldman, R. (1981). Personal involvement as a determinant of argument based persuasion. *Journal of Personality and Social Psychology, 41*, 847-855.

Petty, R.E., Wells, G.L., & Brock, T.C. (1976), Distraction can enhance or reduce yielding to propaganda: Thought disruption versus effort justification. *Journal of Personality and Social Psychology, 34*, 876-884.

Petty, R. E., & Wegener, D. T. (1999). The Elaboration Likelihood Model: Current status and controversies. In S. Chaiken & Y. Trope (Eds.), *Dual process theories in social psychology* (pp. 41-72). New York: Guilford Press.

Pinto, M. B., & Priest, S. (1991). Guilt appeals in advertising: An exploratory study. *Psychological Reports, 69*, 375-385.

Pinto, M. B., & Worobetz, N. D. (1992). Note on guilt appeals in advertising: Covariate effects of self-esteem and locus of control. *Psychological Reports, 70*, 19-22.

Query, J., & Wright, K.(2003). Assessing communication competence in an online study: Towards informing subsequent interventions among older adults with cancer, their lay caregivers and peers [special issue]. *Health Communication, 15*(2), 203-218.

Ragan, S., Wittenberg, E., & Hall, H. T. (2003). The communication of palliative care for the elderly cancer patient {special issue]. *Health Communication, 15*(2), 219-228.

Robinson, J. D., & Turner, J. (2003). Interpersonal and hyperpersonal social support: Cancer and the elderly adult [special issue]. *Health Communication, 15*(2), 229-238.

Rothman, A.J., Salovey, P., Antone, C., Keough, K., & Martin, C.D. (1993). The influence of message framing on intentions to perform health behaviors. *Journal of Experimental Social Psychology*, *29*(5), 408.

Rowan, K., Sparks, L., Pecchioni, L., & Villagran, M. (2003). The CAUSE model: A research supported aid for physicians communicating about cancer risk. *Health Communication, 15*(2), 239-252.

Rubin, A. M., & Rubin, R. B. (1986). Contextual age as a life-position index. *International Journal of Aging and Human Development, 23*, 27-45.

Schaie, K. (1975). Age changes in adult intelligence. In D. Woodruff & J. Birren (Eds.), *Aging* (pp. 111-124). New York: Van Nostrand.

Schaie, K. (1983). The Seattle longitudinal study: A 21 year exploration of psychometric intelligence in adulthood. In K. Schaie (Ed.), *Longitudinal studies of adult psychological development* (pp. 64-135). New York: Guilford.

Schaie, K. (1996). Intellectual development in adulthood. In J. E. Birren & K. W. Schaie (Eds.), *Handbook of the psychology of aging* (4th ed., pp. 266-286). San Diego, CA: Academic Press.

Smith, B. (1996). Memory. In J. E. Birren & K. W. Schaie (Eds.), *Handbook of the psychology of aging* (4th ed., pp. 236-250). San Diego, CA: Academic Press.

Smith, B., Thompson, L., & Michalewski, H. (1980). Average evoked potential research in adult aging: Status and prospects. In L. Poon (Ed.), *Aging in the 1980s* (pp. 135-151). Washington, DC: American Psychological Association.

Sparks, L. (Ed.). (2003a). Cancer communication and aging [special issue]. *Health Communication, 15*(2), 123-258.

Sparks, L. (2003b). An introduction to cancer communication and aging: Theoretical and research insights. *Health Communication, 15*(2), 123-132.
Sparks, L., Pecchioni, L., & Mittapalli, K. (2003). *Health information sources of individuals diagnosed with lung cancer.* A paper presented to the Health Communication Division of the Eastern Communication Association, Washington, DC.
Sparks, L., Pecchioni, L., & Mittapalli, K. (2004). *Health information sources of family caregivers of individuals diagnosed with lung cancer.* Paper presented to the Health Communication Division of the Eastern Communication Association, Boston, MA.
Takeda, S., & Matsuzawa, T. (1985). Age-related brain atrophy: A study with computer tomography. *Journal of Gerontology, 40,* 159-163.
Todorov, A., Chaiken, S., & Henderson, M. D. (2002). The heuristic-systematic model of social information processing. In J. P. Dillard & M. Pfau (Eds.), *The persuasion handbook: Developments in theory and practice* (pp. 195-211). Thousand Oaks, CA: Sage.
Turner, J. W., Grube, J., & Meyers, J. (2001). Developing an optimal match within online communities: An exploration of CMC support communities & traditional support. *Journal of Communication, 51*(2), 231-251.
Verbrugge, L. (1984). A health profile of older women with comparisons to older men. *Research on Aging, 6,* 291-322.
Villaume, W. A., Brown, M. H., & Darling, R. (1994). Presbycusis, communication, and older adults. In M. L. Hummert, J. M. Wiemann, & J. F. Nussbaum (Eds.), *Interpersonal communication in older adulthood: Interdisciplinary theory and research* (pp. 83-106). Thousand Oaks, CA: Sage.
Wells, G., & Harvey, J. (1977). Do people use consensus information in making causal attributions. *Journal of Personality and Social Psychology, 35,* 279-293.
Willeford, J. A. (1971). The geriatric patient. In D. Rose (Ed.), *Audiological assessment* (pp. 281-319). Englewood Cliffs, NJ: Prentice-Hall.
Willis, S. L. (1996). Everyday problem solving. In J. E. Birren & K. W. Schaie (Eds.), *Handbook of the psychology of aging* (4th ed., pp. 287-307). San Diego, CA: Academic Press.
Witte, K. (1992). Putting the fear back in to fear appeals: The extended parallel process model. *Communication Monographs, 59,* 329-349.
Witte, K. (1994). Fear control and danger control: A test of the extended parallel process model. *Communications Monographs, 61,* 113-134.
Witte K., & Allen, M. (2000). A meta-analysis of fear appeals: Implications for effective public health campaigns. *Health Education and Behavior, 27,* 591-615.
Wohlwill, J. F. (1970). The age variable in psychological research. *Psychological Review, 77,* 49-64.

3

Aging Adults and Online Cancer Information

Promises and Pitfalls in an Era of Genomic Health Care

Roxanne Parrott
The Pennsylvania State University

Janice L. Raup Krieger
Ohio State University

Kami Silk
Michigan State University

Nichole Egbert
Kent State University

In the early 1990s, health communicators optimistically forecast the use of computers to fulfill a role in health education (Lieberman, 1992). Even their best case scenario seems likely to have missed the mark. At the beginning of the 21st century, one review put the number of Web sites disseminating health information at 70,000 (Grandinetti, 2000), with online Web searches having become a mainstay of health information provision for millions of Americans. Harris polling data projected that, as of March 2002, 110 million Americans were using the Internet to find information about health, searching an average of three times per month (H. Taylor & Leitman, 2002). In a national survey of 4,764 self-reported Internet users, 40% had sought health information online (Baker, Wagner, Singer, & Bundorf, 2003), with 6 million Americans seeking such information on a typical day (Fox & Rainie, 2002). This use pattern was associated with significant numbers of men and women of most ages, education levels, and races: 72% of women and 51% of men; 53% of 18- to 29-year-olds, 63% of 30- to 40-year olds, and 71% of 50 to 64-year-olds; 44% with less than a high school education, 57% with a high school education, 61% with some college, and 69% of college graduates; and 62% of Whites, 61% of African Americans and 60% of Hispanics (Fox & Rainie, 2002).

Although data representing Internet use for health information demonstrate widespread patterns of search behavior, the same data also reveal patterns associated with nonuse. In particular, for purposes of this chapter, findings related to indirect relationships between age and education for Internet use to search for health information are of particular interest. Since the introduction of SeniorNet in 1986 (Furlong, 1989), aging adults' motivation and ability related to computer technology has spawned a considerable amount of research (e.g., Charness, Parks, & Sable, 2001; Morrell, 2002; Rogers & Fisk, 2002). Access to credible health information via the Web can be beneficial in many ways, especially as one ages (Nussbaum, Pecchioni, Robinson, & Thompson, 2000). With this as the overarching premise of this chapter, we review behavioral health outcomes prominently associated with exposure to online information, specifically referencing cancer and genetics. Our review is situated within a construct commonly associated with cancer communication, perceived control, both behavioral and cognitive. An individual's beliefs about the nature of cancer, its impacts, and level of control play an important role in information-seeking and people's more general pattern of actions related to health (Johnson, 1997). We situate control as a multifaceted construct within a larger theoretical framework, problematic integration (PI) theory (Babrow, 1992), linking aging adults' motivation and ability to seek cancer information online to this macro-view.

AGING ADULTS' MOTIVATION TO SEEK CANCER INFORMATION ONLINE

PI theory (Babrow, 1992) asserts that humans rely on probabilistic and evaluative judgments to help reference and predict future events. When evaluations, whether positive or negative in orientation, diverge from probability of an event, we have difficulty integrating the information. For example, "How likely is it that this cancer medication will relieve my pain, that participation in a cancer clinical trial will benefit me, or that I have inherited a gene related to cancer?" are all questions associated with cancer treatments and therapies that may motivate one to seek information. "How likely is it that Internet information-seeking will answer these questions, that I can access credible and accurate information online, or that it will relate to me?" are questions likely to predict online searches. Related to the likelihood that one will seek information online are also answers to such questions as, "How much do I value relief from my pain, the possibility of benefiting other cancer patients in the future, or knowing that I have a gene that may predict the likelihood that I will get cancer?" PI theory states that integration is inevitable and central to the human experience, but the experience of integration may be either routine or problematic (Babrow, 2001). New information, regardless of whether it is evaluated as positive or negative, likely or unlikely, will be incorporated into a person's set of experiences, intentions, knowledge, and feelings. However, "as integration of probability and evaluation becomes more problematic, it becomes increasingly difficult to form and maintain associated cognitive, affective, and behavioral orientations" (Babrow, 1992, p. 98), contributing to situations in which "integration is often problematic" (Babrow, 2001, p. 5).

Four situations have been identified in which integration is likely to be "problematic":

1. When probabilistic and evaluative orientations diverge (bad things become very likely or good things seem very unlikely).
2. When ambiguity clouds our ability to discern either probability or evaluation.
3. When ambivalence upsets these processes by removing one's choice or erasing evaluative orientations.
4. When impossibility seems imminent, causing probabilistic judgments to be at odds with evaluative orientations (Babrow, 1992; Brashers & Babrow, 1996).

Thus, problematic integration would be likely when (a) an individual's genetic test reveals the presence of a gene that appears in about 5% of cases associated with female breast cancer; (b) the status of knowledge about the gene's role in cancer makes it impossible to determine which women with the gene get breast cancer; (c) one has no control over which genes one inherits; and/or (d) the gene(s) linked to breast cancer if present offers only one primary option to remove uncertainty regarding the formation of breast cancer, prophylactic mastectomy. Adding to that likelihood may be perceptions that online information is inaccurate (divergent case), online information is difficult to access (ambiguous case), online access is unavailable (ambivalent case), or use for aging adults appears physically unlikely (impossibility). These scenarios illustrate the wide range of situations that may impact aging adults' motivation to seek cancer information online. Communication scholars have applied PI theory to breast cancer survivorship (Campbell, 1997; Ford, Babrow, & Stohl, 1996); end-of-life decision making (Hines, Babrow, Badzek, & Moss, 1997); and the conduct of breast self-examinations (Babrow & Kline, 1999). These situations, described as more problematic to integrate, appear likely to be associated with too little or too much perceived cognitive or behavioral control, perhaps affecting aging adults' motivation to seek cancer information online.

OPTIMISM OR PESSIMISM: PERCEIVED COGNITIVE CONTROL

Perceptions of personal risk are likely to result in information-seeking (Viswanath, Kahn, Finegan, Hertog, & Potter, 1993; Yows, Salmon, Hawkins, & Love, 1991). One challenge for cancer communicators is to strike a balance between perceived risk and perceived invulnerability. Too much perceived cognitive control negatively relates to taking personal action on behalf of one's health, a finding that represents an optimistic bias used to explain why people do not behave in health-promoting ways, with inaction attributed to a lack of perceived vulnerability. Optimism decreases with experience, however, also a persistent finding (Renn, Burns, Kasperson, Kasperson, & Slovic, 1992; van der Vedle, Hooykaas, & van der Pligt, 1992), with heredity affording one path to experience with a health problem. In a community-based study of adults between 18 and 65, Weinstein (1987) found that "people usually do take family history into account in formulating ideas of their risk" (p. 494), as illustrated with regard to cancer generally and lung cancer specifically, as well as diabetes, hypertension, arthritis, and heart attacks. Research on optimistic bias has found that heavy smokers overestimate their longevity. Specifically, estimates by heavy smokers that they would live to be at least 75 years old were twice the estimates of what actuarial studies would predict (Schoenbaum, 1997). Adult smokers in another study doubted that they would die from smoking even if they smoked for 30 or 40 years (Arnett, 2000), perhaps relating heredity to health.

Heredity has not been discussed in terms of contributing to a pessimistic bias in which individuals overestimate risk and avoid behaving in health-promoting ways because of fatalistic views. This may be due to the fact that in the past we knew less about the role of inherited genes for health or the role of personal behaviors and social support on the expression of genes in health. With the mapping of the human genome, however, that situation has drastically changed. An era of traditional genetics in which conditions relating to a single gene such as cystic fibrosis and sickle cell disease has been replaced with greater awareness that the leading causes of mortality have genetic components. This includes cancer. "An example is colon cancer, where nine genes have been identified that show a significant degree of correlation with susceptibility to this cancer" (Cole, 1998, p. 61).

In this burgeoning era of genomic health care, however, shortcuts have been observed in research that examined the approach of the news to reporting about advances associated with genetics and cancer, as newspaper and television, for example, use such shorthand phrases and terms as "the breast cancer gene" (Condit, 1999). Our research has demonstrated that genes are perceived to be the most important cause of breast cancer in women by both African American (Duncan, Parrott, & Silk, 2001) and European American women (Parrott, Silk, & Condit, 2003). An increased number of messages from sources other than online cancer information sites associating heredity with cancer may thus lead to both optimistic and pessimistic biases. This may be particularly problematic among aging adults who may perceive that the status of cancer science more often relates to interventions associated with genetics rather than interventions to extend and/or improve the quality of life for aging cancer survivors. This may create situations in which information is difficult to integrate with experience and impedes motivation to seek online information. Moreover, if online information is sought and found to also emphasize the role of genes for cancer and cancer therapies, this may importantly contour behavioral health outcomes associated with aging adults' perceived behavioral control.

BEHAVIORAL HEALTH OUTCOMES AND PERCEIVED BEHAVIORAL CONTROL

Adults who access the Internet for cancer information include a wide range of age groups, averaging early 50s (Chen & Siu, 2001), late 50s (Metz et al., 2001), and mid-60s (Peterson & Fretz, 2003), but including adults into their 70s, 80s, and up to 90 years of age. Online sources provide information seekers with a plethora of prevention, treatment, and coping information found to increase knowledge and levels of hope, but also arouse fear, confusion, or uncertainty (Helft, Hlubocky, & Daugherty, 2003). The exact content producing these outcomes has not been identified. However, research relating genes to cancer affords one path for understanding these seemingly conflicting outcomes.

Knowledge

Human genetics research (HGR) has received widespread and sustained coverage in the popular media (Condit, 1999). This may lead to a lack of accurate understanding about genetics and cancer, and online searches to clarify the confusion (M. Taylor et al., 2001). Women, for example, have increased their efforts to seek information regarding their individual breast cancer risk in the wake of media reports about a breast cancer gene. "Many of these women will not have a family history that suggests the presence of a highly penetrant breast cancer susceptibility gene. However, a small subset of such women will come from families with a striking incidence of breast and other cancers often associated with inherited mutations" (Hoskins et al., 1995, p. 577). Women in the latter group may benefit greatly from awareness of HGR in this regard and their decision to seek testing. Women in the former group, however, may impose undue emotional and financial burdens on themselves and their families. The risk goes as high as 85% that a woman carrying a mutation in either the *BRCA1* (breast cancer 1) or *BRCA2* (breast cancer 2) gene will develop breast cancer by the age of 80 (Breast Cancer Information Center, 2003). More knowledge about the role of genes in disease has been directly related to greater reservations about the wholesale adoption of genetic technology, testing, and screening (Jallinoja & Aro, 2000), suggesting an impact for knowledge on perceived behavioral control.

Response Efficacy

One line of expectancies emerging from discourse about HGR is related to an overly optimistic view about the availability and efficacy of genetic therapies (Parrott, Silk, Krieger, Condit, & Harris, 2004). Online sites relating genes to cancer may reify these impressions as a result of content that suggests the availability and use of genetic technologies and gene therapies for cancer treatment far beyond the actual availability and efficacy of these approaches. Although no research to date has focused explicitly on such content, there are many warnings given about information published on the Internet (Crocco, Villasis-Keever, & Jadad, 2002). Four criteria used to assess Web sites that provided information about alternative/complementary treatments to cancer, for example, identified descriptions of treatment as a "cancer cure" and/or "having no side effects" as "red flags" associated with overstatements of the effectiveness of the proposed therapies; these phrases were found in 90% of the 194 sites reviewed (Matthews, Camacho, Mills, & Dimsdale, 2002).

Self-efficacy

One of the most significant outcomes of individual knowledge and outcome expectancies is one's confidence in the ability to gain and maintain control over inputs to a particular behavior, or self-efficacy (Bandura, 1997). One of the most often underrated aspects of health care, for example, is preparation for tests and/or treatments, with doctors consistently underrating the importance of preparation when compared to patients or nurses (Schofield, Walkom, Ethics, & Sanson-Fisher, 1997). Use of online cancer information may increase individuals' feelings of self-efficacy and control through enhanced perceptions of preparation. One case study, in fact, demonstrated how use of the Internet led to an increase in perceived sense of control for a 51-year-old patient with terminal cancer who used e-mail to express her distress and emotions to her physician, associated with a decrease in the number of hospital and emergency room visits (Strausser, Fisch, Bodurka, Sivesind, & Bruera, 2002). Other patients report that the ability to bring information to consultations and talk with physicians about their treatment options and issues related to cancer has helped them to feel more empowered and in control of their illness (Murray et al., 2003). Although such information appears to enhance feelings of behavioral control and contribute to motivation to seek online cancer information, it also introduces some concerns about the impact of this action on the physician-patient relationship.

PHYSICIAN–PATIENT RELATIONSHIP

Patients who seek online information and present it during medical visits feel that it affects their relationship with their physician more positively than negatively (Murray et al., 2003). One survey of oncologists ($N = 266$) found that 30% estimated that their patients use the Internet to obtain cancer information, with the majority (96%) of oncologists reporting that they always or most of the time discuss information that patients bring with them to medical visits, though it adds an estimated 10 minutes to the meeting (mean = 10, mode = 10, range = 1–37); 54% reported that the Internet had a negative impact on patients and their relationships with patients, whereas 36% of oncologists reported a positive impact (Helft et al., 2003). Reasons for negative impact included inaccurate information from the Internet, greater anxiety, false hope, and lack of understanding of information. Oncologists who reported positive effects stated that relationships were strengthened through discussion of Internet information, awareness of new and appropriate clinical trials, greater patient satisfaction, and patients who could make more informed treatment decisions (Helft et al., 2003).

Research has identified that some patients perceive their physicians as feeling "challenged" if health information is presented by patients during the medical visit (Murray et al., 2003). These patients' perceptions may be accurate, as some oncologists (9%), a group who actively seek health information online themselves (Chen & Siu, 2001), have reported feeling threatened by Internet information (Helft et al., 2003). Most physicians report a neutral or positive attitude toward online information brought to them by patients, and most general practitioners report they would be willing to use computer decision support systems to manage familial cancer care (Braithwaite, Sutton, Smithson, & Emery, 2002). Most patients report that they simply want the physician's opinion about the information rather than anything specific (e.g., treatment referral, order a test, change medication; Murray et al., 2003).

In summary, a diagnosis of cancer creates a situation in which information about treatment, quality of life, and survival may produce instances in which the information is problematic to integrate and thus motivates aging adults to seek information online. The online cancer information searches may contribute to enhanced cognitive and/or behavioral control through information that increases individual knowledge, and self- and response efficacy. Such searches may be inhibited by other information sources that prioritize the role of genes in cancer causation or genetic therapies in treatment. Or, such messages may motivate aging adults to explore online sites to expand their understanding of these and other options related to cancer. One important predictor of the use of this channel to gain information may be aging adults' perceptions associated with the impact on their relationships with their oncologists and other medical caregivers. To enhance perceptions of control in this regard, online cancer sites may explicitly address how to talk to caregivers about information found over the Internet, how to introduce questions that emerge based on such information, and how to assess the credibility of the online information. Each of these issues may contribute not only to aging adults' motivations to seek cancer information online, but also be tailored by related abilities associated with such searches.

AGING ADULTS' ABILITIES RELATED TO SEEKING CANCER INFORMATION ONLINE

A cancer diagnosis has often been identified as the impetus to overcome barriers to seeking health information and enact actions to close the gap between what one usually has available to draw on for information resources and what is actually available (Johnson, 1997). The advantages of Internet health information searches in satisfying these needs include access, interactivity, information tailoring, and the seeming ability to search for information anonymously (Cline & Haynes, 2001). Compared to younger adults, however, older adults spend less time using computers, less time browsing the Web when they do use computers, are less expert at using the

Web, and less comfortable and satisfied with their computer and Internet use (Kurniawan, Ellis, & Zaphiris, 2003). Although adults aged 60 and older are often subject to the negative cultural stereotype that paints the elderly as "computer-phobic" (Kubeck, Miller-Albrecht, & Murphy, 1999, p. 181), several variables besides age may better explain experiences of aging adults.

Accessibility: Availability, Affordability, Use, and Usability

When employed to predict computer use for health information, accessibility relates not only to the actual presence of computers, but to physical and cognitive developmental issues that contribute to use and usability. According to Brodie, Flournoy, Altman, and Blendon (2000), 31% of people under age 60 use computers at home to get health information, compared to only one in ten adults over the age of 60. One characteristic associated with use by older adults, direct computer experience, plays a vital positive role on attitudes, a finding repeated in studies across a decade of research (Baldi, 1997; Cody, Dunn, Hoppin, & Wendt, 1999; Czaja & Sharit, 1998; Jay & Willis, 1992; Kelley, Morrell, Park, & Mayhorn, 1999; Kubeck et al., 1999). One successful experience using the Internet is related to high levels of positive affect toward using it again (Kelley et al., 1999; Williamson, Bow, & Wale, 1997). For all online health information-seekers, barriers relating to health literacy, the skills and motivation to understand and use health information and resources, have been identified (Christensen & Griffiths, 2000; Merriman, Ades, & Seffrin, 2002).

Cognitive dissonance has been applied to computer use to explain the impact of voluntary use and ownership of a computer on computer anxiety, confidence, and liking, with use positively relating to ownership, and both reducing anxiety about computer use together with increased confidence and liking of computers (Parish & Necessary, 1996). Sometimes, training plays a vital role in older adult computer proficiency, directly relating to continued use of the computer (Kelley et al., 1999).

The perceptual, motor, and cognitive demands of using computers and the Internet are often overlooked as potential reasons for Internet access disparities that exist between young-old and older adults. Older adults (75–89 years) have been found to make significantly more motor control errors when using the computer than do young-old adults (60–74 years; Echt, Morrell, & Park, 1998). Use of computers and the Web requires fine motor skills to complete tasks such as positioning the cursor on a particular target. Ergonomic issues such as size of letters on the screen, and difficulty using a keyboard contribute to the effectiveness of this modality in addressing information needs (Baldi, 1997; Czaja & Sharit, 1998; Ellis & Allaire, 1999;

Festervand, Meinert, & Vitell, 1994; Kubeck, 1999; White et al., 1999). Older adults may struggle with the perceptual requirements of many Web sites, as many older adults have difficulty perceiving the differences between certain colors or between light and dark (Stronge, Walker, & Rogers, 2002). Additionally, small fonts have been found to cause difficulties for older adult users (Hutchison, Eastman, & Tirrito, 1997).

Finally, the design of the Web requires particular types of cognitive functioning that tend to decline as we age, such as problem solving, working memory, attention, and concept formation (Jones & Bayen, 1998). The physical decline that accompanies older adulthood for many helps explain why increasing age is positively related to reduced use of the computer (Kamal & Patil, 2003). Williamson et al. (1997) found common problems to include older adults' inability to use a mouse for pointing, clicking, and scrolling as well as the inability to read the screen. When talk-through interfaces that "talk" users through their interaction on the Web are employed for visually impaired users, older adults have been found to have a limited capacity to remember long messages that ask users what functions they would like to perform (Zajicek & Morrisey, 2003).

Personal Relevance: Culture and Gender

Evidence shows that large groups of people share similar patterns of computer and/or Internet non-use. Some studies have shown that when education and income are controlled, African Americans still have a lower rate of home computer ownership and computer access (K. Wilson, Wallin, & Resier, 2003). However, African Americans have also been found to be more likely than White Americans to be aware of and utilize free public access to computers and the Internet (Ervin & Gilmore, 1999; Wilson et al., 2003). One way to explain who is marginalized from participation in online technology is to examine the cultural values inherent in the use of this type of technology. Several critiques of the Internet as it relates to culture have emerged. One type of critique challenges the notion that technology is "neutral" in respect to culture (Bowers, Vasquez, & Roaf, 2000). It has been argued that computers and the Internet are situated within a cultural context of White, Western masculinity (Bowers et al., 2000; Escobar, 1995; F. Wilson, 2003). Proponents of the neutrality of technology point to examples of ways that technology has helped marginalized members of society have a voice in the larger discourse. One example is Santa Monica's Public Electronic Network (PEN), the nation's first city government-sponsored interactive electronic communication system designed to improve access to technology of all residents, particularly the "have-nots" (Schmitz, 1997).

Despite the potential for altruistic applications of technological advancements such as PEN, Escobar (1995) pointed out that computer and

Internet technology was developed and continues to be advanced in the cultural context of military and economic interests. Because of the militaristic and economic forces that drive the proliferation of the Internet, certain values have been subsequently ascribed to its use. For example, Bowers et al., (2000) posited that computers reinforce a "modern, Western pattern of individual-centered relations and forms of consciousness essential to the earlier phase of the Industrial Revolution" (p. 185). Other critiques associate computers and the Internet with dominant values of "rationality, instrumentality, profit, and violence" (Escobar, 1995, p. 412), as well as charges that it alienates women through the construction of technology as masculine (F. Wilson, 2003).

Critiques of computers and the Internet based in cultural values have led some to recommend that certain minority communities take extreme caution in the adoption of computer technology, citing the potential of the Internet to subvert the rich culture of minority communities (Bowers et al., 2000). Still others see eradicating the digital divide as a means of empowering minority communities (Cross, 2001). Everett (2002), for example, argued that the Internet was "elitist, white masculinist" (p. 127), but that certain changes, such as the introduction of a separate category for Afrocentric content on the Yahoo! search engine in 1995, have helped to create a more egalitarian public sphere.

If Web sites devoted to providing the lay public with cancer information associate race or ethnicity with increased incidence, however, this explanation may "naturalize racial and ethnic difference and create a conceptual barrier to developing a research program that explores the complex ways in which social inequality and experiences of racial discrimination interact with human biology to influence patterns of disease" (Braun, 2002, p. 159). Such outcomes could contribute to increased expectations that particular ethnic groups seek therapy as a choice to produce normative outcomes, with norms relating to a Euro-American male as the standard.

Gender disparities also continue to be a concern regarding computer and Internet use. For example, African-American men use the Internet at a higher rate than African-American females (Ervin & Gilmore, 1999). Research has suggested that these disparities can be attributed to women being less experienced, less confident, and less integrated into the computer culture (F. Wilson, 2003). On the other hand, Parish and Necessary (1996) reported that women demonstrate more computer confidence and computer liking than do males. The attention placed on attributes, such as confidence and liking, point to the importance of attitudes toward computers in predicting use. Ervin and Gilmore (1999) found that about two-thirds of the African-American women in the study believed that the Internet and World Wide Web were government-tracking devices, compared to about one-third of African-American males. Better understanding of the attitudes of various populations toward technology is one way to better explain the differential utilization rates.

Assistance With Use

According to one survey, more than 50% of Internet users have found health information online for someone else (Pew Research Center, 2003), demonstrating that health is not a solitary issue, but rather a collective issue in which friends and family are involved. Grandchildren and children have been discovered to assist older adults in their efforts to go online. According to a survey conducted for the American Association of Retired Persons (AARP), 78% of younger respondents have taught older adults how to use the computer, and 87% have helped parents find information online (WirthlinWorldwide, 2003). Specifically, 36% of respondents reported that they help their parents or grandparents find health information online. A previous study has focused on populations such as adult daughters of women who had had breast cancer, finding that these women "monitor" the information environment, tracking available information about breast cancer (Rees & Bath, 2000). Another study conducted at ambulatory cancer care clinics in Canada found that 50% of individuals accessed the Internet for cancer information and 15% of those who performed information searches reported that they conducted searches with the help of family and friends (Chen & Sui, 2001). For older adults who want to use the Internet independently, peer-group teaching has been found to be effective and efficient (Furlong, 1989). Additionally, mentors who are similar in age may help to add validity to claims by the younger generations that the Internet is useful, accessible, and easy to use. However, one's peer group may also serve as a negative influence. For example, one study in a nursing home that developed a training program for residents found that some residents perceived a potential loss in their status within their peer groups and decided not to continue with computer and online training sessions (Namazi & McClintic, 2003).

Technological Features

Technological features of Web sites are critically important in shaping users' abilities to access available information (Rieh & Belkin, 1998). Health information-seekers cite navigational ease and site structure as the primary reasons for revisiting a specific site (Fox & Rainie, 2002). The type of hyperlinking structure offered by a Web site is crucial in determining both cognitive and affective aspects of user reaction to the site (May, Sundar, & Williams, 1997). Moreover, the type and volume of responses obtained by the user from a search engine have significant perceptual consequences (Kalyanaraman, Mahood, Sundar, & Oliver, 2000). Other determinants of navigational ease of use include download speed and interactivity. Download speed influences not only users' physiological arousal during message reception, but also the volume of their clicking activity (Sundar & Wagner, 2002). Increasing the interactivity of a political Web site served to enhance positive user impressions of the candidate featured on the site (Sundar, Brown, & Kalyanaraman, 1999). Multimedia features, on the other hand, serve to complicate navigation in a Web site and lead to cognitively and perceptually inferior outcomes (Sundar, 2000).

Individuals might have a negative attitude toward accessing online cancer information because of their inability to judge the credibility of sources (Bernhardt, Weaver Lariscy, Parrott, Silk, & Felter, 2001; Pew Research Center, 2003). Bernhardt et al. (2001) identified concerns with source credibility, information accuracy, and confidentiality regarding use of the Internet for health information related to genetics research. In contrast, one study of cancer patients using academic, community, or veterans medical centers found that 21% of patients reported using the Internet for health information, with 27% regarding the retrieved information as very reliable and 71% as somewhat reliable (Metz et al., 2001). Attitudes and fears about the accuracy of online cancer information may be merited, as illustrated by a study examining Web sites about melanoma that found that 14% of the 74 Web sites examined contained inaccuracies and often lacked complete basic melanoma information (Bichakjan et al., 2002).

Attitudes may also relate to the challenges associated with identifying the source of information on the Internet. For example, if a piece of medical information appears on WebMD.com, a variety of source attributions are possible: (a) the scientist responsible for discovering the fact, (b) the scientific journal where the fact first appeared, (c) the gatekeepers at WebMD, (d) the Internet itself, (e) the computer from which the information was accessed, (f) the receiver him or herself, or (g) other Internet user(s) as in the case of a chatroom (see also Sundar, 1998). Depending on which one of these is made salient, a different type of heuristic will disproportionately influence processing of the information obtained. For example, if the scientist is made salient, then the expert heuristic will predominate. If the construct of "other users" is more salient, then the bandwagon heuristic in which an individual presumes that agreement is related to being one of the crowd is more likely to operate. In reality, multiple source attributions are simultaneously made salient on the Web, representing a kind of "source layering." Sundar and Nass (2001) distinguished between visible sources such as gatekeepers (WebMD in the example above), technological sources such as the medium (Internet and computer), and receiver sources. Users' inability to parse the various layers may lead to source confusion, thereby complicating the identification of the psychological locus of credibility and other assessments involved in processing the obtained information.

CONCLUSION

> Government, educational institutions, non-profit organizations, community groups, health care institutions (such as nursing homes and assisted-living facilities), libraries and others can work together or separately to address the training and access needs of older adults. (Kawamoto, 2003, p. 6)

The ethical translation of science in an era when targeting and tailoring have become the presumed superior strategies in health communication requires a step back to consider why, when, and how online communication may contribute to targeting dilemmas, in which multiple segments of an audience are identified, but reached differentially with information (Guttman, 1997). Aging adults and online cancer information comprise such a dilemma. This problem represents a "digital divide" of sorts that is not so much related to the accessibility of computers and related technology, but to the usability and accuracy of Internet materials. Forecasts into the future suggest that these concerns will continue unabated, as more homes are likely to have Internet access, and more health-related sites will be made available (Mittman & Cain, 2001).

The future of online communication technology and its impact on aging adults seeking quality health-related information is fraught with uncertainty. From considerations of the accessibility, quality, and impact of Internet information, this area is a rich one for future research. Researchers and designers of online health messages must consider older adults an audience segment with very specific but also diverse needs and characteristics. Therefore, in the future, and in the present, tailoring health messages to this population may require not only tailoring language and images, but the very medium as well. Although not a panacea, health information comprises a foundation on which to build communication to guide informed decisions and actions (Kreps, 2000). Online technology in the form of cancer Internet sites affords one strategy to satisfy these needs.

We posit a situation in which an information-rich resource exists that may motivate aging adults to participate in treatments including clinical trials, extend their life-spans, and enhance the quality of their lives, but may be largely inaccessible due to the characteristics of the technology. Many cancer patients are not even aware of credible, evidence-based online cancer information sources (Sgouin & Jadad, 2002). Older adults are not necessarily at a great disadvantage because they are not computer and Internet savvy. A problem exists however if they would like to be wired and barriers exist that prevent them from accessing the Internet (Kawamoto, 2003).

REFERENCES

Arnett, J.J. (2000). Optimistic bias in adolescent and adult smokers and nonsmokers. *Addictive Behaviors, 25*, 625-632.

Babrow, A.S. (1992). Communication and problematic integration: Understanding diverging probability and value, ambiguity, ambivalence, and impossibility. *Communication Theory, 2,* 95-130.

Babrow, A.S. (2001). Uncertainty, value, communication, and problematic integration. *Journal of Communication, 51*, 553-573.

Babrow, A.S., & Kline, K.N. (2000). From "reducing" to "managing uncertainty": Reconceptualizing the central challenge in breast self-exams. *Social Science & Medicine, 51*, 1805-1817.

Baker, L., Wagner, T.H., Singer, S., & Bundorf, M.K. (2003). Use of the internet and e-mail for health care information: Results from a national survey. *JAMA, 289*(18), 2400-2406.

Baldi, R.A. (1997). Training older adults to use the computer: Issues related to the workplace, attitudes, and training. *Educational Gerontology, 23*, 453-465.

Bandura, A. (1997). Self-*efficacy: The exercise of control.* New York: Freeman.

Bernhardt, J.M., Weaver Lariscy, R.A., Parrott, R.L., Silk, K.J., & Felter, E.M. (2001). Human genetics information and the Internet: Opportunities and obstacles for communication. *Journal of Health Communication, 7*, 325-340.

Bichakjian, C.K., Schwartz, J.L., Want, T.S., Hall, J. M., Johnson, T.M., & Biermann, S. (2002). Melanoma information on the Internet: Often incomplete—A public health opportunity? *Journal of Clinical Oncology, 20*(1), 134-141.

Bowers, C.A., Vasquez, M., & Roaf, M. (2000). Native people and the challenge of computers: Reservation schools, individualism, and consumerism. *American Indian Quarterly, 24*(2), 182-199.

Braithwaite, D., Sutton, S., Smithson, W.H., & Emery, J. (2002). Internet-based risk assessment and decision support for the management of familial cancer in primary care: A survey of GPs' attitudes and intentions. *Family Practice, 19*(6), 587-590.

Brashers, D.E., & Babrow, A.S. (1996). Theorizing communication and health. *Communication Studies, 47*, 243-251.

Braun, L. (2002). Race, ethnicity, and health: Can genetics explain disparities? *Perspectives in Biology and Medicine, 45*, 159-174.

Breast Cancer Information Center. (2003). What are the risk factors for breast cancer? Retrieved November 4, 2003, from http://www.infoaging.org/d-breast-4-risk.html.

Brodie, M., Flournoy, R.E., Altman, D.E., & Blendon, R.J. (2000) Health information, the Internet, and the digital divide. *Health Affairs, 19(6)*, 255-265.

Campbell, R.G. (1997). *Evaluating the potential "threat" of social support among breast cancer survivors: Implications for uncertainty reduction*. Paper presented at the annual meeting of the Central States Communication Association, St. Louis, MO.

Charness, N., Parks, D.C., & Sabel, B.A. (2001). *Communication, technology, and aging: Opportunities and challenges for the future*. New York: Springer, Inc.

Chen, X., & Siu, L.L. (2001). Impact of the media and the Internet on oncology: Survey of cancer patients and oncologists in Canada. *Journal of Clinical Oncology, 19*(23), 4291-4297.

Christensen, H., & Griffiths, K.M. (2000). The Internet and mental health literacy. *Australian & New Zealand Journal of Psychiatry, 34*, 975-979.

Cline, R.J.W., & Haynes, K.M. (2001). Consumer health information seeking on the Internet: The state of the art. *Health Education Research, 16*(6), 671-692.

Cody, M.J., Dunn, D., Hoppin, S., & Wendt, P. (1999). Silver surfers: Training and evaluating Internet use among older adult learners. *Communication Education, 48*(4), 269-286.

Cole, R.D. (1998). The genome and the human genome project. In T. Peters (Ed.), *Genetics: Issues of social justice* (pp. 49-70). Cleveland, OH: The Pilgrim Press.

Condit, C.M. (1999). *The meanings of the gene: Determinism, discrimination, and perfectionism in U.S. public discourse*. Madison: University of Wisconsin Press.

Crocco, A.G., Villasis-Keever, M., & Jadad, A.R. (2002). Analysis of cases of harm associated with use of health information on the internet. *Journal of the American Medical Association, 287*(21), 2869-2872.

Cross, D.E. (2001). For whom does the NET work? *Black Issues in Higher Education, 18*(15), 104.

Czaja, S.J., & Sharit, J. (1998). Age differences in attitudes toward computers. *The Journals of Gerontology, 53B*(5), 329-340.

Duncan, V.J., Parrott, R.L., & Silk, K.J. (2001). African American women's perceptions of the role of genetics in breast cancer risk. *American Journal of Health Studies, 17*, 50-58.

Echt, K.V., Morrell, R., & Park, D. (1998). Effects of age and training formats on basic computer skill acquisition in older adults. *Educational Gerontology, 24*(1), 3-25.

Ellis, R.D., & Allaire, J.C. (1999). Modeling computer interest in older adults: The role of age, education, computer knowledge, and computer anxiety. *Human Factors, 41*(3), 345-355.

Ervin, K.S., & Gilmore, G. (1999). Traveling the superinformation highway: African Americans' perceptions and use of cyberspace technology. *Journal of Black Studies, 29*(3), 398-407.

Escobar, A. (1995). Anthropology and the future: New technologies and the reinvention of culture. *Futures, 27*(4), 409-421.

Everett, A. (2002). The revolution will be digitized: Afrocentricity and the digital public sphere. *Social Text, 20*(2), 125-146.

Festervand, T.A., Meinert, D.B., & Vitell, S.J. (1994). Older adults' attitudes toward and adoption of personal computers and computer-based lifestyle assistance. *Journal of Applied Business Research, 10*(2), 13-22.

Ford, L.A., Babrow, A.S., & Stohl, C. (1996). Social support messages and the management of uncertainty in the experience of breast cancer: An application of problematic integration theory. *Communication Monographs, 63*, 189-207.

Fox, S., & Rainie. L. (2002). Vital decisions: How internet users decide what information to trust when they or their loved ones are sick. Pew Internet & American Life Project. Retrieved July 7, 2007, from www.pewinternet.org/reports/toc.asp?Report=59

Furlong, M. (1989). An electronic community for older adults: The SeniorNet Network. *Journal of Communication, 39*(3), 145-153.

Grandinetti, D.A. (2000). Help your patients surf the Net safely. *Medical Economics, 77*(5), 186-201.

Guttman, N. (1997). Beyond strategic research: A value-centered approach to health communication interventions. *Communication Theory, 7*, 95-124.

Helft, P.R., Hlubocky, F., & Daugherty, C.K. (2003). American oncologists' views of Internet use by cancer patients: A mail survey of American Society of Clinical Oncology members. *Journal of Clinical Oncology, 21*(5), 942-947.

Hines, S.C., Babrow, A.S., Badzek, L., & Moss, A.H. (2001). From coping with life to coping with death: Problematic integration for the seriously ill elderly. *Health Communication, 13*, 327-343.

Hoskins, K.F., Stopfer, J.E., Calzone, K.A., Merajver, S.D., Rebbeck, T.R., Garber, J.E., & Weber, B.L. (1995). Assessment and counseling for women with a family history of breast cancer. A guide for clinicians. *Journal of the American Medical Association, 273*, 577-585.

Hutchison, D., Eastman, C., & Tirrito, T. (1997). Designing user interfaces for older adults. *Educational Gerontology, 23*, 497-513.

Jallinoja, P., & Aro, A.R. (2000). Does knowledge make a difference? The association between knowledge about genes and attitudes toward gene tests. *Journal of Health Communication, 5*, 29-39.

Jay, G.M., & Willis, S.L. (1992). Influence of direct computer experience on older adults' attitudes toward computers. *Journal of Gerontology, 47*(4), P250-P275.

Johnson, J.D. (1997). *Cancer-related information seeking*. Cresskill, NJ: Hampton Press.

Jones, B.D., & Bayen, U.J. (1998). Teaching older adults to use computers: Recommendations based on cognitive aging research. *Educational Gerontology, 24*, 675-689.

Kalyanaraman, S., Mahood, C., Sundar, S.S., & Oliver, M.B. (2000, August). *Priming effects of accidental exposure to internet pornography: An experimental study of construct accessibility in search engine output.* Paper presented to the Communication Technology and Policy Division at the 83rd annual convention of the Association for Education in Journalism and Mass Communication (AEJMC), Phoenix, AZ.

Kamal, M., & Patil, G.D. (2003). Computer access and utilization patterns among older people. *Journal of American Academy of Business, 3*, 319-322.

Kawamoto, K. (2003). Older adults and the Internet. *The Journal of Education, Community, and Values: Interface on the Internet*. Berglund Center for Internet Studies, Pacific University, Forest Grove, Oregon. Retrieved on September 8, 2003, from http://bcis.pacificu.edu/journal/2003/02/kawamoto.php

Kelley, C.L., Morrell, R.W., Park, D.C., & Mayhorn, C.B. (1999). Predictors of electronic bulletin board system use in older adults. *Educational Gerontology, 25*, 19-35.

Kreps, G.L. (2000). The evolution and advancement of health communication inquiry. In W.B. Gudykunst (Ed.), *Communication yearbook* (Vol. 24, pp. 232-254). Newbury Park, CA: Sage.

Kubeck, J.E., Miller-Albrecht, S.A., & Murphy, M.D. (1999). Finding information on the world wide web: Exploring older adults' exploration. *Educational Gerontology, 25*, 167-183.

Kurniawan, S.H., Ellis, R.D., & Zaphiris, P. (2003). Comparing older and younger adults' traversal time in expandable and non-expandable hierarchical structures. Retrieved on September 8, 2003, from http://www.soi.city.ac.uk/~zaphiri/Papers/hfes02.pdf

Lieberman, D.A. (1992). The computer's potential role in health education. *Health Communication, 4*(3), 211-225.

May, M.D., Sundar, S.S., & Williams, R.B. (1997, May). *The effects of hyperlinks and site maps on the memorability and enjoyability of web content.* Paper presented to the Communication & Technology Division at the 47th annual conference of the International Communication Association, Montréal, Canada.

Matthews, S.C., Camacho, A., Mills, P.J., & Dimsdale, J.E. (2002). The Internet for medical information about cancer: Help or hindrance? *Psychosomatics, 44*(2), 100-103.

Merriman, B., Ades, T., & Seffrin, J.R. (2002). Health literacy in the information age: Communicating cancer information to patients and families. *CA: A Cancer Journal for Clinicians, 52*(3), 130-133.

Metz, J.M., Devine, P., DeNittis, A., Stambaugh, M., Jones, H., Goldwein, J., & Whittington, R. (2001). Utilization of the Internet by oncology patients to obtain cancer related information. *Proceedings of the American Society of Oncology, 19*(63a), abstract 1575. www.asco.org/asco/publications/abstract_print_view/0,1148,_12-002324-00_18-002

Mittman, R., & Cain, M. (2001). The future of the internet in health care: A five-year forecast. In R. Rice & J. E. Katz (Eds.), *The Internet and health communication: Experiences and expectations* (pp. 47-73). Thousand Oaks, CA: Sage.

Morrell, R.W. (2002). *Older adults, health information, and the World Wide Web.* Mahwah, NJ: Erlbaum.

Murray, E., Lo, B., Pollack, L., Donelan, K., Catania, J., White, M., Zapert, K., & Turner, R. (2003). The impact of health information on the Internet on the physician–patient relationship. *Archives of Internal Medicine, 163*, 1727-1734.

Namazi, K.H., & McClintic, M. (2003). Computer use among elderly persons in long-term care facilities. *Educational Gerontology, 29*, 535-550.

Nussbaum, J.F., Pecchioni, L., Robinson, J.D., & Thompson, T.L. (2000). *Communication and aging* (2nd ed.). Mahwah, NJ: Erlbaum.

Parish, T.S., & Necessary, J.R. (1996). An examination of cognitive dissonance and computer attitudes. *Education, 116*(4), 565-566.

Parrott, R.L., Silk, K.J., & Condit, C.M. (2004). Diversity in lay perceptions of the source of human traits: Genes, environments, & personal behaviors. *Social Science and Medicine, 56*, 1099-1109.

Parrott, R.L., Silk, K.J., Krieger, J., Condit, C.M., & Harris, T.M. (2004). Behavioral health outcomes associated with religious faith and media exposure about human genetics. *Health Communication, 16*(1), 29-46.

Peterson, M.W., & Fretz, P.C. (2003). Patient use of the Internet for information in a lung cancer clinic. *Chest Journal, 123*(2), 452-457.

Pew Research Center, Washington, DC. (2003, April). *The Internet & American Life Project*. Retrieved September 8, 2003, from, http://www.pewinternet.org/reports/toc.asp?Report=88

Rees, C.E., & Bath, P.A. (2000). The psychometric properties of the Miller behavioral style scale with adult daughters of women with early breast cancer: A literature review and empirical study. *Journal of Advanced Nursing, 32*, 366-374.

Renn, O., Burns, W.J., Kasperson, J.X., Kasperson, R.E., & Slovic, P. (1992). The social amplification of risk: Theoretical foundations and empirical applications. *Journal of Social issues, 48*, 137-160.

Rieh, S.Y., & Belkin, N.J. (1998). Understanding judgment of information quality and cognitive authority in the WWW. *Proceedings of the 61st annual meeting of the American Society for Information Science, 35*, 279-289.

Rogers, W.A., & Fisk, A.D. (2002). *Human factors interventions for the health care of older adults*. Mahwah, NJ: Erlbaum.

Schmitz, J. (1997). Structural relations, electronic media, and social change: The Public Electronic Network and the homeless. In S. Jones (Ed), *Virtual culture: Identity and communication in cybersociety* (pp. 80-101) Thousand Oaks: Sage.

Schoenbaum, M. (1997). Do smokers understand the mortality effects of smoking? Evidence from the Health and Retirement Survey. *American Journal of Public Health, 87*(5), 755-759.

Schofield, M.J., Walkom, S., Ethics, M.A., & Sanson-Fisher, R. (1997). Patient-provider agreement on guidelines for preparation for breast cancer treatment. *Behavioral Medicine, 23*, 36-45.

Segouin, C., & Jadad, A.R. (2002). Awareness of sources of peer-reviewed research evidence on the internet. *JAMA, 287*(21), 2867-2869.

Strausser, F., Fisch, M., Bodurka, D. C., Sivesind, D., & Bruera, E. (2002). E-motions: Email for written emotional expression. *Journal of Clinical Oncology, 21*(9), 98-101.

Stronge, A.J., Walker, N., & Rogers, W. (2002). Searching the World Wide Web: Can older adults get what they need? In W. Rogers & A. Fisk (Eds), *Human factors interventions for the health care of older adults* (pp. 255-270). Mahwah, NJ: Erlbaum.

Sundar, S.S. (1998). Effect of source attribution on perception of online news stories. *Journalism & Mass Communication Quarterly, 75*(1), 55-68.

Sundar, S.S. (2000). Multimedia effects on processing and perception of online news: A study of picture, audio, and video downloads. *Journalism & Mass Communication Quarterly, 77*(3), 480-499.

Sundar, S.S., Brown, J., & Kalyanaraman, S. (1999, May). *Reactivity vs. interactivity: Impression formation effects of message contingency in political websites*. Paper presented to the Communication and Technology Division at the 49th annual conference of the International Communication Association, San Francisco.

Sundar, S.S., & Nass, C. (2001). Conceptualizing sources in online news. *Journal of Communication, 51*, 52-72.

Sundar, S.S., & Wagner, C.B. (2002). The world wide wait: Exploring physiological and behavioral effects of download speed. *Media Psychology, 4*, 173-206.

Taylor, H., & Leitman, R. (2002, April). Patient/physician online communication: Many patients want it, would pay for it, and it would influence their choice of doctors and health plans. *Health Care News, 2*(8).

Taylor, M.R., Alman, A., & Manchester, D.K. (2001). Use of the Internet by patients and their families to obtain genetics-related information. *Mayo Clinic Proceedings, 76*(8), 772-776.

Van der Velde, F.W., Hooykaas, C., & Van der Pligt, J. (1992). Risk perception and behaviour: Pessimism, realism and optimism about AIDS-related health behaviour. *Psychological Health, 6*, 23-28.

Viswanath, K., Kahn, E., Finnegan, J.R., Hertog, J.H., & Potter, J. (1993). Motivation and the knowledge gap: Effects of a campaign to reduce diet-related cancer risk. *Communication Research, 20*, 546-563.

Weinstein, N.D. (1987). Unrealistic optimism about susceptibility to health problems: Conclusions from a community-wide sample. *Journal of Behavioral Medicine, 10*(5), 481-500.

White, H., McConnell, E., Clip, E., Bynum, L., Teague, C., Navas, L., Craven, S., & Halbrecht, H. (1999). Surfing the net in later life: A review of the literature and pilot study of computer use and quality of life. *Journal of Applied Gerontology, 18*(3), 358-378.

Williamson, K., Bow, A., & Wale, K. (1997). Older people and the Internet. The speech project intelligent systems research group. School of Computing and Mathematical Sciences. Oxford Brookes University. Retrieved September 8, 2003 from, http://infotech.monash.edu/itnr/reports/olderp2.html.

Wilson, F. (2003). Can compute, won't compute: Women's participation in the culture of computing. *New Technology, Work, and Employment, 18*(2), 127-142.

Wilson, K.R., Wallin, J.S., & Reiser, C. (2003). Social stratification and the digital divide. *Social Science Computer Review, 21*(2), 133-143.

WirthlinWorldwide. (2003). Generations online. Retrieved September 9, 2003, from www.aarp.org/olderwiserwired.

Yows, S., Salmon, C.T., Hawkins, R., & Love, R. (1991). Motivational and structural factors in predicting different kinds of cancer knowledge. *American Behavioral Scientist, 34*, 727-741.

Zajicek, M., & Morrissey, W. (2003). Spoken message length for older adults. Retrieved September 8, 2003 from, http://www.brookes.ac.uk/schools/cms/research/speech/pubs.htm

4

Connecting Health, Communication, and Aging

Cancer Communication and Older Adults

Jon F. Nussbaum
The Pennsylvania State University

Doreen Baringer
Shippensburg University

Carla L. Fisher
The Pennsylvania State University

Amanda L. Kundrat*

A diagnosis of cancer is devastating to the patient as well as to the formal and informal relationship support networks of those individuals who must cope with this disease. The focus of this chapter is to highlight the significant potential contributions to our understanding of cancer communication that can be made by incorporating scholarship within the broad domain of communication and aging. The diagnosis of cancer simultaneously changes the life course of the older individual with the disease and the life and relational courses of the spouse, adult children, grandchildren, siblings, and friends. Other chapters in this book highlight the importance of competent health care provider communication and the advances in telemedicine and online support groups. Although advances in technology, medical interventions, physical therapy, and the general vitality of the population of older adults have been near miraculous, the fundamental caring and psychosocial adap-

*Deceased.

tations that must occur to ensure a consistent quality of life for the older patient with cancer depend to a great extent on those family and friends who have shared happiness and support throughout life (Nussbaum, Pecchioni, Robinson, & Thompson, 2000).

Three principles guide this chapter's major position that an understanding of successful adaptation and effective management of cancer by older adults cannot be accomplished without the study of the interpersonal communication of older adults. First, the nature and management of cancer for older adults depends on not only biological processes but also on psychological and social processes (Cohen, 2003). Second, the socioemotional selectivity theory advanced by Carstensen (1991, 1992), which proposes that older adults reduce their overall social interactions while maintaining the relationships that provide them with the most emotional support, can enlighten our understanding of where a diagnosis of cancer will be most disruptive in an older adult's relational world. And, third, our understanding of how family and friend relationships function in old age can help us to predict and explain the process of an older individual's successful adaptation to living with cancer.

GERIATRIC MEDICINE AND CANCER

Geriatric medicine is a subdiscipline within geriatrics (the health and social care of older adults) specifically devoted to the medical care of individuals over the age of 65 (Hazzard, Blass, Halter, Ouslander, & Tinetti, 2003). Although the study of how disease may affect older adults differently than infants, children, and young adults is not new, the classification of geriatrics as a subdiscipline of medicine worthy of recognition and special attention within traditional medical education is very recent. Only three departments of geriatric medicine exist within medical schools: Mt. Sinai in New York, The University of Arkansas, and the University of Oklahoma. Additionally, the Department of Medicine at the University of Washington includes a Division of Gerontology and Geriatric Medicine within its 14 divisions of medicine. The trend, however, is for medical and health educators to place great and much needed emphasis on the special health circumstances and needs of older adults. This is typically accomplished within family medicine departments or a department of internal medicine.

As evidenced by this text, it is now commonly recognized that cancer is a major problem for older adults. Cancer is the second leading cause of death after heart disease in the United States (Hoyert, Kung, & Smith, 2005). More than 50% of cancer diagnoses are in adults aged 65 and older, and it is the leading cause of death in men and women between the ages of 60 and 79

(National Comprehensive Cancer Network, 2005, p. MS-1). A comprehensive geriatric model has been advanced to help formal and informal caregivers understand the process of cancer within the elderly population (Cohen & Demarca, 1986). This model emphasizes specific interventions to manage cancer as well as the biological, psychological, and social dimensions of the disease. Although the type of cancer (prostate, colon, pancreas, urinary, stomach, rectum, and lung are the most common for older adults) and the specific therapeutic modalities (surgery, radiation, chemotherapy, and hormonal therapy) create unique circumstances, the biology of cancer and the medical intervention used to manage cancer by far receive the most attention within geriatric medicine. The psychological and social factors surrounding cancer in older adulthood have been less studied and less understood.

The first position of this chapter is that the psychological component and the social component of cancer within an older population are as important to investigate, describe, and understand for the competent management of cancer as are the biological or medical intervention components. Of special importance within this fundamental position are the communicative behaviors and functions of the patient and those family and friends who will care for the older adult diagnosed with cancer. Cancer survivors and family caregivers like Jan Dravecky, who cared for her husband Dave Dravecky, a former pitcher for the San Francisco Giants who is now in remission, speak and write eloquently concerning the importance of close relational support during the cancer caring process.

Nussbaum et al. (2000) advanced the notion that our communicative behaviors, and the functions that these behaviors serve, change across the life span. Our close relationships that are defined and maintained by our communication are not stagnant in nature because each individual as well as each relationship ages. The marriage relationship; our sibling relationships; the relationships we maintain with our children, parents, and grandparents; and our friendship relationships are in a constant state of flux as we negotiate and adapt to age-related biological, economic, psychological, and social circumstances. At times throughout the life span, the intimacy and power dimensions of the parent–child relationship appear to dominate our lives, whereas at other points in the life span, our marital and friendship relationships dominate with a much diminished role for our parents and siblings.

Laura Carstensen (1991, 1992) posited the socioemotional selectivity theory of aging to better explain the interactive world as we pass into our 70s and 80s. Briefly, socioemotional selectivity theory predicts that as we age beyond 65, we will begin to interact less frequently with those who are not within our closest interactive networks. At the same time, we will begin to devote more of our emotional resources to much fewer but intensely close relationships. Thus, as we age into our 70s, we tend to leave behind our large interactive and support networks of those with whom we worked, those who were our neighbors, or those with whom we interacted because they were friends of friends. We surround ourselves and begin to exclusively interact with our spouse, our children and grandchildren, our siblings, and those whom we pay to care for our health needs. Thus, the quality of our lives in old age is dependent on our ability to maintain several very close relationships (Nussbaum et al., 2000). Furthermore, Lockenhoff and Carstensen (2004) posited that "an intact social network serves as a buffer against physical and psychological stressors" (p. 1402).

The second position that we explicitly take is that our interactive world will change dramatically as we age and these changes will affect the very nature of the relationships most relied on by the older cancer patient. This proposition expands on the first by focusing more narrowly on communication implications as influenced by a diagnosis of cancer. Nussbaum, Hummert, Williams, and Harwood (1996) reviewed the existing literature that concentrates on the many cognitive, language, and relational changes that occur as we grow old. Many of these normal age-related changes will directly affect our ability to communicate effectively and, thus, maintain close relationships. These transformations include such things as changes in working memory, in our ability to process information, in language performance, and in the beliefs, attitudes, and stereotypes by and about older adults. The deaths of close friends and family also affect our ability to satisfy our interactive as well as physical needs. Nussbaum et al. (1996) maintained, "Our physical as well as psychological well-being is often dependent upon our ability to adapt to these changes and to produce language and maintain relationships that accomplish those goals necessary to our survival" (p. 39).

Cancer is a disease whose effects and treatments can be devastating to older patients and may require substantial supportive care (Cohen, 2003). Support such as effective pain management; maintenance of appropriate nutritional support; the supportive role of nursing; the importance of patient, family, and physician discussions; and the utility of hospice care are of great concern to both formal and informal caring networks. This is not to state that those who are not physicians, nurses, or therapists will provide the great majority of care. Rather, family and friends will care for the older patient with cancer in ways that at times appear heroic. Keeping in mind that socioemotional selectivity theory informs us that fewer, more intense relationships are part of the normal aging process, an understanding of competent communication within these important, caring relationships can help us to understand how appropriate caring can be accomplished. For example, according to Lockenhoff and Carstensen (2004), changes in the health care system have increased the amount of choice one has, yet, with that, is the need for an actively involved patient to make a well-informed decision. This could be problematic for older adults as cognitive decline and memory loss can inhibit sound decision making. Additionally, as we age, our individual goals and emotions change as well. Collectively, these changes affect older adults' desires to seek information that is potentially negative, and as a result, they may avoid or defer decision making. For that reason, the family caregiving support system is vitally important in maintaining older adults' health care. Furthermore, Lockenhoff and Carstensen (2004) stressed the importance of adapting one's communication of health care information in accordance with older individuals' specific needs and strengths.

The third position taken within this chapter is that interpersonal communication scholars are well positioned to investigate the changing nature of relationships in old age and then to work with health scholars and health practitioners to help older patients manage their cancer. Nussbaum et al. (2000) addressed the changing nature and various functions of the marital relationship, the parent–child relationship, the sibling relationship, and friendship for older adults. It is highly likely that the primary caregiver for the older patient with cancer will be a spouse or a daughter (Cicirelli, 1992; Prohaska & Glasser, 1996). In cases where the spouse or adult children are not available to provide care, a sibling, a friend, and, more frequently in our society, a grandchild will provide care. Edwards (2001) also demonstrated that spousal and filial caregiving may be significantly different due to the nature of the relationship. Children may care for their parents in different ways than spouses because of the negotiated meaning of "appropriate and effective care" within a parent–child relationship versus a marital relationship. For instance, adult children often report more rewards from the caregiving experience, such as satisfaction and an improved relationship, than spousal caregivers (for a brief review see Raschick & Ingersoll-Dayton, 2004). According to Raschick and Ingersoll-Dayton, this may be because spouses tend to have more demanding caregiving responsibilities in comparison to adult children. For instance, Pinquart and Sorensen (2003) found that longer duration of care as well as physical and behavioral problems were strongly associated with caregiver burden in spousal versus adult children caregivers. Additionally, although most research has concentrated on the costs rather than rewards of caregiving, gender differences in caregiving exist in both realms. Women often report more caregiving burden than men, and husband caregivers more often report that their spousal relationship has improved since caregiving began. Clearly, gender and relationship type clearly affect the nature of the caregiving experience (Pinquart & Sorensen, 2005; Raschick & Ingersoll-Dayton, 2004). Thus, it is reasonable to assume that not all spouses, daughters, sons, friends, and grandchildren will be effective or even willing to provide the care needed to manage cancer successfully.

Additionally, at times, the family or friend caregiver will be overwhelmed by the demanding care the older cancer patient needs. The family or friend caregiver frequently has the added responsibility of interacting with the various physicians, nurses, therapists, and insurance providers. Caregivers often serve as a liaison or a companion entrusted with looking after the priorities of the cancer patient. Many treatments for cancer are exhausting, radical, and lengthy, and significant caring could last for years. Edwards (2001) demonstrated that numerous stressors occur for family members who are caring for an ill older adult. These stressors can be related to such factors as the amount of care given, the length of time the care must be given, and the quality of the relationship between the caregiver and older patient. Previous studies have found that spousal caregivers experience more distress than adult children, and gender affects caregiving outcomes (e.g., wives and daughters experience more stress than husbands and sons; Raschick & Ingersoll-Dayton, 2004; Schultz, O'Brien, Bookwala, & Fleissner, 1995; Walker, Pratt, & Eddy, 1995). Furthermore, ethnicity affects the caregiving experience. Pinquart and Sorensen (2005) found that Hispanic and Asian-American caregivers experience more depression than White caregivers, and African-American caregivers experience less depression and caregiver burden than their White caregiving peers.

These factors point not only to the importance of effective family and friend relationships in our old age but to the complexities of successfully maintaining and managing the treatment of cancer for an older adult, given that care is dependent on family and friend caregivers. To ensure the well-being of the older adult cancer patient, interpersonal communication scholars can help each individual involved in the older adult's life sustain healthy relationships and provide effective medical care. Literature in realms such as patient counseling and behavioral medicine can further inform and assist us in our endeavors to educate others about communicative challenges related to a diagnosis of cancer.

PRAGMATIC IMPLICATIONS

The positions stated in this chapter posit that a diagnosis of cancer for an older adult has significant consequences, not only on the physiology of the patient but also on the social and relational world of those who make up the close support network of family and friends who must care for the ill individual. Health care models and practitioners, who must deal with the medical consequences of the disease, have recognized the social and relational nature of cancer for an older adult. However, health care professionals well trained in physiology, biology, pharmacology, surgery, and even psychology are often not able to comprehend the enormous importance of understanding and incorporating the close, support network of those family and friends who will provide the day-to-day care for the cancer patient.

Interpersonal communication scholars who study the very nature of these family and friend relationships across the life span are in a unique position to inform these formal health care providers and, in many cases, the informal caregivers as to the relational consequences of a diagnosis of cancer. Additionally, our research can provide very valuable information as to whether a particular relationship or a network of relationships is well suited to handle such a tremendous burden given the history and dynamics of that family. Interpersonal communication scholars can make a substantial contribution to our overall understanding of cancer and communication by incorporating significant external dynamics such as a diagnosis of cancer into our understanding of how the nature of relationships changes over time. Often, our theories of interpersonal communication ignore or downplay the environmental constraints imposed on relationships, and therefore, may not easily help us to incorporate the fundamental descriptions of interpersonal behavior into real-life crises. Future theories of interpersonal communication need to specifically address the changing nature and functions of our relationships once a diagnosis of cancer has been received.

In addition, health communication scholars can do a much better job of translating interpersonal theories and literature into the lives of cancer patients and caregivers. Interpersonal theories of relationship development and processes are wonderful building blocks for those interested in using sound empirical evidence to help explain the essential ingredients of a successful relationship that is devastated by news that a cherished family member or friend must now cope with cancer. Numerous factors such as the type of cancer diagnosed, the age at which the diagnosis occurs, and the existing support network of family and friends need to be studied as predictors of successful management strategies for the cancer patient and the caregivers. Interpersonal researchers interested in communication dynamics of health must collect information directly from individuals who are actively coping with cancer. Studies need to be designed that capture the changes in our relational lives from diagnosis through the various medical interventions and to the death process. These studies must not ignore the support network of family, friends, and formal care providers who manage this journey with the cancer patient. Our interpersonal theories should inform us as to the necessity of investigating the entire communicative world of the cancer patient.

A diagnosis of cancer for an older adult will most likely be formally managed by an interdisciplinary care team set up by a hospital, a clinic, an extended care unit, a rehabilitation center, or a long-term care facility (Nussbaum, Pecchioni, & Crowell, 2001). This interdisciplinary team may include oncologists, family physicians, nurses, social workers, various therapists, nutritionists, pharmacists, and psychologists. Jon Nussbaum served as a member of such teams within a large veteran's hospital. It became apparent that the care team, when confronted with an older adult who presented with multiple chronic as well as acute conditions (often including cancer), could manage the diagnosis and treatment quite well as long as the patient remained institutionalized. However, the team was often confused as to how to manage the various treatments and interventions within a context of the family and friend caregivers when the patient moved home or to a less restrictive living environment. The role of a team member schooled in interpersonal communication and relationship development across the life span can help the interdisciplinary team move away from their confused state and can indicate how the family and friend caregivers can optimally care for the older patient. This often requires the team to incorporate the needs, views, and wishes of the patient and family caregivers into the management decisions. Furthermore, ethnic differences also affect intervention needs, and thus, should be considered (Pinquart & Sorensen, 2005).

Effective communication between the interdisciplinary team, the older patient, and the family and friend caregivers is a necessity. Cancer communication becomes a vehicle by which the team can meet the needs of the patient in a context of both formal and informal relationships. As mentioned previously, various cancers require different and varying degrees of radical medical interventions. Changes in diet, exercise, and sexual habits are only a few of the many factors that will greatly affect existing, close relationships. The consequences of these relational changes due in large part to a diagnosis of cancer for an older adult will have direct effects on numerous quality-of-life issues.

Previous studies have indicated that team-approached health care is beneficial to the patient and their health. Blanchard, Albrecht, and Ruckdeschel (2000) asserted that patient health care interventions are concurrently family interventions. Their discussion examined a partnership model of the physician–patient–family relationship, which encourages shared decision making and promotes patient and family participation. As cancer patients experience fear and cancer-associated stigma, the communication process involving the physician, patient, and family must be attuned to the patient's needs and individual context. Social support must also be encouraged. A partnership model advocates patient and physician involvement through an effective partnership that enables sound decision making. Furthermore, empirical studies have shown that when various types of health care patients are treated via this type of communication model of health care, their emotional health improves (Blanchard et al., 2000; Quill & Brody, 1995; Stewart, 1995).

The overall well-being of the patient and the individuals within the support network of the patient should be of great interest to scholars studying interpersonal communication because of the direct link between effective communication, satisfying relationships, and quality of life. Interpersonal researchers should not be shy in their attempts to join these interdisciplinary teams as professionals educated in the understanding of effective and satisfying relationships. The mere presence of a communication researcher on such teams directs the focus of care planning toward social issues that would never emerge in the rather sanitized medical context within which these meetings occur. There is no better way to inform the health care community of our knowledge than to engage in actual formal care.

REFERENCES

Blanchard, C.G., Albrecht, T.L., & Ruckdeschel, J.C. (2000). Patient–family communication with physicians. In L. Baider, C.L. Cooper, & A. Kaplan De-Nour (Eds.), *Cancer and the family* (2nd ed., pp. 477-495). Chichester: Wiley.

Carstensen, L.L. (1991). Socioemotional activity theory: Social activity in life-span context. *Annual Review of Gerontology and Geriatrics, 11,* 195–217.

Carstensen, L.L. (1992). Social and emotional patterns in adulthood: Support for socioemotional selectivity theory. *Psychology and Aging, 3,* 331–338.

Cicirelli, V.G. (1992). *Family caregiving: Autonomous and paternalistic decision making.* Newbury Park, CA: Sage.

Cohen, H.J. (2003). Oncology and aging: General principles of cancer in the elderly. In W.R. Hazzard, J.P. Blass, J.B. Halter, J.G. Ouslander, & M.E. Tinetti (Eds.), *Principles of geriatric medicine and gerontology* (5th ed., pp. 671-683). New York: McGraw-Hill.

Cohen, H.J., & Demarca, L. (1986). Special problems of the elderly. In J. Lazlo (Ed.), *Physician's guide to cancer care complications* (pp. 120–127). New York: Decker.

Edwards, H. (2001). Family caregiving, communication, and the health of care receivers. In M.L. Hummert & J.F. Nussbaum (Eds.), *Aging, communication, and health: Linking research and practice for successful aging* (pp. 203–224). Mahwah, NJ: Erlbaum.

Hazzard, W.R., Blass, J.P., Halter, J.B., Ouslander, J.G., & Tinetti, M.E. (Eds.). (2003). *Principles of geriatric medicine and gerontology* (5th ed.). New York: McGraw-Hill.

Hoyert, D.L., Kung, H.C., & Smith, B.S. (2005). *National vital statistics reports: Deaths: Preliminary data for 2003.* Washington, DC: U.S. Department of Health and Human Services, National Center for Health Statistics, Center for Disease Control and Prevention, National Vital Statistics System.

Lockenhoff, C.E., & Carstensen, L.L. (2004). Socioemotional selectivity theory, aging, and health: The increasingly delicate balance between regulating emotion and making tough choices. *Journal of Personality, 72*(6), 1395-1424.

National Comprehensive Cancer Network. (2005). Senior adult oncology, version 1.2005. *Clinical Practice Guidelines in Oncology*, MS1-MS8.

Nussbaum, J.F., Hummert, M.L., Williams, A., & Harwood, J. (1996). Communication and older adults. In B. Burleson (Ed.), *Communication yearbook* (Vol. 19, pp. 1–48). Thousand Oaks, CA: Sage.

Nussbaum, J.F., Pecchioni, L., & Crowell, T. (2001). The older patient–health care provider relationship in a managed care environment. In M.L. Hummert & J.F.

Nussbaum (Eds.), *Aging, communication, and health: Linking research and practice for successful aging* (pp. 23–42). Mahwah, NJ: Erlbaum.

Nussbaum, J.F., Pecchioni, L.L., Robinson, J.D., & Thompson, T.L. (2000). *Communication and aging*. Mahwah, NJ: Erlbaum.

Pinquart, M., & Sorensen, S. (2003). Associations of stressors and uplifts of caregiving with caregiver burden and depressive mood: A meta-analysis. *The Journals of Gerontology, 58B*(2), 112–128.

Pinquart, M., & Sorensen, S. (2005). Ethnic differences in stressors, resources, and psychological outcomes of family caregiving: A meta-analysis. *The Gerontologist, 45*, 90–106.

Prohaska, T.R., & Glasser, M. (1996). Patient's views of family involvement in medical care decisions and encounters. *Research on Aging, 18*, 52–69.

Quill, T.E., & Brody, H. (1996). Physician recommendations and patient autonomy: Finding a balance between physician power and patient choice. *Annals of Internal Medicine, 125*, 763–769.

Raschick, M., & Ingersoll-Dayton, B. (2004). The costs and rewards of caregiving among aging spouses and adult children. *Family Relations, 53*(3), 317–325.

Schultz, R., O'Brien, A.T., Bookwala, J., & Fleissner, K. (1995). Psychiatric and physical morbidity effects of dementia caregiving: Prevalence, correlates, and causes. *Gerontologist, 35*, 771–791.

Stewart, M.A. (1995). Effective physician-patient communication and health outcomes: A review. *Canadian Medical Association Journal, 152*, 1423–1433.

Walker, A.J., Pratt, C.C., & Eddy, L. (1995). Informal caregiving to aging family members: A critical review. *Family Relations, 44*, 402–411.

5

Cancer, Aging, and Social Identity

Development of an Integrated Model of Social Identity Theory and Health Communication

Lisa Sparks
Chapman University

Jake Harwood
University of Arizona

In Harwood and Sparks (2003), we argued for the general applicability of Social Identity Theory (SIT: Tajfel & Turner, 1986; see also Harwood & Giles, 2005) to the health communication literature, and most specifically to issues surrounding cancer diagnosis, treatment, and recovery. SIT is a broad sociopsychologically grounded theory of intergroup relations, which focuses particularly on the importance people ascribe to their identities, the ways in which they protect them, and the ways in which they respond when their identities are threatened. It deals primarily with identification with large social groups (age, culture, sexuality, etc.), but can also be applied to smaller and more specialized groups (an alma mater, a family, a victim of a particular disease).

In the earlier article, we specified three levels of identity. At the primary level, individuals identify with large-scale social groups, and those identifications influence their susceptibility and coping with cancer. For instance, highly identified women might, under some circumstances, be more likely to attend to breast cancer risks and engage in appropriate prevention strategies. At the secondary level, identifications with particular behaviors will influence cancer communication processes. For instance, identifying strongly as a smoker will likely make it harder to quit. At the tertiary level, identification with cancer-specific identities come into play (e.g., patient, victim, survivor, etc.). For example, as individuals identify more strongly with being a survivor rather than a victim (and despite perhaps very similar prognoses), we might predict a better outcome for the survivor. In all cases, the issue here is that particular conceptualizations of self within the cancer realm have the capacity to change psychological orientation and behaviors related to cancer, and hence to influence concrete outcomes. Given the parameters of the current book, the first and third levels of identity are the most pertinent. Age identities fall into the first level and cancer identities fall into the third. Although in the previous chapter we dealt largely with the independent effects of different types of identity, in this article we plan on elaborating their interdependence. As has been noted by many other scholars, perhaps most notably in Hecht's recent work (e.g., Hecht, Jackson, & Pitts, 2005), identities can be understood as layered and complex in terms of their interactions. Therefore, we examine the cancer identity, how individuals experience "having cancer" and being a member of that (inherently stigmatized) group, and in particular how that identification might be experienced differently for an older person.

First, we present a mathematical model of the interconnections between various identifications, including the cancer identity. This provides a preliminary framework within which future scholars can examine identity change. Afterwards, we apply this mathematical model to (a) a social identity-based schema for responding to a stigmatized identity such as cancer, and (b) a broader model of response to identity threat developed from work on responses to terrorism.

THE MATHEMATICAL MODEL OF SOCIAL IDENTITY AND HEALTH COMMUNICATION

Our mathematical model provides a method for describing lifelong changes in group identities. We believe that it can be used to model group identity (and especially its changes over time) in a quantitative way, thus giving the researcher the opportunity to apply knowledge of identity change to other life developments. In the current example, we are particularly concerned with responses to cancer as a stigmatized identity. Following the description of the model, we describe how it might apply to two more specific existing theoretical perspectives.

Our mathematical mode is consistent with the ideas of functional data analysis (see Ramsay & Silverman, 2002). The key idea behind functional data analysis is that longitudinal data can be interpolated as if they were samples from a continuous function. One can then use the instruments from analysis of continuous functions to obtain results that would not be apparent or easily detected from discrete data. Ramsay and Silverman (2002) present several examples of how this technique can be applied to social sciences, in particular when the researchers are interested in detecting patterns of behaviors among large populations. The description we offer in this chapter is intended as a first step in that direction.

For the sake of simplicity, let us model group identities through set theory. So, each identity for a given individual is represented by a set (the set of women, the set of scholars, the set of cancer patients, the set of cancer survivors), and so, at every given moment, the identity of an individual is described by a finite collection of sets. For example, Jane Doe, on June 25, 2004, has the following identities: woman, mother, daughter, marathon runner, spouse, and attorney. These identities did not all appear simultaneously, nor will they remain forever in Jane's consciousness. For example, Jane only acquired the identity of marathon runner in her 23rd year of life, when she ran her first marathon. Similarly, she acquired the identity of spouse only in her 27th year of life, and her identity of attorney in her 30th year of life. Some of these identities will remain forever (e.g., she will always identify with women). Other identities will disappear with time (perhaps being a marathon runner). So, we can think of group identity for a given individual as a function (F) which associates to any instant of time (t) the collection F(t) of all identities that are perceived by the subject at that time.

From our point of view, however, looking at which identities are present at a given time is only part of the story. We are interested in which identities are more or less salient for the subject, and how these rankings change through time. For example, a natural question is to ascertain whether in fact these changes are predictable (are the same for all individuals in a given population) or at least whether possible patterns can be established (we could discover, e.g., that the functions associated to the individuals in a given population have variations that are described accurately by a fixed number of possible behaviors). So, we need to refine a bit the description we have given in the previous paragraph.

Let us assume that, for a given individual, at a given instant t, the value of the function F is $F(t)=\{A,B,C\}$, where A, B, and C are three sets describing the major relevant identities of the individual. These identities are not, at time t, all equally relevant for the individual we are studying, and we are interested in ranking them. So, we can assume that A is the primary (most important), C is the secondary, and B is the tertiary identity. We can then refine our description of group identity for this given individual by incorporating the rankings and so our new descriptive function will be F(t)={(A,1),(B,3),(C,2)}, which indicates both the identities and their rankings. The function F, therefore, has values that are collections of ordered pairs, the first element of a pair being a set, and the second being an integer.

Things are, however, a bit more complex, as we saw before that sets come in and out from a person's identity, and we need to account for that. For example, if set D was an important identity at time t-1, and is not any more relevant at time t, we need to be able to capture this information, which on the other hand escapes the description in the previous paragraph.

We propose the following further improvement on our model. Consider an individual, and the collection of all the identities which the individual will experience throughout his or her life. Then we order all the corresponding sets as S1, S2, S3, ... into a finite collection. We now define F(t) to be, at each instant, the collection of integers which represent the respective salience of identities S1, S2, S3, and so on, at that instant. In this way, we need to consider also the sets which, at a given instant, may not be relevant. In that case, we are able to also keep track of the sets which come in and go out of the individual consciousness. To do so, we will attribute value zero to those sets which are not a consideration at a given moment. Within this framework, the function F (which we think of as the function "group identity" for a given individual) associates to each time t a collection of integers.

As we indicated at the beginning of this section, this function F has a purely descriptive value. By looking at F(t) we see, graphically if necessary, how identities change throughout the life of an individual. We suggest, however, that the use of this numerical description may be amenable to statistical analysis. We are thinking, for example, of applying the instrument from functional data analysis, as described in Ramsay and Silverman (2002). For example, one may follow a small number of individuals through time. We can then look at the behavior of their corresponding functions to see if in fact one can detect emerging patterns. The fact that some sets appear and disappear, and that the function can assume value zero, may actually make this analysis amenable to even more modern treatments, involving the study of singularities for such functions. At this stage it is premature to see how much can in fact be inferred from these data, but the model we propose does have the advantage of making our discussion numerical.

We acknowledge that self-categorization theory (SCT) has pursued a similar goal to our mathematical model (e.g., Turner et al., 1987). SCT has focused on rather micro-level fluctuations in identity salience, driven by accessibility and fit of identities to an immediate context. Our model has a broader goal of understanding macro-level life-span changes in identity. Nevertheless, we do suspect that there are connections between the two approaches, and that they may be complementary. The description of the model is rather abstract right now. Next we apply it in two areas of interest to the study of cancer and aging. First, we consider the responses individuals may have to threatened identities. Second, we consider the broader identity management process based on a recent model of responses to terrorism.

Social Identity and the Response to a Stigmatized Identity

In Harwood and Sparks (2003) we paid only minimal attention to the consequences of identity threat, an area that is a major focus of SIT. Specifically, SIT suggests that when an identity does not provide rewards to an individual, three potential routes are available. The choice between these is grounded in the level of identification an individual has with the group, the degree to which boundaries between the group and other groups are open or closed, and the degree to which the power structure is viewed as legitimate and stable.

Social Mobility. In situations of low identification and open boundaries, the path of least resistance is for an individual to leave a stigmatized or unrewarding group (social mobility). This may take the form of actually leaving (e.g., ceasing to pay membership dues in a union; changing nationality) or of psychologically "passing" (e.g., closeted gay people).

In terms of a cancer identity, the mobility option can be exercised in two ways. First, there is an obvious desire for a cancer patient to move towards health, and in so doing to leave the cancer identity behind. In the long term, regaining full health and getting rid of the cancer is a form of social mobility. A residual sense of the cancer-based identity is however likely in such situations—while the body is cancer-free, the identity of being a survivor, or of having had cancer, may remain. This mobility strategy is obviously differentially available depending on the type and severity of the cancer: Some cancers are simply more survivable than others. Beyond this issue, however, the extent to which this strategy is perceived to be available may differ. In particular, older people may perceive this strategy to be more difficult to achieve, and/or those around them may be less likely to view it as an option. Older adults may treat certain symptoms with less concern (e.g., attributing them to "age"), or vigorous treatment options may be denied or downplayed by physicians compared to their treatment of younger people (e.g., because of stereotyping). Effectively, the boundaries to the "healthy" identity may be less open than they are for younger people.

Certain communication practices may perpetuate such inequities. Everyday talk may emphasize the limited social mobility options for older adults. Physicians may express age-related reservations about vigorous treatment ("you're too old to take it"), or age-graded prognosis estimates ("a 25-year-old might have 2 years, but I doubt you have that long"). More generally, discourse surrounding the inevitability of decline and illness in old age (Coupland, 2004) may well lead to a less militant approach to fighting the illness. Communicatively, for instance, older people may block their own attempts at effective treatment by age-related accounting practices ("I've had a good run—at 83 you can't expect much better"), and the plethora of discursive turns available to older adults for justifying illness and tolerating the marginalized status of being unhealthy. Indeed, it is the case that poor health may be viewed by some older adults in certain contexts as a valuable discursive resource that is available to share with younger people (Coupland, 2004). Unfortunately, these discursive strategies block constructive action like requesting more aggressive treatment, doing research on therapy options, dealing assertively with health providers, and the like.

The residual "survivor" identity resulting from successfully battling the disease may also have some interesting age-related facets. In particular, the experience of "having been sick" may take different forms depending on age. If the illness is interpreted as a sign of impending decline, then even middle-aged survivors may reorient to their own aging and mortality in interesting ways. For older adults, even survival may be viewed as a brief reprieve from the inevitable, as opposed to a "new start." In other words, the experience of surviving the illness may have profound effects on the nature of age and aging identity.

In the more immediate term, failing to disclose diagnosis, concealing side-effects of treatment, and lying about absences from work, and so forth, can also be understood as social mobility strategies. Cancer patients concerned about the stigma associated with a cancer diagnosis may pursue numerous strategies to avoid such stigma while they are fighting the disease. Obviously, these activities are unlikely with the immediate social support network, but they may be common in other contexts (e.g., in protecting vulnerable family members from concern, avoiding discrimination at work, etc.). Age probably changes the affordances for such strategies, in particular inasmuch as sickness and decline are perceived as normative and hence less distressing when the victim is older.

The social mobility option is not effective for individuals who value their group membership strongly (they are simply unwilling to abandon the group). Hence, we see a place here for our mathematical model. Put simply, the model can predict when individuals may be willing to disidentify with their group by monitoring life-span changes in group identification. When identification is high, mobility is unlikely and one of the other options (described later) will be adopted. When identity is low, mobility may indeed be the preferred option. Mobility is also unlikely in situations where the boundaries are closed (people simply are unable to leave because other groups will not accept them). This suggests that the permeability of group boundaries might be an influential factor in future theorizing here. When mobility is not an option, individuals will engage in social creativity or social competition.

Social Creativity. If the power structure is viewed as legitimate (i.e., the low status of the ingroup is justified), then people will engage in social creativity. Social creativity generally involves one of two strategies. People may seek out some dimension on which their group is valued, despite its generally low status (e.g., Asian Americans gaining positive identity from academics when other forms of status are unavailable). Alternatively, members of low-status groups can find other (even lower) status groups with which to compare themselves and obtain positive intergroup comparisons (e.g., African Americans gaining positive identity through comparisons with Korean Americans).

Seeking positive dimensions of the cancer identity seems unlikely from our perspective. It is a highly stigmatized identity, and in contrast to other identities does not appear to yield the opportunity for seeking alternative dimensions on which to make comparisons. The identity is defined by the health dimension, and it is negatively valenced on that dimension.

More likely, however, is the targeting of alternative outgroups. For instance, there is already a literature illustrating the ways in which people target other, less well off, ingroup members in order to achieve positive identities. For instance, Coupland, Coupland, and Giles (1991) described the ways in which older people target other elders as a comparison group—in particular, elders suffering physical decline will talk about older people with dementia as a salient outgroup against whom they compare themselves positively ("At least my brain box is still working!"). For patients with cancer, people with more negative cancer prognoses and/or cognitive problems, and the like, may be a salient outgroup. They may also target groups whose illness is perceived to be more "their fault, for example, nonsmokers who have breast cancer may be able to achieve positive comparisons relative to smokers with lung cancer ("I'm an innocent victim, they brought it upon themselves!"). Blameworthiness, in this regard, is certainly an interesting prospect for further work both in terms of how people understand their own cancers, but also in terms of sympathy and support provided to cancer patients.

As noted previously, older adults have already been shown to target other disadvantaged groups in discourse; indeed, they may have a greater range of (real or imagined) "less well-off" outgroups to target, given the age of their peers and the social representations available for their peers' health. For younger people with a wide array of largely vital peers, such positive comparisons may be more difficult to achieve.

For people who have recovered, the "survivor" identity may well be intrinsically a highly rewarding identity, of course, and hence there would be no reason to pursue any mobility/creativity strategies. Age may again moderate responses to survivors—a young cancer survivor may be viewed as a hero, whereas an older survivor may still carry some residual aura of illness and decline—postponed, perhaps, but looming. Our mathematical model is one route to teasing apart some of these complexities. For instance, the model might be able to track over time the ways in which a "survivor" identity was associated with either an age and/or a cancer identity. Such patterns would yield information on whether and how identification with being a survivor displaces or complements other identities, and hence the ways in which identifying with those other groups provides salve to the threat of the cancer identity.

Social Competition. In contrast to social creativity, when the power structure is seen as illegitimate or unstable, people will engage in social competition: collective action, social protest, political agitation, and the like. The formation of political pressure groups like the National Association for the the Advancement of Colored People or the American Association of Retired Persons is sometimes the most visible means for such struggle, although more confrontational forms emerge at certain times in certain groups (e.g., the Nation of Islam, ACT UP, etc.).

At the level of social competition, people are publicly seeking a change in the status quo that lends more status and resources to their group. Campaigns and awareness programs all fall into this area—perhaps the most visible is the pink ribbon campaign. Relative to other group memberships, these campaigns are interesting in that the primary goal is not to achieve more respect or status for people currently in the group, but rather to raise the status of group membership as an issue (primarily to support research that would prevent future people becoming members of the group!). Along these lines, social competition in the area of cancer is quite a bit different from civil rights movements surrounding ethnic identities, for instance.

Interestingly, older adults seem largely invisible in programs such as the pink ribbon campaign. It is possible that the organizers behind those kinds of campaigns deliberately avoid older adults. Given the broadly accepted links between old age and ill health, people may be less responsive to campaigns featuring older people who are unhealthy, effectively responding with "we all know that older people get sick, so what's the big deal?" An audience may only be shocked into donating money when it is relatively younger people getting sick. In other words, the options for patients with cancer to campaign for resources, or even for basic levels of dignity and equal treatment, may be limited by increasing age. Using our mathematical model, we can examine individuals' involvement with these causes. To what extent does identification as a cancer patient predict involvement in social action surrounding the cause, and to what extent does this interact with age identity? For instance, the model might be able to demonstrate that younger individuals who are heavily identified with their cancer tend to focus on treatment issues and avoid concerning themselves with broader social action. In contrast, older adults might perhaps adopt a more society-oriented approach. The model might even be extended to predict how/why family members of cancer patients engage in action. Building on the previous article (Harwood & Sparks, 2003), and the arguments above, we finally introduce a social identity model of cancer communication. The model aims to elaborate on the role of social identity processes in determining prevention, preparation, and response strategies to cancer.

Development of the Social Identity Model of Cancer Communication

Lance Armstrong, a well-known cancer survivor, won the grueling 2,290 mile *Tour de France* road race seven consecutive times from 1999 to 2005. Although younger than most individuals diagnosed with cancer, Armstrong survived what many consider a dramatic comeback from his diagnosis of advanced testicular cancer with large metastasis to the lungs and a less than 40% survival rate. At time of diagnosis (1997), Armstrong asked himself, "If I live, who is it that I intend to be?" Little did we know that he would become the first person to win the *Tour de France* seven times and become

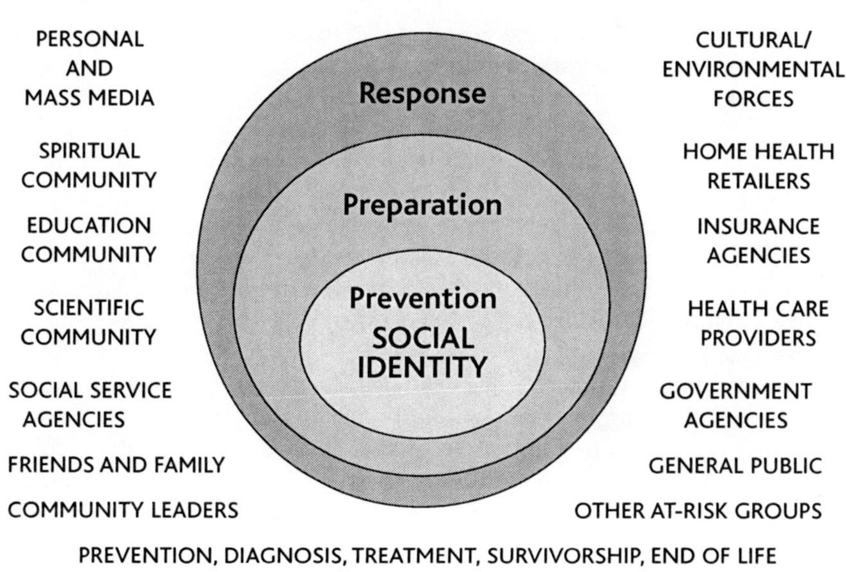

FIG. 5.1. The Social Identity Model of Cancer Communication.

recognized as the top cyclist in the world! Certainly, he is a rare case. Cancer tends to be an older adult disease and survivors of cancer tend to also be older adults. Whether experiencing cancer through a friend, family member or a personal experience, it is our various relationships and/or conversations about the cancer experience across the continuum of care from prevention, diagnosis, treatment, survivorship, to end of life that continually reinforce, renegotiate, and bring about shifts in our social identities across the life span.

Moving forward, we present a model to reflect and integrate some of the identity shifts that are perpetuated via communicative and biological experiences related to the disease. The model reflects how the continuum of cancer care from prevention to diagnosis, treatment, survivorship, end of life, and especially the talk with others throughout is central to such shifts in identity. The three stage "Social Identity Model of Cancer Communication" considers preventing, preparing for, and responding to a cancer diagnosis. The model builds, in part, on Kreps et al.'s (2005) efforts to develop relevant communication strategies toward bioterrorism contexts. In addition, it draws on our (Harwood & Sparks, 2003) conclusion that social identity shifts depending on a variety of communicative interactions with friends, family, health care providers, and the like, all of whom participate in co-creating identity shifts for the patient. As with the earlier sections, we see our mathematical model as crucial to the further examination of this model. As is elaborated here and in Harwood and Sparks (2003), the relative salience of different identities will dramatically influence preparation, prevention, and response strategies. For instance, the mathematical model might reveal low salience for age identity in an individual at risk for an age-related cancer. The low level of age identification would be a cue that simple messages of age-related risk might not work for this individual. Hence, messages might be designed that either framed the health risk in some alternate way, or that increased age identification to a point where the age-related message gained power.

The model focuses on prevention of cancer as the central and constant communication activity for cancer prevention efforts. Prevention is defined as the reduction of cancer mortality via reduction in the incidence of cancer (National Cancer Institute, 2006). Prevention can be accomplished by avoiding a carcinogen (e.g., not smoking) or altering its metabolism; pursuing lifestyle or dietary practices that modify cancer-causing factors or predispositions (e.g., changing diet); and/or medical intervention (e.g., chemoprevention). Preparation is different in that it focuses on a more global approach to cancer preparedness that tends to be policy-oriented including participation in legislation, ethics, health policy, health care finance, population health and health outcomes, and social and organizational policy to discuss current cancer prevention programs and key elements of change in social and political systems (NCI, 2006).

Prevention, we would argue, can be partially attained via relationships and embedded health behaviors—all of which contribute to shaping one's social identity. However, even the best prevention efforts cannot help avert all cancer threats, and communication activities must also be geared towards preparing key high-risk groups to mobilize actions to respond effectively to those who receive cancer diagnoses not linked to lifestyle choices and/or embedded health behaviors (e.g., smoking, etc.). Strategic communication is needed to prevent, prepare for, and respond effectively to cancer diagnoses. By understanding how social identity plays a role, particular support networks can be better prepared to use strategic and relational communicative strategies when talking with those diagnosed with cancer.

The outer circle of the model describes the critical communication activities needed to effectively respond to a patient once a cancer diagnosis occurs. Generally, these response activities are intended to activate the potential plans developed during preparation (e.g., not smoking, using sunscreen, getting regular and early check-ups, etc.), for example, recently developed smoking cessation campaigns for toddlers, elementary and junior high school kids, and the 5-a-day fruits and vegetables National Institute of Health campaign to reduce cancer risk. I also recently heard a talk by Dr. Claudio Belluco who is an MD/PhD connected with the Italian version of NIH who had this a on breast cancer (see Table 5.1) that tells us that prevention behaviors (and likely some elements of health campaigns along these lines, which are communication-based) are paying off to some degree. Cancer prevention, that is, in terms of early detection.

However, responsive health risk communication must be able to adjust to changing conditions and shifts in diagnoses (e.g., due to chemotherapy regimens, radiology efforts and when appropriate surgery). Scholars of chaos theory suggest that logical planning does not always reflect the unpredictable and equivocal nature of health risks and crises, and crisis communi-

TABLE 5.1

BREAST CANCER	INCIDENCE	MORTALITY
• World	1,150,000	411,000
• United States	213,000	41,000
• EC	350,000	130,000
• Italy	30,000	11,000

cation in the interpersonal arena must take into account unexpected events and suggest novel response strategies (Sellnow, Seeger, & Ulmer, 2003). Surrounding the concentric circles of the "Social Identity Model of Cancer Communication" are examples of the many interdependent groups who must coordinate activities and share information in cancer prevention, preparation, and response efforts.

Communication is a critical process in preventing, preparing for, and responding to serious cancer threats and diagnoses. Effective health risk communication requires a high degree of health care provider, friend, family, and community collaboration and poses special challenges to developers of effective health communication campaigns and practitioners. Communication is essential to coordinate groups of health professionals, friends, family members, and community members affected by cancer. Cancer communication requires advanced research by scholars and practitioners, in terms of preparation as well as constant and accurate updating during such crisis times of diagnosis to end of life. Multiple channels of human and mediated communication (including the use of new information technologies) must be strategically coordinated in order to help prevent cancer threats in the best ways possible; continue to identify the risks of such threats (e.g., smoking cessation); prepare for cancer diagnoses once they arise and understanding the differences in stages of cancer, metastatic diagnoses, cancer types; and to coordinate effective, evidence-based responses to such differential diagnoses.

CONCLUSION

Cancer communication audiences must be carefully analyzed, messages finely crafted, and channels appropriately selected to meet the needs of diverse groups. Care must be taken to identify credible spokespersons and work cooperatively with health care providers, friends, family, community leaders, and even media representatives to ensure that accurate and timely information is delivered to those most affected. In crafting such messages, researchers must begin to consider how emerging patterns in identities can be described and tracked via theoretical and mathematical models. Such models can serve as useful tools for beginning to systematically understand how messages function in terms of social identity negotiation, renegotiation, and the like in health communication contexts.

REFERENCES

Adelman R., & Greene M. (2000). Communication between older patients and their physicians. *Clinics in Geriatric Medicine, 16,* 1-24.

Allport, G.W. (1954). *The nature of prejudice.* Reading, MA: Addison-Wesley.

Amir, Y. (1976). The role of intergroup contact in change of prejudice and race relations. In P. A. Katz (Ed.), *Toward the elimination of prejudice* (pp. 245-280). New York: Pergamon.

Anderson, N.B. (1989). Racial differences in stress-induced cardiovascular reactivity and hypertension: Current status and substantive issues. *Psychological Bulletin, 105,* 89-105.

Armstrong, L., & Jenkins, S. (2000). *It's not about the bike: My journey back to life.* New York: Putnam Publishing.

Arora, N., & McHorney, C. (2000). Patient preferences for medical decision making. *Medical Care, 38*(3), 335-341.

Arrington, M. (2000). Thinking inside the box: On identity, sexuality, prostate cancer, and social support. *Journal of Aging and Identity, 5*(3), 151-158.

Banker, B.S., & Gaertner, S.L. (1998). Achieving stepfamily harmony: An intergroup-relations approach. *Journal of Family Psychology, 12,* 310-325.

Bourhis, R.Y., & Giles, H. (1977). The language of intergroup distinctiveness. In H. Giles (Ed.), *Language, ethnicity and intergroup relations* (pp. 119-135). London: Academic Press.

Branscombe, N.R., Schmitt, M.T., & Harvey, R.D. (1999). Perceiving pervasive discrimination among African Americans: Implications for group identification and well-being. *Journal of Personality and Social Psychology, 77,* 135-149.

Brashers, D.E., Neidig, J.L., Haas, S.M., Dobbs, L.K., Cardillo, L.W., & Russell, J.A. (2000). Communication in the management of uncertainty: The case of persons living with HIV or AIDS. *Communication Monographs, 67,* 63-84.

Brewer, M.B., & Miller, N. (1988). Contact and cooperation: When do they work? In P.A. Katz & D.A. Taylor (Eds.), *Eliminating racism* (pp. 315-326). New York: Plenum Press.

Charmaz, K. (1999). From the "sick role" to stories of self: Understanding the self in illness. In R.J. Contrada & R.D. Ashmore (Eds.), *Self, social identity, and physical health: Interdisciplinary explorations* (pp. 209-239). New York: Oxford University Press.

Chew, F., Palmer, S., & Kim, S. (1998). Testing the influence of the health belief model and a television program on nutrition behavior. *Health Communication, 10*(3), 227-245.

Cole, S.W., Kemeny, M.E., Taylor, S.E., & Visscher, B.R. (1996). Elevated physical health risk among gay men who conceal their homosexual identity. *Health Psychology, 15*(4), 243-251.

Contrada, R.J. (1989). Type A behavior, personality hardiness, and cardiovascular responses to stress. *Journal of Personality & Social Psychology, 57,* 895-903.

Contrada, R.J., & Ashmore, R.D. (1999). Introduction: Self and social identity: Key to understanding social and behavioral aspects of physical health and disease? In R.J. Contrada & R.D. Ashmore (Eds.), *Self, social identity, and physical health: Interdisciplinary explorations* (pp. 3-21). New York: Oxford University Press.

Coupland, J. (2003). Ageist ideology and discourses of control in skin care product advertising. In J. Coupland & R. Gwyn (Eds.), *Discourse, identity and the body* (pp. 127-150). London: Palgrave.

Coupland, N. (2004). Age in social and sociolinguistic theory. In J.F. Nussbaum & J. Coupland (Eds.), *Handbook of communication and aging research* (pp. 69-91). Mahwah, NJ: Erlbaum.

Coupland, N., Coupland, J., & Giles, H. (1991). Telling age in later life: Identity and face implications. *Text, 9,* 129-151.

Creagan, E.T. (1997). Attitude and disposition: Do they make a difference in cancer survival? *Mayo Clinic Proceedings,* 72(2), 160-164.

Crocker, J., & Major, B. (1989). Social stigma and self-esteem: The self-protective properties of stigma. *Psychological Review, 96,* 608-630.

Deimling, G., Kahana, B., & Schumacher, J. (1997). Life threatening illness: The transition from victim to survivor. *Journal of Aging and Identity, 2*(3), 165-186.

Dion, K.L., Dion, K.K., & Pak, A.W. (1992). Personality-based hardiness as a buffer for discrimination-related stress in members of Toronto's Chinese community. *Canadian Journal of Behavioral Science, 24,* 517-536.

Dryden, C., & Giles, H. (1987). Language, social identity, and health. In H. Beloff & A.M. Coleman (Eds.), *Psychology survey* (pp. 115-138). Leicester: British Psychological Society.

Eckes, T. (1994). Explorations in gender cognition: Content and structure of female and male subtypes. *Social Cognition, 12,* 37-60.

Edwards, C.C., & Harwood, J. (2003). Social identity in the classroom: An examination of age identification between students and instructors. *Communication Education, 52,* 60-65.

Eysenck, H.J. (1994). Cancer, personality and stress: Prediction and prevention. *Advances in Behaviour Research and Therapy, 16*(3), 167-215.

Eysenck, H.J. (1995). The causal role of stress and personality in the aetiology of cancer and coronary heart disease. In C.D. Spielberger & I.G. Sarason (Eds.), *Stress and emotion: Anxiety, anger and curiosity* (pp. 3-12). Philadelphia, PA: Taylor & Francis.

Falomir, J.M., & Invernizzi, F. (1999). The role of social influence and smoker identity in resistance to smoking cessation. *Swiss Journal of Psychology, 58*(2), 73-84.

Fitzpatrick, M.A., & Vangelisti, A. (2001). Communication, relationships, and health. In W. P. Robinson & H. Giles (Eds.), *The new handbook of language and social psychology* (pp. 505-530). Chichester, England: Wiley.

Ford, S., Fallowfield, L., & Lewis, S. (1996). Doctor-patient interactions in oncology. *Social Science and Medicine, 42*(11), 1511-1519.

Garstka, T.A., Branscombe, N.R., & Hummert, M.L. (2001). *Age group identification in young, middle-aged, and older adults.* Unpublished manuscript, Gerontology Center, University of Kansas, Lawrence.

Gascoigne, P., Mason, M.D., & Roberts, E. (1999). Factors affecting presentation and delay in patients with testicular cancer: Results of a qualitative study. *Psycho-Oncology, 8*(2), 144-154.

Gazmararian, J., Baker, D., Williams, M., Parker, R., Scott, T., Green, D., Fehrenbach, S.N., Ren, J., & Koplan, J. (1999). Health literacy among medicare enrollees in a managed care organization. *Journal of the American Medical Association, 281*(6), 545-551.

Giles, H., & Coupland, N. (1991). *Language: Contexts and consequences.* Pacific Grove, CA: Brooks/Cole.

Greene, M.G., & Adelman, R.D. (2001). Building the physician-older patient relationship. In M.L. Hummert & J.F. Nussbaum (Eds.), *Aging, communication, and health: Linking research and practice for successful aging* (pp. 101-120). Mahwah, NJ: Erlbaum.

Grossarth, M.R., Eysenck, H.J., Boyle, G.J., Heep, J., Costa, S.D., & Diel, I.J. (2000). Interaction of psychosocial and physical risk factors in the causation of mammary cancer and its prevention through psychological methods of treatment. *Journal of Clinical Psychology, 56,* 33-50.

Hamel, M.B., Lynn, J., Teno, J.M., Covinsky, K.E., Wu, A.W., Galanos, A., Desbiens, N.A., & Phillips, R.S. (2000). Age-related differences in care preferences, treatment decisions, and clinical outcomes of seriously ill hospitalized adults: Lessons from SUPPORT. *Journal of the American Geriatrics Society, 48*(5), S176-S182.

Harwood, J., & Giles, H. (2005). *Intergroup communication: Multiple perspectives.* New York: Peter Lang.

Harwood, J., & Roy, A. (2005). Social identity theory and mass communication research. In J. Harwood & H. Giles (Eds.), *Intergroup Communication: Multiple perspectives* (pp. 189-212). New York: Peter Lang.

Harwood, J., & Sparks, L. (2003). Social identity and health: An intergroup communication approach to cancer. *Health Communication, 15,* 145-160.

Harwood, J., Giles, H., & Ryan, E.B. (1995). Aging, communication, and intergroup theory: Social identity and intergenerational communication. In J.F. Nussbaum & J. Coupland (Eds.), *Handbook of communication and aging research* (pp. 133-159). Hillsdale, NJ: Erlbaum.

Harwood, J., Hewstone, M., Paolini, S., & Voci, A. (2005). Grandparent-grandchild contact and attitudes towards older adults: Moderator and mediator effects. *Personality and Social Psychology Bulletin, 31,* 393-406.

Harwood, J., Soliz, J., & Lin, M.-C. (2006). Communication accommodation theory: An intergroup approach to family relationships. In D.O. Braithwaite & L.A. Baxter (Eds.), *Engaging theories in family communication: Multiple perspectives* (pp. 19-34). Thousand Oaks, CA: Sage.

Hecht, M.L. (1993). 2002—a research odyssey: Toward the development of a communication theory of identity. *Communication Monographs, 60,* 76-82.

Hecht, M.L., Jackson, R.L., & Pitts, M. (2005). Culture. In J. Harwood & H. Giles (Eds.), *Intergroup communication: Multiple perspectives* (pp. 24-47). New York: Peter Lang.

Herd, D., & Grube, J. (1996). Black identity and drinking in the U.S.: A national study. *Addiction, 91,* 845-857.

Hewstone, M., & Brown, R.J. (1986). Contact is not enough: An intergroup perspective on the contact hypothesis. In M. Hewstone & R. J. Brown (Eds.), *Contact and conflict in intergroup encounters* (pp. 1-44). Oxford: Basil Blackwell.

Hogg, M., & Tindale, S. (2005). Social identity, communication, and influence within small groups. In J. Harwood & H. Giles (Eds.), *Intergroup communication: Multiple perspectives.* New York: Peter Lang.

Hummert, M.L., & Ryan, E.B. (2001). Patronizing. In W.P. Robinson & H. Giles (Eds.), *Handbook of language and social psychology* (pp. 253-270). Chichester: Wiley.

Hummert, M.L., Garstka, T.A., Shaner, J.L., & Strahm, S. (1994). Stereotypes of the elderly held by the young, middle aged, and elderly adults. *Journal of Gerontology: Psychological Sciences, 49,* 240-249.

Kaplan S., Gandek B., Greenfield S., Rogers W., & Ware J. (1995). Patient and visit characteristics related to physicians' participatory decision-making style. *Medical Care, 33(12),* 1176-1187.

Kreps, G., & O'Hair, D. (Eds.). (1995). *Communication and health outcomes.* Cresskill, NJ: Hampton Press.

Kreps, G.L., Alibek, K., Bailey, C., Neuhauser, L., Rowan, K., & Sparks, L. (2005). Emergency/risk communication to promote public health and respond to biological threats. In H. Haider (Ed.), *Global public health communication: Challenges, perspectives, and strategies* (pp. 349-362). Sudbury, MA: Jones & Bartlett.

Krieger, N. (1990). Racial and gender discrimination: Risk factors for high blood pressure? *Social Science and Medicine, 30,* 1273-1281.

Kruijver, I.P., Kerkstra, A., Bensing, J.M., & Van de Wiel, H.B. (2001). Communication skills of nurses during interactions with simulated cancer patients. *Journal of Advanced Nursing, 34*(6), 772-779.

Leets, L. (2001). Response to Internet hate sites: Is speech too free in cyberspace? *Communication Law and Policy, 6,* 287-317.

Lester, D. (1992). The stigma against dying and suicidal patients: A replication of Richard Kalish's study twenty-five years later. *Omega: Journal of Death and Dying, 26,* 71-75.

Levy, B. (1996). Improving memory in old age through implicit self-stereotyping. *Journal of Personality and Social Psychology, 71,* 1092-1107.

Maass, A., Salvi, D., Arcuri, L., & Semin, G. (1989). Language use in intergroup contexts: The linguistic intergroup bias. *Journal of Personality and Social Psychology, 57,* 981-993.

Maguire P. (1998). Breaking bad news. *European Journal of Surgical Oncology, 24,* 188-199.

Manderson, L. (1999). Gender, normality and the post-surgical body. *Anthropology and Medicine, 6,* 381-394.

Mastro, D. (2003). A social identity approach to understanding the impact of television messages. *Communication Monographs, 70,* 98–113.

McGee, R. (1999). Does stress cause cancer? There's no good evidence of a relation between stressful events and cancer. *British Medical Journal, 319*(7216), 1015-1016.

Mears, J.B. (1997). The cultural construction of breast cancer. *Dissertation Abstracts International Section A: Humanities and Social Sciences, 58*(6-A), 2273.

Morman, M.T. (2000). The influence of fear appeals, message design, and masculinity on men's motivation to perform the testicular self-exam. *Journal of Applied Communication Research, 28*(2), 91-116.

National Cancer Institute, National Institutes of Health. Retrieved April, 04, 2006 from, http://www.cancer.gov/cancertopics/pdq/prevention/overview/health-professional

National Center for Health Statistics (1994). *Health, United States 1993.* Hyattsville, MD: U.S. Department of Health and Human Services.

National Center for Health Statistics (2000). *Health, United States, 2000.* Hyattsville, MD: US Department of Health and Human Services.

Ng, S.H., Giles, H., & Moody, J. (1991). Information-seeking triggered by age. *International Journal of Aging and Human Development, 33,* 269-277.

Noone, I., Crowe, M., Pillay, I., & O'Keeffe, S.T. (2000). Telling the truth about cancer: Views of elderly patients and their relatives. *Irish Medical Journal, 93*(4), 104-105.

Nordin, A., Chinn, D., Moloney, I., Naik, R., de Barros Lopes, A., & Monaghan, J. (2001). Do elderly cancer patients care about cure? *Gynecological Oncology, 81*(3), 447-455.

Oakes, P.J., Haslam, S.A., & Turner, J.C. (1994). *Stereotyping and social reality.* Oxford: Blackwell.

Ogden, J., & Nicoll, M. (1997). Risk and protective factors: An integration of the epidemiological and psychological approaches to adolescent smoking. *Addiction Research, 5*(5), 367-377.

Ong, L., Visser, M., Kruyver, I., Bensing, J.M., Brink-Muinen, A., Stouthard, J., Lammes, F., & de Haes, J. (1998). The Roter Interaction Analysis System (RIAS) in oncological consultations: Psychometric properties. *Psycho-oncology, 7,* 387-401.

Ong, L., Visser, M., Lammes, F., & de Haes, J. (2000). Doctor-patient communication and cancer patients' quality of life and satisfaction. *Patient Education and Counseling, 41,* 145-156.

Parsons, T. (1951). *The social system.* Glencoe, IL: The Free Press.

Pechmann, C. (2001). A comparison of health communication models: Risk learning versus stereotype priming. *Media Psychology, 3*(2), 189-210.

Pederson, L.L., Koval, J.J., & O'Connor, K. (1997). Are psychosocial factors related to smoking in grade-6 students? *Addictive Behaviors, 22,* 169-181.

Peters, L., den Boer, D.J., Kok, G., & Schaalma, H.P. (1994). Public reactions towards people with AIDS: An attributional analysis. *Patient Education and Counseling, 24,* 323-335.

Pettigrew, T. (1998). Intergroup contact theory. *Annual Review of Psychology, 49,* 65-85.

Phinney, J.S. (1990). Ethnic identity in adolescents and adults: Review of research. *Psychological Bulletin, 108,* 499-514.

Postmes, T., & Baym, N. (2005). Intergroup dimensions of the internet. In J. Harwood & H. Giles (Eds.), *Intergroup communication: Multiple perspectives.* New York: Peter Lang.

Postmes, T., & Spears, R. (1998). Deindividuation and antinormative behavior: A meta-analysis. *Psychological Bulletin, 123,* 238-259.

Postmes, T., Spears, R., & Lea, M. (1998). Breaching or building social boundaries? SIDE-effects of computer-mediated communication. *Communication Research, 25,* 689-715.

Raman, P., Weis, D., Harwood, J., Miller, G., & Anderson, J. (2004, June). *Older adult portrayals in Indian and US magazine advertisements.* Paper presented at the ninth International Conference on Language and Social Psychology, State College, PA.

Ramsay, J.O., & Silverman, B.W. (2002). Applied functional data analysis. In *Methods and case studies.* New York: Springer-Verlag.

Rayburn, T.M., & Stonecypher, J.F. (1996). Diagnostic differences related to age and race of involuntarily committed psychiatric patients. *Psychological Reports, 79,* 881-882.

Reicher, S. (1986). Contact, action and racialization: Some British evidence. In M. Hewstone & R. Brown (Eds.), *Contact and conflict in intergroup encounters* (pp. 152-168). Cambridge, MA: Basil Blackwell.

Reicher, S.D. (1987). Crowd behavior as social action. In J.C. Turner, M.A. Hogg, P.J. Oakes, S.D. Reicher, & M.S. Wetherell (Eds.), *Rediscovering the social group: A self-categorization theory* (pp. 171-202). Oxford: Blackwell.

Roberts, C.S., & Cox, C.F. (1997). Medical and psychosocial treatment issues in breast cancer in older women. *Journal of Gerontological Social Work, 28,* 63-74.

Robin, M. (1999). Explanations of ethnic and gender differences in youth smoking: A multi-site, qualitative investigation. *Nicotine and Tobacco Research, 1,* S91-S98.

Robinson, W.P. (Ed.). (1996). *Social groups and identities: Developing the legacy of Henri Tajfel.* Boston, MA: Butterworth Heinemann.

Ruscher, J. (2001). *Prejudiced communication.* New York: Guilford Press.

Sellnow, T.L., Seeger, M.W., & Ulmer, R.R. (2003). Chaos theory, informational needs, and natural disasters. *Journal of Applied Communication Research, 30*(4), 269-292.

Sheeran, P., & Abraham, C. (1996). The health belief model. In M. Conner & P. Norman (Eds.), *Predicting health behaviour: Research and practice with social cognition models* (pp. 23-61). Bristol, PA: The Open University.

Siminoff, L.A., Ravdin, P., Colabianchi, N., & Sturm, C.M.S. (2000). Doctor-patient communication patterns in breast cancer adjuvant therapy discussions. *Health Expectations, 3,* 26-36.

Soliz, J. (2004). *Shared family identity, age salience, and intergroup contact: Investigation of the grandparent–grandchild relationship.* Unpublished dissertation, University of Kansas, Lawrence.

Stott, C., & Reicher, S. (1998). Crowd action as intergroup process: Introducing the police perspective. *European Journal of Social Psychology, 28,* 509-529.

Tajfel, H., & Turner, J.C. (1986). The social identity theory of intergroup behavior. In S. Worschel & W.G. Austin (Eds.), *The social psychology of intergroup relations* (2nd ed., pp. 7-24). Chicago: Nelson-Hall.

Takayama, T., Yamazaki, Y., & Katsumata, N. (2001). Relationship between outpatients' perceptions of physicians' communication styles and patients' anxiety levels in a Japanese oncology setting. *Social Science and Medicine, 53*(10), 1335-1350.

Turner, J.C. Hogg, M.A., Oakes, P.J., Reicher, S., & Wetherell, M. (1987). *Rediscovering the social group: A self-categorization theory.* Cambridge, MA: Basil Blackwell.

Uncapher, H., & Arean, P.A. (2000). Physicians are less willing to treat suicidal ideation in older patients. *Journal of the American Geriatrics Society, 48*(2), 188-192.

Van Knippenberg, D. (1999). Social identity and persuasion: Reconsidering the role of group membership. In D. Abrams & M.A. Hogg (Eds.), *Social identity and social cognition* (pp. 315-331). Malden, MA: Basil Blackwell.

Walker L., Kohler R., Heys S., & Eremin O. (1998). Psychosocial aspects of cancer in the elderly. *European Journal of Surgical Oncology, 24,* 375-378.

Williams, D.R., & House, J.S. (1991). Stress, social support, control, and coping: A social epidemiologic view. In B. Badura & I. Kickbusch (Eds.), *Health promotion research: Towards a new social epidemiology* (pp. 157-172). Copenhagen: World Health Organization.

Williams, D.R., Spencer, M.S., & Jackson, J.S. (1999). Race, stress, and physical health: The role of group identity. In R.J. Contrada & R.D. Ashmore (Eds.), *Self, social identity, and physical health: Interdisciplinary explorations* (pp. 71-100). New York: Oxford University Press.

Word, C.O., Zanna, M.P., & Cooper, J. (1974). The nonverbal mediation of self-fulfilling prophecies in interracial interaction. *Journal of Experimental Social Psychology, 10,* 109-120.

PART II

COMMUNICATING ABOUT CANCER SURVIVORSHIP AND AGING

Issues of Comfort, Healing, and Social Support

6

Comforting Episodes

Transcendent Experiences of Cancer Survivors

Athena du Pré
University of West Florida

Eileen Berlin Ray
Cleveland State University

> Whether you live a long life or a short one, it's out of your control. All you can do is make sure it will be a richer one.
>
> —Brett (2003a, p. B1)

Conventional wisdom suggests that good health is ideal and sickness a threat to be avoided. Although no one wishes to face a health crisis, some cancer survivors and their loved ones achieve a heightened sense of peace and understanding (Callahan & Kelly, 1992; LeShan, 1989). In this chapter, we examine how some people use communication to find new meaning in life while coping with the uncertainties presented by cancer.

It is often difficult to determine what having cancer means. Will it be an acute event, treated by surgery and/or chemotherapy or radiation and then essentially cured? Will it be a chronic illness, managed by medications but with an optimistic long-term prognosis? Or will it be untreatable and terminal? No matter which of these scenarios occurs, no one who has been given a cancer diagnosis remains the same. Answers to personal and fundamental questions such as "Why did this happen to me?" "Why now?" "What does this say about me?" "How will my relationships be affected?" and "What will life (and perhaps death) be like?" are elusive. The evolving meanings that arise from such queries are personal, social, and cultural. Answers lie more in the realm of social interaction (communication) than in biomedicine.

One objective is to achieve greater understanding about the way people cope with health crises. Such knowledge will be useful to professionals and laypersons. But coping is not the whole story. The stories presented here support that some cancer survivors not only endure; they gain something from the difficult circumstances in which they find themselves.[1] We characterize these experiences as transcendent in that the people who experience them come to see themselves and their relationships in new ways. Victor Frankl (1959) described *transcendence* as a supra-meaning that makes sense of and reframes an experience, and in so doing, provides a higher level of understanding or awareness. In lay terms, people in health crises often prioritize differently after being forced to confront their mortality. As a survivor of a rare lung disease said:

> I am no longer concerned that someone might see me in the same outfit and I no longer have to have the same sweater in every color. I can now not finish reading a book if I don't like it. Every day is a guessing game. But that's okay. I'm still here to talk about it. (Brett, 2003b, p. B1)

Margaret Newman's (1986, 2000) theory of health as expanding consciousness provides a theoretical framework for exploring these ideas by addressing the link between transcendence and health experiences. Newman proposed that health crises are not simply regrettable deviations from the norm, but meaningful episodes that can yield important insights. From this perspective, the uncertainty surrounding a health crisis provides the impetus to expand one's consciousness and to develop more complex and adaptive ways of interacting with the world. As they struggle to make sense of their lives

[1]Narrative accounts by people experiencing health crises appear throughout this chapter. As indicated, some of these experiences have been published. Others were obtained through open-ended interviews with people who have been diagnosed with chronic illnesses (usually cancer) and/or their loved ones. Interviews were conducted after securing Institutional Review Board approval and the written consent of all participants

in light of a cancer diagnosis, many people find a deeper understanding of life and its meaning (Charmaz, 1999). As one cancer survivor noted:

> We cannot afford to live passively. We do not have the luxury of complacency, because we do not know how many good days or years we may have left. It was amazing to me how little everyday annoyances mattered—no need for road rage, impatience in a slow-moving checkout line, or irritation at telemarketers. I have a newfound appreciation for my family, my friends, my job, and my life. (Brett, 2003b, p. B1)

Newman maintained that meaning is important, it is attainable, and the way to identify that meaning is through engaged dialogue with caring others.

We use the term *cancer survivor* in this chapter to refer to people who have been diagnosed with cancer, whether or not they still have cancer. Some in this category are undergoing treatment. Others are not. For some, the prognosis is for a long life. For others, their condition is considered terminal. In this context, we believe the term survivor is preferable to cancer patient or victim or sufferer in that it emphasizes the lived experience of dealing with cancer even if no cure is available, not the narrower role of patienthood or a sense of being victimized or punished by the disease.

This chapter provides a description of theory and literature about transcendent health experiences. We begin by discussing the uncertainty surrounding cancer and the quest for meaning that typically arises from this sense of disorder or chaos. Then we describe transcendence in terms of a supra-meaning (Frankl, 1959) that makes sense of and reframes an experience, and in so doing, provides a higher level of understanding or awareness. We argue, from the perspective of Newman's theory, that transcendent experiences—because they are based on an appreciation of complex life patterns—are particularly accessible to people as they grow older.

UNCERTAINTY

Whether the prognosis is encouraging or not, individuals diagnosed with cancer typically find themselves in a netherworld of diagnosis, treatment, and unknown outcomes. Each person responds differently, and even when cancer is removed from the body, the threat of recurrence lingers. Thus, uncertainty is always present, sometimes in the forefront, sometimes in the background. A cancer diagnosis upsets the equilibrium of our daily life, forces us to redefine who we are, and becomes a significant turning point in our lives. However, out of this upheaval often comes a quest for meaning in a context of uncertainty.

Uncertainty and the Quest for Meaning

> No one tells you normal is gone forever. But in some ways, that's a change for the better. (Brett, 2003a, p. B1)

Uncertainty is typically viewed as something to be reduced as much as possible. In the case of cancer, however, uncertainty always exists. Ann Hilton (1988) found that cancer survivors reported several areas of uncertainty, including the inability to foretell the future, feeling unsafe and not secure from danger, being in doubt, being undecided, having perceptions of vagueness, and not being able to rely or count on someone or something. Uncertainty exists throughout diagnosis, treatment, and prognosis. Merle Mishel (1984) noted that uncertainty caused by living with an illness is characterized by ambiguous, vague, unpredictable, unfamiliar, inconsistent, and unknown factors that may overlap but do not necessarily occur simultaneously. The degree of uncertainty results from three attributes: (a) probability, or the chance of a particular outcome occurring; (b) temporality, or how long, fast, and often to expect illness-related occurrences; and (c) perception, or the extent to which the survivor perceives the situation as uncertain (Mishel, 1984, 1990). Thus, at issue is not the ability to reduce the uncertainty but to successfully *manage* it (Babrow, Kasch, & Ford, 1998). There are numerous ways survivors can manage their uncertainty. Leigh Ford, Austin Babrow, and Cynthia Stohl (1996), for example, conceptualized supportive communication as uncertainty management. Uncertainty is also managed through survivors' unexpected transcendent experiences. It is through these experiences that uncertainty may be transformed from having a negative outcome to being a positive opportunity (McCormick, 2002).

Transcendence

When we stand
on the low rungs
of the ladder of sorrow,
we cry.
When we come
to the middle
we're silent.
But when we climb
to the top
of the ladder of sorrow,
we convert sadness into song.

—ancient Hebrew poem, in Rich (1999)

The term *transcendence* rarely appears in health communication literature. However, it is widely recognized in other forms of scholarship and has an avid audience among nurses and nurse educators, particularly those who have followed the work of theorists Martha Rogers and Margaret Newman. (For treatises on these scholars' work, we recommend Malinski, 1986, and Newman, 1995, 2000.)

Before narrowing the definition for the purposes of this chapter, it should be acknowledged that *transcendence* is defined many ways across disciplines. A search for "transcendent or transcendence" in a popular general academic index yielded 934 hits. The majority of these sources are addressed to some form of religious transcendence, but others are secular. For instance, there is research about the transcendent power of nature (Williams & Harvey, 2001), athletic competition (Murphy & White, 1995), and organizational life (Eisenberg, 1990)—the latter two characterizing transcendence as being "in the zone," a state of heightened confidence and unity in which remarkable accomplishments are attainable.

In using the term *transcendence*, we do not limit the scope to religious experiences, although there is often a spiritual element to the stories people tell, including contact with another world, spiritual beings, and loved ones who have died (Callahan & Kelley, 1992; Geist-Martin, Ray, & Sharf, 2003). Many people described do not speak of being "in the zone" per se, but often note the same sense of slow motion or timeliness (e.g., Bentov, 1988).

An influential concept of transcendence emerged from the work of Victor Frankl, whose ideas developed from his experience as a prisoner in Nazi concentration camps in the 1940s. Frankl (1959) observed that, even within the harsh and seemingly hopeless conditions, some prisoners experienced lives of "inner riches and spiritual freedom" (p. 35). In other words, they found meaning beyond the immediate threats that faced them. For many, the will to live was supported by anticipation of seeing loved ones again or resuming favorite activities (Frankl, 1959).

Frankl, who trained as a psychiatrist prior to the war and corresponded regularly with Sigmund Freud, disagreed with Freud's assumption that sex is the primary motivation for human action. Instead, Frankl believed people are motivated primarily by the search for meaning. In his view, transcendence may be defined as the discovery of a supra-meaning beyond one's previous understanding. This supra-meaning is transformational in that it makes sense of events that might otherwise seem senseless or unthinkable. From Frankl's perspective, transcendence is not denial of one's circumstances, but an awareness that those circumstances exist within the framework of something more meaningful than one might previously have imagined.

Consider the experience of Alison, a college instructor interviewed for this study, who recalls a transcendent experience prior to the death of her grandfather. As a college student, Alison drove home nearly every weekend to spend time with her grandfather, who was dying. She would rent old movies, lie beside him on the hospital bed in her parents' home, and the two would laugh and talk for hours.

One day, Alison's grandfather mentioned a pleasant visit from a relative Alison knew to be long-since deceased. "I was a little spooked at first, but he was so alert and lucid otherwise, I soon began to accept it when he would talk about all the people who 'visited' him," she recalls. "He was so happy about these visits." She did think it odd, however, her grandfather never mentioned visits by his late mother, to whom he was very close.

The mystery was solved and the circle completed when, one day, in the presence of Alison and her parents, her grandfather looked toward the corner of the room and said with delight: "Mother!" He died that day. "My grandmother's birthday was the next day," Alison says. "I know people might think we were crazy, but we had a party! We felt like celebrating. It was okay. Everything was right."

This experience represents transcendence in that the participants' understanding of the situation was transformed by a new type of sense-making. Although Alison acknowledges people might have considered them "crazy" for feeling joyous, the family members were overcome by an unexpected and joyous sense of things being "okay" and "right." (For other instances of near-death awareness and families' reactions, see Callahan & Kelley, 1992.)

Pamela Reed (1991, 1996) theorized that self-transcendence is an experience of expanded boundaries. One is able to see beyond oneself while at the same time becoming more self-aware. The past and present are integrated in a higher level of understanding and connectedness. Reed (1996) proposed that such experiences are often evident in situations in which people are confronted with aging, serious illness, or death.

In the following quote, one woman recalls the process of her mother's death as immense yet profoundly detailed:

> It's about paying attention to every word and story that you tell because this thing, this dying process that is going on and you can't stop this current, it's so big and so vast in contrast to all these tiny things you're dealing with and feeling every moment. . . . And I have to say, looking back a month after my mom's death, it has real beautiful aspects to it. . . . This is it, this is the last big dance and you either join in or you lose this incredible experience. (Geist-Martin et al., 2003, p. 245)

This sense of living in two dimensions—the immense and the minute—is common in personal narratives of chronic illness and death.

A high-profile examination of cancer and transcendence was published in *The Journal of the American Medical Association*. In the article, Susan D.

Block (2001) described how a 77-year-old man with incurable pancreatic cancer was able to find a heightened sense of meaning and pleasure in life during his final years. Commenting on his outlook, the patient said, "What this last year has provided me with is the occasion to be deliberately open to receiving other people's love and care . . . and I'm delighted when it happens" (p. 2898). Block, a psychosocial oncologist, observed that, "not every patient will seek or be able to invest emotionally in the possibility of discovery and transcendence in the dying process. But it is not rare" (p. 2898). She suggested that physicians and loved ones can help cancer survivors transcend a sense of helplessness by attending to their physical comfort, helping them maintain a healthy sense of self, maintaining rewarding relationships, and helping them preserve a sense of control. Block suggested a list of questions such as, "What would allow you to feel that going through this has a purpose?" to help people accept and make sense of life-threatening health concerns and, if necessary, the dying process.

THEORY OF HEALTH AS EXPANDING CONSCIOUSNESS

In Newman's (1986, 2000) perspective of health as expanding consciousness, illness is a meaningful and integral part of personal development. Newman views life as an ongoing pattern characterized by openness and interconnection with other people and one's environment. A person's life pattern develops as he or she encounters disorder, experiences disequilibrium, and advances to new levels of understanding and consciousness.

Although it is natural to dread the temporary chaos of disharmony, it is a vehicle for expanding consciousness, which Newman (1986) defined as the evolving capacity of a system to interact effectively with its environment. She proposed that a sense of being "thrown off balance" (p. 27) forces a person to go beyond previous assumptions and ways of being, thus expanding the person's repertoire of responses. As Newman (2000) said, the imperative is to let go of the "old rules" and open one's mind to a new order (p. 47). This viewpoint is reminiscent of Frankl's. In defining a system of logotherapy (based on the Greek word for meaning, logos), he wrote:

> I consider it a dangerous misconception of mental hygiene to assume that what man [sic] needs in the first place is equilibrium or, as it is called in biology, "homeostasis," i.e., a tension-less state. What man [sic] actually needs is not a tension-less state but rather the striving and struggling for some goal worthy of him [*sic*]. (Frankl, 1959, p. 107)

Like Newman, Frankl believed spiritual growth is accelerated by challenge.

Illness is one such challenge. Or worded another way, it is natural part of the cycle in which people encounter uncertainty and (hopefully) transcend previous consciousness. Long-term or identity-threatening illnesses such as cancer bring people to crisis points in which previous ways of thinking and behaving are no longer functional. Faced with this, people may avoid transformation—by denying changes, feeling depressed, or suffering long-term loss of identity—or they may progress from chaos into a new sense of order. Newman (2000) said that it is impossible to know the outcomes of change in advance, but once made, the effects are profound.

From Newman's perspective, the objectives of caregivers are not to simply make disease go away, but to help people identify the patterns in which disease has occurred and the promise it holds for expanding consciousness. She proposed that illness may occur when the pattern of a person's life become so disharmonious that "sickness" provides a needed "shock that reorganizes the relationships of the person's pattern in a more harmonious way" (Newman, 1986, p. 20). In other words, disease can bring attention to issues and patterns previously ignored. In fact, "disease may be the only way a person can get in touch with his or her pattern" (p. 26).

Newman draws upon David Bohm's (1980) premise that elements of the physical world (the explicate order) are, in reality, manifestations of an implicate order below the surface. Although the explicate order seems more "real" because it is directly observable, Bohm maintained that the underlying implicate order is actually more fundamental and consequential. Newman proposed that disease is one way in which these underlying patterns are revealed, with the consequence that people achieve new awareness and perspective—not only of the current moment but of patterns and meanings in their lives that transcend the here and now.

One implication of health as expanding consciousness is that senior citizens—because they have rich life histories—are particularly well qualified to identify and learn from their patterns. Martha Rogers, a health theorist and mentor of Newman's, writes that "aging is not a disease," but a process of ever greater development (Rogers, 1986, p. 7). As an evolution toward greater complexity, aging is a process of growth and expansion. Newman (2000) observed that elements of the life pattern often become more clear over time, thus older people have an advantageous perspective. Moreover, varied experiences give them a "greater repertoire of responses" and more experience adapting to their environments (Newman, 1986, p. 34).

Newman's theoretical framework provides a basis for Frankl's (1959) concept of transcendence as the realization of an overarching meaning and Reed's (1991) description of a transcendent process in which people expand personal boundaries. Central to both definitions is a sense of discovery and sense-making. Through transcendence, people find meaning in the midst of difficult situations. Often, the sense of transformed understanding is euphoric and pleasurable. Based on studies of cancer survivors, some people experience transcendence without expecting it whereas others work consciously to transform the meaning of their lives.

Lawrence LeShan (1989), a psychologist who has worked with cancer survivors for several decades, said that cancer can be a turning point when people discover what is most meaningful to them. He asks clients to imagine a life custom made to their passions and joys, a life in which the world adjusts to them. In his experience, those who seek that life find that it is not as difficult, unobtainable, or socially unacceptable as they initially believed. Whether their cancer is cured or not, they begin to see their lives as "a pattern and a symphony in which the themes swell and recede and the whole makes a real and organic whole" (LeShan, p. 25). This approach, although compatible with biomedicine, offers something different and additional and is facilitated almost entirely by communication. LeShan has found that cancer survivors who can describe their experiences and hopes aloud often find meaning in the telling and stimulate the cooperation of people around them. In this way, communication serves to identify and create meaningful experiences while reducing the sense of uncertainty and helplessness.

Ardath Rodale (1998), a breast cancer survivor, remembers a turning point when she bought a puppy and began walking him through nearby fields. The daily contact with nature was an inspiration:

> I looked with wonder at the artistry of the seasons, and the music of the birds filled my ears. My thoughts were filled with peace and what was happening at the moment. . . . On my drives to radiation therapy, I tried to discover something new each day: great cloud formations, the beautiful blue of the sky, sometimes blessing the drip of the rain on the roof of the car, and looking for interesting people. I shared all of this with the technicians. We laughed and actually looked forward to seeing each other! (Rodale, 1998, p. 192)

Her experience was both personal and social, appreciated alone and shared with others.

Some cancer survivors achieve transcendence by focusing on nature, others by serving the community, or identifying another means of awareness. In Doris Coward's (1990) study of women with Stage IV breast cancer, one woman described a transcendent experience following a devastating mastectomy and the loss of her husband. She underwent training to answer calls at a crisis line and was able to help a man who was contemplating suicide:

> I put my whole self into this call. All my energies, compassion, and understanding were at a very high level. When I finally got him to make

> a "contract" with me, to wait until the next day to make a decision, I was ecstatic. I felt such an accomplishment. I felt I was needed and my feeling of self-worth was at its highest pitch—the highest I could remember in a long time. My body felt light. My shoulders felt free of burden. I actually walked lighter and more easily—almost floating—but not really. I stepped out into the night, the sky was clear, stars bright and twinkling. To inhale felt good. To breathe felt like a heavenly experience. (p. 164)

In this narrative and others by women with advanced-stage breast cancer, the sense of rising beyond oneself was exhilarating and transformational.

Most cancer survivors interviewed by Newman (1995) felt that cancer provided them an unprecedented opportunity to focus on relationships and spirituality, not just on tasks to be accomplished. The participants in her study described being unhappy in early life and subsequently disconnected from the people around them. In dealing with cancer, several participants felt liberated from this destructive pattern. One woman in the study said, "I used to worry about the future, but now since I got the cancer, I live one day at a time. . . . I am happy now" (p. 167).

In Newman's (2000) view, responding to a life pattern may or may not involve eradicating disease. As a nurse and nurse educator, she does not consider that disease is necessarily negative or undesirable, nor does she engage in a reductionistic examination of symptoms or causes. Instead, Newman treats disease as the reflection of a dynamic process involving a person and his or her interplay with the environment. She wrote that "transcendence of the limitations of the disease does not necessarily mean more freedom from the disease; it does mean more meaningful relationships and greater freedom in a spiritual sense" (p. 65).

Needless to say, this is a radical shift from considering disease as the antithesis of health or a condition to be abolished without actively engaging the patient. Newman (2000) recognizes the value of biomedical care but considers that it is equally or more important to address patients' life context. She wrote:

> If we view illness as something discrete, something to be avoided, diminished, or eliminated altogether, we may be ruling out the very factor that can bring about the change in the life process that the person is naturally seeking. Illness may accomplish for people what they secretly want but are not able to acknowledge, even to themselves. (p. 20)

This idea hit home for one author (Athena) when, halfway through preparing this chapter, her father suffered a stroke.

> Previously fascinated with Newman's work, I suddenly found myself sitting in the intensive care waiting room wondering how she could have been so wrong. It was absurd to think Dad was experiencing a state of expanded consciousness. His brain was badly damaged. We were not even sure he knew where or who he was. A gifted artist throughout his life, his drawing hand was now paralyzed. I railed in my mind for several days. Then, upon entering my father's hospital room one time, it dawned on me: "I have never seen Dad look so relaxed." He has nearly always worked two or more jobs, more to satisfy an inner drive than for the money. In the last few years, he has worked 60 hours a week and been the primary caregiver for his bedridden mother, who died several months prior to this stroke. Contemplating his 65th birthday later this year, Dad had begun to talk about retirement and the many things he would like to do. Everyone in the family wondered if he would actually retire, and if so, if he could find a means to relax rather than keep up his customary pace. We seriously doubted it. It dawned on me: The stroke provided what he was unable to provide for himself—a slower pace, a simpler outlook, and much needed rest. No one would have chosen this method, but it suddenly seemed meaningful in the scheme of his life, and therefore easier to accept and learn from.

In the following section, we present implications for the ideas presented here as they apply to the study and practice of health-related communication.

IMPLICATIONS, RESEARCH DIRECTIONS, AND APPLICATIONS FOR HEALTH COMMUNICATION

With the literature and theory presented here, we suggest an expanded conceptualization of health communication. More specifically, we invite greater consideration of health crises—not merely as episodes to be avoided or curtailed—but as meaningful components of life and personal and relational development. Considering health as a means of personal evolution is not meant to downplay the difficulty of dealing with cancer. Rather, we suggest that cancer is not only (or even primarily) a condition to be "battled" or "tamed," but an experience to be explored and understood. As one woman who survived cancer, responding to another survivor's recommendation of the book *The Battle Against Cancer*, said,

> I stopped reading illness books that have the words battle or war in the title. . . . It's such a militaristic way of looking at it. So long as you think of yourself in battle with cancer, you'll never transcend cancer. You'll always be engaged with it. (Rich, 1999, p. 227)

Implications

There are several implications of this perspective for the study of health communication. One is that cancer is not merely a cellular anomaly but an experience with far-reaching implications for what it means to be happy, healthy, and human. Defining health in purely physical or reductionistic terms sometimes suits the goals of science and diagnosis, but it may distract people from seeing the overall patterns that contribute most profoundly to their well-being and development. Ignoring broader implications of disease may impede people's ability to cope with—and even benefit from—health crises they experience. Likewise, if disease is a natural and meaningful part of life, "fixing" a health concern without identifying underlying patterns that define it is an incomplete operation. This viewpoint gains credence as evidence mounts that health is defined by the interplay of many factors including physical activity, stress levels, relational life, and more.

The second implication is that there are valuable experiences to be had even within supposed chaos. In the conception of health that emerges from this analysis, periods of disequilibrium are crucial for developing increased understanding and development. As a number of scholars have observed (e.g., Pascale, 1999; Prigorine, 1976), open systems (such as humans) respond to stimuli in any number of ways and, through a process of self-organization, evolve in novel ways to suit their environments. Instability, within bounds, provides the impetus for change and improvement. Appreciating the uncertainty and quest for meaning among cancer survivors seems especially important. The people quoted in this chapter who feel they have benefited from cancer share an important quality: They feel their lives have more meaning as a result of the experience. The process by which they transcended the uncertainty of the disease to arrive at new meanings is worth our attention.

Third, because people are open systems profoundly influenced by their environments, their ability to cope is affected by the people around them. In short, we are all in this together. There are mutual benefits to participating in people's coping experiences. Callahan and Kelley (1992) observed that people are sometimes uncomfortable with the experiences of very ill loved ones, and consequently write off transcendent experiences as hallucinations or confused thinking. Although it is natural to be wary of the unfamiliar, ignoring these experiences can make the individual feel isolated, misunderstood, and unable to communicate important goals and experiences. Moreover, people experiencing health crises have valuable lessons to share about the meaning of life and what it means to die peacefully (Callahan & Kelley, 1992).

Finally, viewing aging as a process of decline obscures part of the picture, perhaps the most important part. People within Western cultures are typically familiar with the loss of physical capacity as the body ages, but they tend to overlook the opportunities for inner development and complexity. From the perspective outlined here, people with rich life experiences have varied repertoires and patterns from which to draw, provided their understanding is not diminished by denial, depression, or cognitive impairment. Respecting and nurturing the inner resources of people with life-altering and life-threatening illnesses may help them find meaning within the experiences and share their insights with others.

Research Directions

This perspective suggests several applications to the study of health communication. First, health communication scholars should broaden the scope of their literature and theory reviews. Research in nursing and other fields, although highly relevant, is too often overlooked.

Second, communication scholars should seek multiple vantage points when studying health experiences. The literature and theories reviewed here illustrate the insights to be gained from a phenomenological examination of health-related experiences. In analyzing transcendent experiences, the goal is not to prove or disprove their occurrence, but to recognize them as lived experiences with consequences for the way people deal with health crises.

Third, in exploring health experiences alongside the people living them, health communication scholars become part of a reflexive process. If we wish to embrace the idea of health as an open and interconnected experience, as presented in this review, we must acknowledge that we are, to some degree, part of that experience. This interactive process of meaning-making challenges assumptions that social science should be aimed at generalizable or objective conclusions. However, it seems to reflect a natural process of discovery in the social world, and is therefore not only revealing in a scientific sense, but immediately meaningful to the people who participate in it.

Applications

Acknowledging transcendent experiences as a means of managing uncertainty has repercussions for the way we think and talk about health. Much of the meaning surrounding a cancer diagnosis is socially constructed. That is, the significance of personal identity, life, and death are weighed and negotiated through dialogue and storytelling.

From this perspective, describing health experiences is more than a means of relaying diagnostic information or collecting research data. Sharing one's stories can be both informative and cathartic (Pennebaker, 1995). Jane Neill (2002) reflected, "The research is not therapy in the sense of advice to people or intervention in the way they lead their lives, but the process of pattern recognition allows people to see their situations differently and illuminates action for transforming their lives" (p. 32). Through the interview process, survivors are given a voice; hearing themselves speak can be transformative and become a way of knowing (Varallo, Ray, & Ellis, 1998). In other words, these individuals do more than cope. They discover truths and resources that exceed the lessons of everyday life. In Newman's terms (2000), they achieve "expanded consciousness."

Listening to survivors' stories can also be a profound experience for others. When physician and athlete George Sheehan learned he had prostate cancer, he was disappointed in the literature available. "The New Jersey Cancer Association gave me a pile of books on my disease," he said, "But none of their authors was sick. I think that should be a prerequisite" (Moore, 1993, p. 3). Sheehan (1996) chronicled his experiences in *Going the Distance: One Man's Journey to the End of His Life*, a project friends say gave him a reason for dying. When asked how her father was dealing with cancer, Sheehan's daughter once said, "Oh, he loves it. He talks about it all the time" (Moore, 1993, p. 80). Stories such as Sheehan's reduce some of the uncertainty surrounding cancer and provide multiple perspectives about living and dying.

Practically speaking, counselors, caregivers, and loved ones should keep in mind that cancer survivors are likely to feel overwhelmed by uncertainty and motivated by the need to make sense of their experiences. In telling their stories, people may boost their sense of control, understanding, and acceptance. Finding new meaning in life can be a joyous experience. However, people may be unwilling to share their feelings with those who seem judgmental or skeptical. Remarkable insights sometimes arise from unexpected experiences. People unable to accept or share those experiences may lose valuable opportunities for coping and developing.

Understanding the rewards sometimes found in the most unlikely circumstances is likely to change the way we regard cancer, aging, coping, and death. The stories presented here provide lessons about the power of faith and emotional strength. They are important in the telling, both for the teller and the listener. If there is one overall lesson to be learned, it is this: No experience is entirely good or bad. Miracles occur within the most heart-wrenching moments and serenity sometimes arises from pain. As one participant interviewed for this study said, "It wasn't the worst thing that could happen. It wasn't the best. It was just part of living, and you can work with that."

REFERENCES

Babrow, A. S., Kasch, C. R., & Ford, L. A. (1998). The many meanings of uncertainty in illness: Toward a systematic accounting. *Health Communication*, *10*(1), 1-23.

Bentov, I. (1988). *Stalking the wild pendulum.* Rochester, VT: Destiny Books.

Block, S. D. (2001). Psychological considerations, growth, and transcendence at the end of life. *Journal of the American Medical Association, 285*(22), 2898.

Bohm, D. (1980). *Wholeness and the implicate order*. London: Routledge & Kegan Paul.

Brett, R. (2003a, February 16). Illness teaches a lot about living. *The Plain Dealer*, p. B1.

Brett, R. (2003b, February 21). Life's great, say area survivors. *The Plain Dealer*, p. B1.

Callahan, M., & Kelley, P. (1992). *Final gifts: Understanding the special awareness, needs, and communications of the dying.* New York: Poseidon.

Charmaz, K. (1999). "Discoveries" of self in illness. In K. Charmaz & D. A. Paternati (Eds.), *Health, illness, and healing: Society, social context, and self* (pp. 72-82). Los Angeles: Roxbury.

Coward, D. D. (1990). The lived experience of self-transcendence in women with advanced breast cancer. *Nursing Science Quarterly, 3*(3), 162-169.

Eisenberg, E. M. (1990). Jamming: Transcendence through organizing. *Communication Research, 17*(2), 139-164.

Ford, L. A., Babrow, A. S., & Stohl, C. (1996). Social support messages and the management of uncertainty in the experience of breast cancer: An application of problematic integration theory. *Communication Monographs, 63*(3), 189-207.

Frankl, V. (1959). *Man's search for meaning* (I. Lasch, Trans.). Boston: Beacon Press.

Geist-Martin, P., Ray, E. B., & Sharf, B. F. (2003). *Communicating health: Personal, cultural, and political complexities.* Belmont, CA: Wadsworth/Thomson Learning.

Hilton, B. A. (1988). The phenomenon of coping with uncertainty for women with breast cancer. *Issues in Mental Health Nursing, 9*, 217-238.

LeShan, L. (1989). Cancer as a turning point. *Noetic Sciences Review, 11*(3), 22-28.

Malinksi, V. M. (Ed.). (1986). *Explorations on Martha Rogers' science of unitary human beings.* Norwalk, CT: Appleton-Century-Crofts.

McCormick, K. M. (2002). A concept analysis of uncertainty in illness. *Journal of Nursing Scholarship*, *34*(2), 127-132.

Mishel, M. H. (1984). Perceived uncertainty and stress in illness. *Research in Nursing and Health*, *7*(3), 163-171.

Mishel, M. H. (1990). Reconceptualization of the uncertainty in illness theory. *Image: Journal of Nursing Scholarship*, *22*, 256-262.

Moore, K. (1993). Death has no sting. *Sports Illustrated, 79*(12), 80.

Murphy, M., & White, R. A. (1995). *In the zone: Transcendent experiences in sports.* New York: Penguin.

Neill, J. (2002). Transcendence and transformation in the life pattern of women living with rheumatoid arthritis. *Advances in Nursing Science, 24*(4), 21-47.

Newman, M. A. (1986). *Health as expanding consciousness*. St. Louis, MO: C. V. Mosby.

Newman, M. A. (1995). *A developing discipline: Selected words of Margaret Newman*. New York: National League for Nursing Press.

Newman, M. A. (2000). *Health as expanding consciousness* (2nd ed.). Boston, MA: Jones & Bartlett.

Pascale, R. T. (1999). Leading corporate transformation: Are you up to the task? In J. A. Conger, G. M. Spreitzer, & E. E. Lawler, III, (Eds.), *The leader's change handbook: An essential guide to setting direction and taking action* (pp. 195-220). San Francisco: Jossey-Bass.

Pennebaker, J. W. (1995). Emotion, disclosure, & health: An overview. In J. W. Pennebaker (Ed.), *Emotion, disclosure, & health* (pp. 3-10). Washington, DC: American Psychological Association.

Prigogine, I. (1976). Order through fluctuation: Self-organization and social system. In E. Jantsch & C. H. Waddington (Eds.), *Evolution and consciousness: Human systems in transition* (pp. 93-133). Reading, MA: Addison-Wesley.

Reed, P. G. (1991). Toward a nursing theory of self-transcendence: Deductive reformulation using developmental theories. *Advances in Nursing Science, 13*(4), 64-77.

Reed, P. G. (1996). Transcendence: Formulating nursing perspectives. *Nursing Science Quarterly, 9*(1), 2-4.

Rich, K. R. (1999). *The red devil: To hell with cancer—and back*. New York: Crown.

Rodale, A. (1998, November). Winning over cancer. *Prevention, 50(*11), 192.

Rogers, M. E. (1986). Science of unitary human beings. In V. M. Malinski (Ed.), *Explorations of Martha Rogers' science of unitary human beings* (pp. 3-14). Norwalk, CT: Appleton-Century-Crofts.

Sheehan, G. (1996). *Going the distance: One man's journey to the end of his life*. New York: Random House.

Varallo, S., Ray, E. B., & Ellis, B. H. (1998). Speaking of incest: The research interview as social justice. *Journal of Applied Communication Research, 26*, 254-271.

Williams, K., & Harvey, D. (2001, September). Transcendent experiences in forest environments. *Journal of Environmental Psychology, 21*(3), 249-260.

7

Finding Hope and Healing

Composing and Re-Composing Survivor Identities

Jennifer Ott Anderson
Mission Hospital

Patricia Geist-Martin
San Diego State University

> I have thought long and hard about illness, the reason for it, and of course, the age-old question of "Why me?" When battling a disease, the question, the huge question that I dealt with was, "Does this illness define the person that I am?" I began to feel like a cancer, I was a thyroid, and it was a fight to remember that I am a whole [person]—and where does this cancer fit into the scheme of things, into my life?
>
> —Ivy, cancer survivor

Facing the possibility of death associated with a critical illness produces an emotional life-changing experience for those affected by its anguish. When an individual receives the news that his or her time may be limited, attitudes change, questions are asked, reactions intensify, and emotions heighten, not only for the patient, but also for family and friends. Frank (1991) explained that "illness takes away part of your life, but in doing so, it gives you the opportunity to choose the life you will lead, as opposed to living out the one you have simply accumulated over the years" (p. 1). What happens when a person survives a life-threatening illness such as cancer? What communication processes shape survivors' identities when they have faced death and recovered? What part do family interactions play in the development of survivor identities? Finally, how can others identify with and understand the experience of life-threatening illness?

This study investigates the narratives of one family who lived through life-changing events following a cancer diagnosis. We explore the narratives of the cancer survivor and her family members as they struggle to cope with their situation, provide support for one another, and consider their changing personal identities. Benjamin (1987) argued that communication is a key component in survivorship if individuals can talk about having hope even if they do not. The rationale for this study is threefold. First, this study advocates the need for learning about the composition of survivor identities over the course of a life-threatening illness. Second, this study seeks to understand how illness survivors and their family members use narratives as a method of communicating their changing identities. Finally, communicating about illness is often perceived as "taboo," and this study may encourage others to be a part of the participants' stories and learn more about why those stories are often concealed.

Specifically, this research addresses the communication dilemmas that often occur when family members, friends, and healthcare providers do not know how to respond to an individual diagnosed with cancer. Even more important than knowing how to respond is listening to stories and understanding how survivor identities are composed and recomposed through communication. We begin with a discussion of illness identities, followed by a rationale for studying narratives. Then, we describe the methodology used for conducting this research. Next we present the narratives of Ivy, who was diagnosed with thyroid cancer, her husband, and her adult son. Finally, we offer conclusions and implications. The ultimate goal of this research is to share the stories of one illness survivor and her family, and to invite readers to think with, not just about their story (Frank, 1995).

QUIET MARGINS, DISQUIETED CENTER: ILLNESS IDENTITIES IN FLUX

> A story houses us. Often more utterly than does our flesh. . . . We all live in this way: in a story, in and out of place; living and dying in this way, speaking in search and prevention of ourselves, in places and alien to

> them, given to and taken from a family, suspecting, betraying and worshipping that great space that dwells within the story and the storyteller. (Ronan, 1982, p. 7)

> The story of a life is less than the actual life, because the story told is selective, partial, contextually constructed and because the life is not yet over. But the story of a life is also more than the life, the contours and meanings allegorically extending to others, others seeing themselves, knowing themselves through another's life story, re-visioning their own, arriving where they started and knowing "the place for the first time." (Richardson, 1997, p. 6)

In sickness and in health, we tell, listen to, and construct stories about our bodies—their functioning, malfunctioning, and even goals that we have for changing the shape, strength, and capacity of our bodies and ourselves. Such stories confirm, disconfirm, and challenge our identities; they offer advice, remedies, and motivation; and they build and question the guiding philosophies for living life and surviving illness and loss. When we are sick, diagnosed with a particular disease, or are in some way disabled, we and others define our bodies as damaged and changed, implying they are less than whole, complete, able, or "perfect." Any visible "flaws" become scars for the world to see. We may fear that our "invisible flaws" will be discovered, or we may expend a great deal of energy denying the "flaw" in our body—our flaws become the basis upon which we (and others) reject our own bodies as different. Undoubtedly these changes, these "flaws," may alter our communication in ways that intensify dys-appearance and dis-embodiment. Leder (1992) explained dys-appearance in this way:

> Dys is from the Greek prefix signifying "bad" "hard," or "ill" and is found in English words such as "dysfunctional."... However, dys is also a variant spelling, now somewhat archaic, of the Latin root dis. This originally had the meaning of "away," "apart," or "asunder."... The body in dys-appearance is marked by being away, apart, or asunder. (p. 87)

Essentially, our bodies in dys-appearance or disembodiment can be experienced in two ways: as a reversal of a normal or desired state, and as away, apart from self, as an alien thing or painful prison or tomb one is trapped in (Leder, 1990). In this way, illness is perceived as a "negative achievement" in our culture that results in "failure to adequately fulfill interpersonal commitments and, in due course, failure to receive the support and esteem required from others" (Gerhardt, 1989, pp. 21-22). The social stigma surrounding illness may be based on both actual and perceived negative responses about others' thoughts and feelings.

Goffman (1963) coined the term *passing* to describe what people do when they keep invisible from the public's gaze what is spoiled about their identities. Spoiled identities create crises in communication that lead people to engage in strategies to feel more in control and to become embodied in ways that manage their "sick" identity. Frank (1991) said, "when I wear the lapel pin of my own cancer support group I am doing a kind of reverse passing, proclaiming my identity to be spoiled even though I could easily pass" (p. 32). Although people cannot change their illnesses, this "coming out" informs others that they are doing something about this spoiled identity and thus becomes a form of control. Coming out in this way, through lapel pins, bumper stickers, T-shirts, support groups, Internet chatrooms, and health-oriented classes provides opportunities to share stories and learn about others' "spoiled identities" and strategies for communicating.

Embodiment and disembodiment are natural processes that operate every day, habitually, often unconsciously. Most of us experience a tolerable, even comfortable, ebb and flow of our "healthy" and "sick" identities. Yet when sick or diseased identities become all-encompassing and everything we do, everything we say becomes centered on our illness (whether it be an injury, a chronic illness, or a disease) we may find that our communication with others can intensify self-consciousness to the point that our dys-appearance is uncomfortable.

Leder (1990) suggested that this uncomfortable intensification of self-consciousness often relates to a discrepancy in power. When we are sick, ill, or diseased, others have the power to heal, to provide care, to offer ways of helping us feel whole again.

Cancer and other life-threatening illnesses may lead individuals into a maze of different identities, such as the sick role (Parsons, 1978), a victim, a warrior, or a survivor. The different roles are not sequential, and an individual may assume any or all of them at any time. Many issues and experiences affect those identities, such as confronting death, coping with the illness, dealing with the social expectations that guide emotional expression, and even being labeled a patient. The process of composing and re-composing identities is rooted in the communication between ill individuals and their family, friends, and providers. Disclosure of diagnosis, discussions about treatment, shared fears and hopes, responses to physical changes, confronting death, talking about surviving death, and avoidance of discussions about the illness all affect the shaping and reshaping of identities. Composing identities in the face of uncertainty, pain, stress, stigma, and in some cases, the prospect of death, is an ever-changing process over the course of the illness. A broad range of research has focused on the identity work of members of varied cultural communities as they face injury, illness, and disease, including athletes (Sparkes, 1996, 1997, 1998), chronically ill individuals (Charmaz, 1983, 1987, 1991, 1994, 1995), and individuals diagnosed with cancer (Frank, 1991; Lorde, 1980; Ott, 1999), or generally the healing powers of the stories we tell over the course of illness (Pennebaker, 1992; Pennebaker & Beall, 1986; Pennebaker, Kiecolt-Glaser, & Glaser, 1988).

Communication that occurs during a life-threatening illness and survivorship, the narratives that are told and heard, are the heart of identity. Families embark on their cancer journeys by responding to the dilemmas that arise with a cancer diagnosis, such as the initial diagnosis, confronting mortality, dealing with uncertainty in responding to the ill loved one, addressing the outside social expectations placed on emotional expression and behavior, and attempting to find and resume their "normal" lifestyle. Those responses shape ill individuals' conception of self as well as the overall dynamics of family interactions. Coping with the illness means families may develop a strategy for adjusting and adapting to a new lifestyle. Immediate relatives and friends play a large part in addressing ill individuals' feelings of abandonment or isolation, as well as validating their role in the family structure.

How can we learn about illness survivorship, identity composition, and communication among families? One answer is through narratives. Storytelling may help individuals cope with the social stigma surrounding their illness as well as aid in determining its meaning of their illness as it relates to their life, their relationships, and their communicative behaviors. In the following section, we articulate the value of focusing on narratives to explore one family's stories of cancer.

CONSTRUCTING NARRATIVES: DIFFERENT VERSIONS OF DIFFERENT STORIES

Learning about communication of identity in illness is best understood through narratives. Brody (1987) suggested that stories may be helpful in ascertaining explanations for illness, which is important for both patients and their families. Geist and Dreyer (1993) explained that accounts let us "discover new ways to talk about and account for ourselves, our relationships, and the contexts within which we manage our identities" (p. 97). This understanding of accounts can be applied to the stories told and heard throughout the illness experience. Each time the story is told, identities are altered, changed, discovered, or abandoned as a result of the interaction. One recounting of the story may render individuals' self-images as victimized, whereas another recounting later that same day may render them warriors. Sometimes individuals are active constructors of their narratives, whereas other times they may be passive recipients of others' versions of those narratives. Identity is based on interaction and through the telling of illness stories that contribute to the larger narratives of the illness experiences. The following sections discuss how survivors tell others about their illness, the cathartic effects of sharing the illness experience, and the self-changes that occur from shared narratives.

Telling Others about Illness

> Renewal is easiest if it is a shared process. (Frank, 1991)

Every day of their lives, individuals decide who to tell and who not to tell about their illness. Although some individuals may only tell their relatives and a few close friends, others may find solace in inviting many people to share in their experiences. Benjamin (1987) advises patients with cancer to "tell everyone you want to know, and don't tell anyone you don't want to know" (p. 173). However, this approach implies that constructing and telling stories about the illness experience is an easy task to achieve.

Some individuals may have reservations about disclosing their illness experience. For instance, some people may endure changes in their physical appearance, such as hair loss, the amputation of a limb, or weight loss that lead to feelings of insecurity or self-consciousness. In these cases, it may be easier to fabricate a story that accounts for their mysterious appearance or avoid the subject altogether. Other individuals who do not undergo physical changes may maintain the impression that the illness experience is simply a personal, private subject disclosed only to certain people. In these cases, we may hear edited versions of the stories, although these versions are no more untruthful or invalid than a longer, detailed narrative.

The constraints placed on stories of the illness experience affect individuals' identities. For example, people who feel victimized may shy away from full disclosure of their story because avoidance helps them deal with their feelings of stigmatization. On the other hand, warriors (see e.g., Lorde, 1980; Metzger, 1992) may feel that telling more people about their illness will help in their fight to conquer the disease. The individuals responding to the illness stories may shape the context for future disclosure; if people feel their stories are validated and acknowledged by a family member or close friend, they may be willing to share more in the future. In contrast, a negative experience in sharing an illness story may hinder future disclosure.

Acknowledging Narrative's Health Effects

For many of us, illness is an opportunity to pay more attention to the signals of our bodies to help us and "actually learn something from illness that helps to bring us back into alignment with our potential wellness" (Rossman, 1989). Brody (1987) contended that "storytelling as an activity is central to medicine" (p. 12), and that "suffering is produced, and alleviated, primarily by the meaning that one attaches to one's experience. The primary human mechanism for attaching meaning to particular experiences is to tell stories about them" (p. 5). Writing about illness may also help reduce health problems and actually promotes health (Pennebaker & Beall, 1986; Pennebaker, et al., 1988). In other words, narratives serve as a method of working through the anguish and suffering brought on by life-threatening illness.

Narratives may function as a paradox in the illness experience. Some individuals may find that telling their account repeatedly only increases the stress and anxiety brought on by the illness. Some authors argue that survivors' voices need to be heard and that storytelling is a way to achieve recognition (Lorde, 1980). Lorde explained this paradox as she discussed the strain of wanting to feel strong and talk about her cancer, but at times feeling only sorrow and weakness. In those times of weakness, storytelling may prove harmful rather than beneficial. Individuals may feel cornered and obligated to disclose their narrative in every interaction. They may feel that they are becoming less of a person and more of a disease. These paradoxical feelings and the constant obligation to tell the story may leave the patient stressed, anxious, and in pain. Benjamin (1987) suggested that "when cancer patients discard the feelings of shame and embarrassment, they tear down another barrier to living life as it was before the illness" (p. 76).

On the other hand, narratives may function as medicine for some ill people. Telling their stories becomes a form of control for these individuals, allowing them to gain greater understanding of themselves and their relationships (Brody, 1987). Turning illness into story is not only a form of control, but also an opportunity for others to communicate caring and understanding. It is compassion, in the sense of experiencing with and sharing another's perspective, that allows us each to become transformed into real, dimensional, embodied selves, and not defined solely by a physical characteristic, an illness, or a disease (Leder, 1990). Communication can be a vehicle for transformation, for experiencing compassion, for crossing the boundaries between embodied and disembodied selves. Resisting disembodiment through communication can transform interaction in ways that help to build understanding and compassion. Transformation from disembodiment to embodiment may ease tensions of difference/indifference, stimulate interest in understanding those afflicted in ways we have not personally experienced, and, thus, transcend the "othering" (distancing) that routinely occurs for persons who are ill, disabled, or feel disembodied for any reason.

Responding to Self-Changes in Narratives

One of the most difficult components of the illness experience is attributing validity to self-changes. Frank (1993) contended that "people change their lives through telling them in narratives" (p. 42). Illness may be perceived as an epiphany that provides an opportunity to "[stake] a public claim on a new identity" and the only method of claiming that identity is by sharing the illness experience with others by means of narrative (p. 42). Lorde (1980) supported this notion that "it is necessary to teach by living and speaking those truths which we believe and know beyond understanding" (p. 14). The "truth" that Lorde speaks of is not medical truth, not the truth that others agree on, but the truth that individuals create for themselves, or the narrative truth (Ellis, 1996). Learning a new truth is part of the illness experience and acknowledging that truth means recognizing identities prior to the illness, during the illness, and even in recovery.

Frank (1993) explained that illness creates an occasion for individuals to discover not only who they have been, but also who they may become. Illness narratives may be an opportunity to reinforce and redefine self-concept, or a moment to expand to a new emerging self, or maybe a combination of both. For instance, if patients undergo amputation, they may become more rooted in who they were before the illness as a means of coping with the loss of a body part. In this sense, individuals may perceive the amputation not just as a removal of a physical attribute, but more as a mental, emotional, or spiritual amputation. With illness comes the need to reconstruct the self in order for the individual to go on living (Frank, 1993).

Self-changes may indeed help determine meaning in illness narratives. However, as Frank pointed out, illness narratives may also reinforce the "reluctant Phoenixes" or those narratives that illustrate how illness has not changed the self, or if it has, those changes are deemed insignificant (p. 47). For instance, some individuals may feel that because they did not choose to have their illness, self-changes that occur from illness should not be included as part of their new identity. In other words, illness was something that happened to them, and their self-concept that ensues does not include their experience.

Healing Stories: Communicating Transformation

> Illness is the night-side of life, a more onerous citizenship. Everyone who is born holds dual citizenship, in the kingdom of the well and in the kingdom of the sick. Although we all prefer to use only the good passport, sooner or later each of us is obliged at least for a spell, to identify ourselves as citizens of that other place. (Sontag, 1989, p. 3)

The power of story to reflect and affect people's dual citizenship should never be underestimated. Such narratives give voice to the concerns of persons who are usually not heard because of the stigma of their "spoiled identities." More often than not, our society privileges those who have undamaged bodies and minds to speak with a stronger voice than "others."

Narratives reflect people's lives and the changes in identity they experience when they become ill or as they grapple with their "spoiled identities," allowing others to glimpse the experiences and emotions of persons who feel embodied or disembodied in some way. Stories as identity work represent an overarching type of narrative that might also be described as a journey (Jackson, 1989), a performance (Denzin, 1997), a ritual of community (Richardson, 1997). Identity work for individuals who are ill involves articulating what it means to live a life circumscribed by illness (Mathieson & Barrie, 1998). From the moment they are diagnosed with an illness or begin some type of physical or psychological therapy, individuals are faced with a process of composing and renegotiating their identities with family, friends, coworkers, and health care providers (Mathieson & Stam, 1995).

Narratives of health and illness are, more often then not, complicated by the politics of interaction, among family members or friends, providers with dissimilar specialties or ideologies, or our own identity struggles. What people care about, attend to, elicit, ignore, refute, embrace, or even withhold information about is enmeshed in the story of their life experiences with health and illness. In this sense, narratives become a framework for understanding the personal, cultural, and political complexities of communication in health and illness in diverse contexts—in homes, health care settings, policy and legislation, and mass media campaigns (Geist-Martin, Ray, & Sharf, 2003). Vital to understanding and theorizing about communicating in health and illness is understanding these complexities as revealed in narratives that consumers and providers construct when they talk to each other, to families, to colleagues, and to us as researchers.

Narratives become the primary means for negotiating our way through the demanding moments of our personal lives and our changing identities (Hanne, 1994). Through stories, we explain, exemplify, recount, and account for our decisions (Fisher, 1987). We can think of narratives as something we construct for ourselves and with others to make sense of our lives (Bruner, 1987; White, 1981). Narrative is a mode of reasoning that we utilize to make sense of or apprehend the world, and it is a mode of representation we use to tell about the world (Richardson, 1997). On a daily basis, we utilize the two primary and complementary forms of reasoning—narrative and logico-scientific—each relying on different communication codes to get messages across. Narrative reasoning is designed to understand the whole by integrating parts of our experience, often in ways we cannot "prove" but we know intuitively. Logical reasoning, on the other hand, is based on structured observations that "prove" what we experience. The boundaries between narrative and scientific knowledge are permeable and both forms of reasoning arrive in packages that are inseparable aspects of the same thing—both frame and picture (Czarniawska, 1997).

There is a great deal we can learn from juxtaposing narratives and the process of interaction surrounding the construction of narratives in diverse contexts. We often see in this comparison how stories reveal that meanings are "incomplete, tentative, and revisable according to contingencies of our present life circumstances . . . stories rearrange, redescribe, invent, omit, and revise" (Ellis & Bochner, 2000, p. 745). Considering the communication between illness survivors and their families we might ask the following questions: How do individuals explain their illnesses? How is identity composition revealed in the ways ill individuals share their experience? Who participates in the construction of narratives of health and illness? What forms do these narratives take? What can we learn by juxtaposing family narratives? These are the questions this research is designed to consider.

METHODOLOGY

Keeping the previous review of literature in mind, we turn now to one family's experience with cancer. This single case study is part of a larger corpus of family narratives about cancer survivorship (Ott, 1999). In order to maintain the rich text desired for this research, in-depth interviews were used as the method of data collection. In the original study, a total of 20 interviews were conducted of 9 survivors of illness and 11 family members of survivors over an 8-months period. By focusing on family units to learn about the experience of life-threatening illness, we are able to investigate the multiple truths that exist in other people's lives (Emerson, Fretz, & Shaw, 1995). Participants were asked to first tell stories about their illnesses. Follow-up questions targeted specific topics, such as the emotional toll of the illness experience, perceptions of identity changes, and perceptions about the illness after sharing it for the purpose of this research. Each interview was transcribed and revised to read much like a story with a beginning, middle, and end.

For the purposes of this chapter, we present excerpts from one family's narratives. By editing the original narratives, we were able to more closely identify the occasions for healing through the illness journey, and the impact that the experience had on each family member's aging process. Additionally, we were able to reduce the redundancy, which made for cleaner, clearer pieces presented in this chapter. By juxtaposing the narratives, we are able to see the similarities and differences in perceptions about the illness experience, the moments of strained and stressed communication, the epiphanies that arose, and reflective feelings about the experience as a whole. In the paragraphs following each narrative, we identify the moments in each person's experience in which he or she found opportunities for healing, learned to use the illness experience to make life changes, and recognized the impact that an experience like cancer survivorship has on our aging processes.

Presenting these three narratives side by side achieves two goals. First, we see how shared stories serve as catharsis for those who have suffered from life-threatening illnesses. Lindlof (1995) stated that "the qualitative interview creates an event in which one person (the interviewer) encourages another person to articulate interests or experiences freely" (p. 163). Survivors of illness and their families need to tell their stories and this study provided the outlet. People who have had similar experiences may find themselves identifying with the participants. Second, we were able to triangulate the experiences of a survivor and her family members in order to examine communicative processes in the family unit as a whole. These narratives permit discovery of what would be otherwise difficult, and even impossible, to obtain (Hammersley & Atkinson, 1995).

The three narratives presented in this chapter provide access to the participants' experiences and meanings (Nijhof, 1997). First, we present the narrative of Ivy who is a survivor of thyroid cancer. Jack, Ivy's husband, is the second voice in this story. Finally, we present the voice of Ivy and Jack's son Brandon, who was geographically separated from his parents during his mother's experience with cancer. Juxtaposing the voices of Ivy, her husband, and her son, we discover the paradoxes and contradictions that arose in the family's communication. As such, it was important that each family member become part of the multivoiced text that shares Ivy's experience with thyroid cancer.

REVEALING CHANGING IDENTITIES: BRAVE SOULS, SHARED STORIES, AND CHANGED LIVES

There's Strength in Ivy

It was a regular GYN appointment. The nurse practitioner sat across the room. She looked at me.

"So tell me about your neck."

I said, "What about my neck?"

"You seem to have an area that's a little larger."

She came around and she felt it. She sent me back to my physician who referred me to an endocrinologist (the thyroid doctor). He sent me to the hospital to have a scan and there they said 90% of those lumps are benign. The doctor wanted to do a needle biopsy, which is about 90% accurate. I was sent to nuclear medicine for what they called an iodine uptake scan and to see if there was cancer in the lump, and how much. I was scheduled for surgery to remove the lump.

I became very organized before surgery because I thought I was dying. I cleaned drawers and cupboards and put my clothes in order because I wanted things to be right and taken care of. I really did think the chances of my dying during surgery were very great. I had no control over what was happening to me. If something like that can happen to me without my control, what happens with control? Why should I take care of myself, why should I eat properly, why should I do any of these things when something like that happens?

Even though I could not control what was happening to me, I could control my son, Brandon. I didn't want to give him a lot of information because I didn't want him to worry. I sensed that there was nothing he could do and he knew there was nothing he could do. I remember that if I was going to leave my son, I wanted him to be okay.

A mother's role is to protect her child. Brandon was at an age where he really didn't need protecting. But what I needed was to protect him by not giving him a lot of information. I feel very close to my son. I think that I've always known that he loves me. I know he was worried about me. I think I protected him as much as I could. But how do you tell your son this is what's happening? I couldn't protect him from the knowledge of it, but I <u>could</u> protect him from the details.

I wrote out some letters to Brandon and my husband, Jack. I put a note on Jack's pillow. I think it said "if I die, please read this otherwise please don't." The only way I could have control was to write these letters saying what I wanted done if I die. I haven't looked at the letters since then. I should have. I'm sure I will.

I remember waking up after the surgery. Jack just kind of bent down and said, "You're okay but it's cancer." I think I'm kind of a pessimistic person. I just knew it was going to be cancer. The doctors thought they'd only have to take half of my thyroid. But they did the biopsy and the surgery showed that it was cancer. It was starting to go into the muscle tissue as well so they removed it all. It was almost a relief to know what I had, to know what was wrong so we could take care of it. I was worried, thinking about what my future held. I had no thyroid, something that you need very badly.

A doctor said the word cancer and my life did change. It's just not in one part of your body. It's in your mind, in your emotions, it's in your physical being. It's your life all of a sudden. The bad part of it is that other aspects that were important to me were way down the list of importance. The things I enjoyed doing didn't matter. It was like, "I'll get time for it later. Right now I've got to think about this."

Cancer was something that was within myself and that I had to deal with. On the outside, I looked like everyone else and so much was happening to me that I felt very much, I felt like no one could reassure me that everything was okay. Jack said it a lot to me and to believe it and he needed me to say it, that would make it so. But I couldn't make it so for myself. I was afraid.

I became very self-centered. It's a way of coping. There was a disease within me and that disease was all encompassing. Every other instance or thing of importance in my life took second place. I ate a lot. I gained weight. I cried a lot, I shed a lot of tears and I talked a lot, I really did talk a lot. I got angry with myself; almost self-loathing. This cancer was inside me. How dare I allow it to happen? I blamed myself. I guess I felt that there was something wrong within me. It didn't last long but I felt that I should have had control of this.

There was a time when I thought I was never going to be well again. But there was also part of me that said, "I'm still gonna grow that garden and that's important to me." I think I was motivated because we moved in the new house about 6 months before I got cancer and moving to the country was our dream. Everything in our home is the way we want it and this is our new life. Then this happened so soon after moving in.

Despite my motivation, I was worried about my future. If something else happens is it going to be just one thing too much or will I be stronger because of what I've gone through and be able to deal with the future?

I thought long and hard about illness, the reason for it and of course the age-old question of "why me?" When battling a disease, the question, the huge question, that I dealt with was "Does this illness define the person that I am?" I began to feel like a cancer, I was a thyroid and it was a fight to remember that I am a whole—and where does this cancer fit into the scheme of things, into my life?

Being without the thyroid, all I felt like doing was staying in bed. I could not walk around the house or the outside of my house. The emotions went up and down, up and down. One day you're fighting and the next day it was like, I'm just tired, I can't do this.

I talked to Jack and he listened. What I needed was someone just to hear my voice. Our relationship has always been solid but it's even been closer now. Our communication has been really good. We're just on the same wavelength, completing each other's sentences. And he understands what I'm talking about when I talk.

There was a point where Jack's optimism got to me. It was like stop, you're not listening to me. I could die, stop. But Jack needed to hear, "I'm really gonna fight, I'm really gonna conquer this, I'm gonna go forward." I needed to be a warrior for Jack.

I've chosen to be more alone and aloof. During this time I regretted not having more friends to be comfort and say, "You're going to be okay." To just be there to share the experience. I guess through other people you're validated and I needed that. If you have other people reminding you that you're still there, you're okay, and yes, it's a terrible thing that's happened to you but you know what? You're going to make it.

Some people, like my neighbors, saw me. But they didn't want to know because it was too personal. They don't want to be that close to other people. They would ask, "How are you doing?" But it was kind of like greeting somebody. I would say how I was feeling and I'd explain to them a little bit. I realized they didn't care.

They kept me off all thyroid medication for about a month after the surgery. I got really, really weak and very tired. I didn't feel good. The hormone level was as low as they could get it so I could have another iodine scan. The next week I went to the hospital for 2 or 3 days. Being in a hospital and staying in a hospital was a very hard thing for me to do. My mother had a stroke in a hospital during a diagnostic test. From that, and from other experiences in my past, hospitals were NOT good places to be.

I was put into a room. There were signs on the door that everyone who went into the room had to sign their name and how many minutes they were in the room. They put paper on the floor and I could only walk on the paper. None of the nurses wanted to come into the room because I was radioactive. The people who came in to bring me food would literally throw it onto the table and they would go. From the outside they would say, "Is there anything you need or anything you want?" But it was like "don't tell me you need anything, don't tell me you want anything, but I have to ask."

It was really dehumanizing and very lonely. Whatever I brought into the room, it had to be thrown out. I remember I had to throw away my underpants because they were radioactive. It was really hard being isolated because no one could come into my room. Jack had to stay in the hall and we talked to each other back and forth without him coming close to me.

The guy who measured the radioactivity in my body, whose name was also Jack, brought a "humanness" to the whole process that was just so cold. That man was very important to me. He was kind of like a link. I remember his ties. He wore real fancy ties. The man connected with me. He took his time when he probably shouldn't have for his own safety. He asked me personal questions about my life. I think he was concerned about how I was doing. I think he knew this was really hard for me. He was not afraid of me.

Jack, my husband, was able to show me the humor in it all because there IS humor in this. So in spite of everything, we were laughing together. Him being out in the hall and me being in this room that was lined with lead, and talking back and forth. There was humor in everything and that helped.

The iodine treatment came back negative. But after the treatment, I started losing my hair. I looked down in the sink one day and there was a lot of hair there. Part of that was probably due to not having the thyroid medication as well as the iodine treatment.

It took quite a while to get my thyroid medication regulated. A year later I had to be scanned again to see if there was cancer growing again. They had to take me off the thyroid medication. Again, I became very tired and weak. Now they have a treatment where I won't have to go off the medication. So I have to have another scan in another year. Then I wait years. After the 2 years if that one's clean then I wait 5 years.

I learned a lot about human nature through this. I learned that people are afraid of exposing themselves and being exposed to someone in pain. All of us wear our skin tight around us. When somebody is near you and they're needy, it frightens people. They don't want to see that neediness and they don't want to expose themselves to it. I was very needy. I felt like I needed arms around me. I needed mothering. Only one person really gave me that and that was Jack.

I've become more withdrawn and inward. I talk less now than I used to. I don't know if that has anything to do with cancer, but I'm a more quiet person now. I'm really thoughtful, full

> *of thought. I try not to have so much control over all the details around, to let go. I tried not to care so much about things anymore. It was a humbling experience. I guess it taught me that I need to not take things so seriously, I need to relax, I need to just breathe.*
>
> *I wear my scar as a badge of courage but I've never thought of myself as a courageous person. But I am, I am a courageous person. People notice the scar. But you know I don't mind the scar, I really don't mind it at all. I've gone through bad things in my life and have survived before and to have survived this I have to be a courageous person. I feel, looking back, I feel like I did the best that I could do and I'm proud of that.*
>
> *Years ago, I decided that I wanted to change my name, to pick out who I wanted to be. Ivy came to mind because I liked the plant. It's a vine, it is strong, you can cut it down and it comes back. There's a lot of strength in Ivy. I want to be like Ivy so no matter how many times I might be cut down I'm coming back. I'm not there yet. It's a life process. Becoming Ivy's a life process.*

Controlling Destiny: Negotiating Identity in the Face of Illness. One of Ivy's big concerns with cancer was control. She could not control what was happening to her body, but she needed to find ways to somehow control the situation. She did this first prior to the surgery by organizing all of her items at home and writing letters to Jack and Brandon. She also controlled the amount and type of information that she shared with Brandon as a means of retaining her role as a mother. Even beyond the surgery and recovery from the surgery, she faced instances where she was stripped of her control, and in each instance, she looked for something that she could control as a way to begin her healing from this experience.

Prior to having cancer, Ivy never saw herself as being courageous. The experience taught her that if she could survive cancer, she could survive anything. She learned that enduring all of the treatment made her a courageous person. She perceives her surgery scar as a symbol of her courage. She learned that she faced one of the most uncertain and frightening illnesses that anyone can face, and moved beyond it. It will always be a part of her.

Ivy found healing in her relationships with certain people. She was able to rely on her husband for daily support. He was there to listen to her, provide words of encouragement, serve as a sounding board, be the target of her frustration and emotions, accompany her to each and every appointment and treatment session, and help her when she physically could not help herself. That relationship has since strengthened, and they both attribute their increased closeness to this experience. Ivy also found healing in Jack, the technician who measured her levels of radioactivity during her iodine treatments. Jack was not afraid to come into contact with her, and she perceived his willingness to do so as being more concerned with how she was doing emotionally, not just physically. But, even in relationships that were not "close," Ivy found a place for healing. She had to learn that some people simply would not care much about her condition, or they didn't know what to say to her. Juxtaposed with the supportive relationships, Ivy learned in whom she could confide, and to whom she could turn for anything.

One thing that Ivy learned through the experience was that bad things can happen, but we do what we can to get through them. She has discovered that she does not need to worry about insignificant things in life, that there are more important issues that need her attention. This was a large part of her healing process. She was able to, in some ways, redefine what was really important in her life: her relationships with her family, being able to grow her garden, and finding her strength and courage.

Jack: Discovering Ivy's Strength

> *I remember the day she came home and she said she had some nodules. I wasn't thinking that it was anything bad. It didn't really alarm me. I was just, "Oh, you know, okay, it's just one more thing we have to take care of." I wasn't real alarmed at that point in time.*
>
> *The worst emotional strain for me was the fact that Ivy had to go through another crisis. She had previously dealt with so much else. I was distressed that she had to deal with another trying experience. She was quite afraid that she wasn't ever going to come home. And in fact she wrote something to both Brandon and me that was to be opened only after she died. And I still have yet to see that.*
>
> *She was really nervous about the general anesthesia. I had been through one before so I felt fairly comfortable with it. I felt fairly confident that it wasn't a big deal. She had had hernia surgery previously and she demanded not to be put out. And it has to do with some of the other problems that we've gone through earlier in life. Also with the fact that her mother had big problems with surgery one time. She has a real problem with losing control.*
>
> *We went into surgery thinking it was 90% chance that it wasn't anything bad. But the surgery day was hard. But we went in early and again, the thinking early in the day was let's get through the surgery, get half the thyroid out, it'll be benign, and we'll worry about the rest later.*
>
> *I was with her for pre-op and the anesthesiologist came in, we discussed things and I could tell she was really, really nervous but she did fine. He gave her some sedations right there and then*

when they took her in she was really funny. It was almost like she was drunk. As they wheeled her away she just sort of . . . I'm going one way and she's going the other way and she just sort of lifted her hand up and said, "Bye!" That's the last I saw her till afterward.

Jennie (my sister) and Laurie (my niece) stayed with me. The surgery took about 3 hours and I think after a couple hours I started to get a little more concerned because I think he told us it would be a couple hours. And after the second hour, he still didn't come down, still didn't come down.

After about 3 hours, he came down and he said, "She's doing fine. She's in post-op." Then he was about to leave! I said, "Well, was it benign?" And he said, "Oh, no, it was cancer." Very matter-of-factly. These guys deal with it every day. We went to the surgeon specifically because we liked him. But surgeons don't have the best bedside manner because they're used to working on people that are asleep.

I was just devastated. He asked me, "Do you want me to tell her or do you want to tell her?" So I said, "I probably should tell her." Some tears dropped. Jennie and I went for a walk. When we could get in, we went in to see her. It was very hard to tell her, and when I told her, she was very down.

Being a fairly positive thinking person, I didn't worry too much that she may not survive. There are three different kinds of thyroid cancer. The most common kind is the one she has which is just a "garden variety"-type thing. It's 100% curable. Three different physicians separately told us that. But there are two other kinds and one is sort of a medium danger and one is very, very bad. Both of the two bad categories are like 1 to 2% of all the cancers that are found in thyroids. So, we just kept trying to reassure ourselves that what they said is going to be true and we'd get through it.

Jennie and Laurie were extremely supportive. Jennie especially. I mean she had to drive 60 miles for this. Just the fact that they would be there for it. Jennie helped talk me through after we first heard. They were very supportive with calls, and they both took the day off work. I called the rest of the family and my office. The rest of the family was just like, "Oh, well, that's too bad." But we've always sort of set ourselves up to take care of ourselves. We just don't ask for help. Most people didn't know what to say, so they generally didn't say much. Those that were close to us were similar, but sometimes they would say something which often was not appropriate, at least in our opinion.

Ivy and I tried to not dwell on it any more than necessary, which she's one to do. Just tried to always think positively. With the reassurances of all the physicians, we were well founded in that things would turn out fine. I tried to keep a fairly normal schedule at the office other than when she had appointments. I went with her to all of her appointments. We either tried to schedule them around my schedule or I just blocked time out.

The impact on myself personally was just a need to cope with the situation. I tried to keep life as normal as possible while dealing with the problem, which is probably the best way for me to cope. I tried to be as positive as possible. It's very easy to go right down the dunker and for both of us to be depressed. I tried to keep her up as much as we could. We talked a lot about it. I was her sounding board, which has not been an unusual role for me.

The biggest problem occurred between surgery and the scan. It was about a month between them, and she didn't have any thyroid medication. As the month went along, she got to the point where she could hardly do anything. She'd wake up in the morning and take a shower, and she'd have to sit down and rest for an hour before she could dress herself. That's how bad it was. That left some more things for me to do which she did in our normal every day life.

She was off the thyroid for a month because they want any thyroid tissue that's left in her body to be hungry and looking for something so that it can create thyroid hormone. Without hormone production, our brain keeps sending out what's called thyroid-stimulating hormone. That's really how they measure her thyroid hormone; they actually measure the thyroid- stimulating hormone. So when your level's down, your brain puts more of it out saying, "Hey we need some more of this stuff so get it going!" Whereas if it has enough or too much, you don't see any or just a little.

In that scan they computed somehow how much thyroid tissue was left in her body. And we're talking 1% or more and you've got to do something. After the scan, the doctors decided that she needed to be treated; that there was enough thyroid tissue left that she had to be treated. She went into the hospital for a radioactive iodine treatment. The thyroid uses iodine to produce the hormone. This was a special kind of iodine that the thyroid tissue reads as being regular iodine, but yet when it takes it up then it kills the tissue.

It was like she was a leper. Nobody wanted to be in contact with her and they weren't supposed to be because she was radioactive. Each nurse when they brought the food or some-

> *thing, they signed their name, time in, time out. It was a minute or less. They didn't fool with her.*
>
> *I couldn't come in and see her. I could only talk to her through the door. The door was open, but there was a curtain across the door and we could talk through the curtain. It was hard to leave her there, because she really did feel like an outcast. She spent 2 days with virtually no other person being around her. And as soon as she had a low enough level of radiation, then they let her go.*
>
> *This illness and the treatments were completely foreign to us. It's what they call nuclear medicine. All these scans and everything are all done with nuclear fluids. What was nice about that was when she was done with that then she could get on thyroid hormone and start building herself back up which took some time.*
>
> *We learned a lot about illness. We're the type that when something presents us, we find materials to read about it. We did that. I learned a lot about thyroid cancer, which hopefully we'll never need to know about again. More importantly, I think I just learned how resilient she is, more so than I think she realizes or will admit to. It even strengthened our relationship more going through it.*

Needing to Fight: Becoming a Warrior for Ivy. Jack is a rather logical, solution-oriented person. His approach to the experience was that this was just something they would have to get through. He discovered that for his own healing, he had to maintain a positive outlook. He could not let himself become depressed or let his guard down for two reasons: First, he needed to stay positive to cope with his wife's cancer, and second, he needed to be strong for Ivy. Part of staying positive was to keep their daily lives as normal as possible. By not changing how they lived their lives, the cancer was not going to "win." In some ways, Jack needed to take on a warrior identity to indicate his strength. Much literature posits that the person affected by the illness often assumes a warrior identity. In this case, Jack needed to portray this role in order to find his own opportunities for healing, and, in his mind, to help Ivy heal as well.

Much like Ivy, Jack's healing came through supportive relationships with his niece and his sister. They were both there through the surgery and during treatment. They were the two family members who significantly impacted his healing—he saw things such as taking the day off work, helping at home to feed the animals the day of the surgery, and taking a walk with him after the diagnosis as extremely supportive and caring. It was through those gestures, even if they were small, that he was able to find his own strength to pass on to Ivy.

One part of Jack's healing came through information gathering. Throughout his narrative, he discusses many of the "technical" aspects of thyroid cancer, from the different types to the various treatments and their purposes. By learning about the disease, he was able to better cope with what they were experiencing.

Brandon: Discovering What Ivy Needed

> *When I first heard the diagnosis, I wasn't really sure what I should do. Along with the diagnosis came a statement from a doctor that said that thyroid cancer was one of the easier cancers to treat. My natural instinct told me that I shouldn't be 1,000 miles away from my mom, that I should go home and spend time with my parents and help my mom through this. But some other part of me told me that my mom and dad would be able to work through this together.*
>
> *Initially, I think it was easy for me to be somewhat detached from the situation. I was always genuinely concerned and worried about my mom, but I don't think the situation became "real" until I was told that my mom was going to have surgery to remove her thyroid. This time was when I was the most scared and worried about my mom. I was able to curb some of that fear by telling myself that the removal of a thyroid gland is a relatively simple procedure, and this will probably be a solution.*
>
> *The thought of either of my parents being gone hadn't really even crossed my mind. Once this became a very real possibility, I started really valuing my relationship with my family and really feeling like I needed to start spending more time with them. I never feel like spending more time with them because I SHOULD, I genuinely wanted to spend more time with them. I think going through this illness with my mom has made me realize this.*
>
> *The few years prior to the diagnosis had been tough for my mom for other reasons, and I felt like the cancer diagnosis was coming at a time when she was just starting to be happy again. My biggest concern was for my mom mentally. I think fighting cancer really takes a mental toll over time. I was always scared that fighting this illness was mentally overwhelming for her, and that she would be thrown into depression.*
>
> *I remember I just kept thinking that my mom was the ONE person who didn't deserve to have this happen to them right now. I think that was what always bothered me the most. I think that I always knew through this whole ordeal that she was going to be*

physically okay. But I had always felt that my mom had been through enough in her life, and I that this wasn't fair to her.

I think I was always convinced that my mom would be okay. However, I think this was something I used to keep myself from even thinking about alternatives. I don't think I was able to even fathom what life would have been like without my mom, so I think I was constantly convincing myself that everything would be okay. I tend to look at things on a factual, logical basis, and all of the information that I found regarding thyroid cancer told me that this was one of the easier cancers to treat assuming it was diagnosed early on. I am "solution-oriented," and I remember wishing that I could do something to make these treatments easier for my mom. Of course, there wasn't anything I could do. This was incredibly frustrating for me.

A lot of the time, my feelings kept me from anything but surface-level discussion of my mom's illness with my parents. I was so worried about her, but I didn't want to talk to my parents about it because I didn't want to upset my mom. My feelings were, "hey, my mom is fighting cancer here . . . the last thing she needs is for me to be constantly bringing it up."

Whenever I would talk to them on the phone, I always mentally filtered out any thoughts or worries I had. I always tried to keep an upbeat mood and didn't want my mom to think that her illness was affecting my life negatively. I felt that she had enough to worry about, and she didn't need to be concerned with my feelings at that time. Looking back, this internalization of my feelings was probably one of the worst things that I could have done for my mother.

One day on the phone, my mom just came out and asked me why I never asked her anything about her illness. She said that it seemed like I didn't really care that much about it. It was then that I realized that by editing my conversations and keeping them on a surface level, I appeared (to my mom) like I was not concerned and couldn't care less about her illness.

Up until that point, I had not asked any questions about her illness, nor had I asked her how she felt, because I did not want to bring up topics that might be upsetting to her. Up until that point, my mom had not brought up any information about her illness or really shared how she felt because she didn't think I was interested.

There was this giant catch 22 between us. My mom needed to talk with me about what she was going through. This whole time I had been refraining from talking to her about her illness because I wanted to help her by not upsetting her. But this whole time the thing she needed most from me was to talk with me about her illness.

I knew that my dad was a huge help to my mom during this ordeal. There were many times when she was upset with him for some reason or another. I think we all knew that a large portion of that was just emotional release. I think that was one of my dad's largest contributions; he was always there for my mom, no matter what she said or how bad she felt.

I always knew that I couldn't just quit the semester and go home, but for the rest of college, I think a little part of me always felt like I should have been there in some capacity other than just holidays and the times I visited.

I think going through my mom's illness helped me become more comfortable with the idea that my parents wanted (needed) to hear from me. Before her illness, I always felt like my mom had other issues to deal with, and didn't need to be bothered with my problems or concerns about anything. I, of course, carried these feelings over into this situation. Once I realized that it was important to my mom to hear from me and hear my feelings about her illness, I instantly felt much more comfortable speaking with both my parents about my feelings about any topic.

Defying Logic: Discovering the Power of Contradiction. One of Brandon's main tools for coping with the situation was, like his father, to find information about thyroid cancer to put his mind at ease. He did his own research and learned that thyroid cancer was virtually curable, and that helped him approach the situation more calmly and rationally.

Brandon, as he explains, is a very logical person. Provide him a question or puzzle, and he figures out a logical, feasible solution. He applied his own personality traits to his mother's experience with cancer—if you have cancer, you take it out and treat it so it will not come back. Keeping this mindset helped him in his own healing process. He was able to keep the solution in mind rather than focusing on the problem. He was frustrated that he could not provide the solution personally, but he knew that the doctors could.

A major turning point in Brandon's healing came during the phone call in which Ivy asked why he never wanted to know about her experience. Throughout the surgery and treatment, Brandon felt that bringing it up would upset her, and he did not want to cause any additional emotional pain. He felt his mom had faced enough and by constantly hounding her for details, he would exacerbate her anguish. Ivy, on the other hand, felt as though he did not care about her or her illness. Upon confronting the situation, he explained his approach, to which she provided her take on his avoidance of talking about her cancer. By working through this catch 22 (as he called it), he was able to better understand what she was experiencing. Although he still lived 1,000 miles away, conversations about her illness improved once they discussed this issue.

Brandon didn't always feel that his parents (specifically his mom) wanted and needed to hear from him, not only about Ivy's cancer, but about anything. Part of his healing came through this discovery. He felt more comfortable sharing his feelings about the situation, and feels that his relationship with both of his parents has become closer. Brandon needed that closeness in order to move along his own path of healing.

Communicating through Illness: Implications for Healing

The stories shared in this chapter provide insight into the power of narratives as an opportunity for healing. Each person's story brings us one step closer to understanding the impact that a cancer diagnosis has on the communication among family members, the difficult and enlightening moments throughout the journey, and how those moments impact our perceptions of self as we grow older. Surviving cancer was not a linear process for Ivy and her family. Many moments throughout the journey came about unexpectedly, by surprise. The juxtapositioning of voices leaves us with three emotional, rich, and detailed narratives from which we can draw our own insights. We offer the following questions as we turn now to a discussion of what we have learned through these narratives: What contradictions and alignments arose during the family's experience with cancer? How did the family members determine their roles? How did Ivy handle the family's identity expectations? Overall, what have we learned from their experiences?

DISCUSSION: THE PARADOX OF COMMUNICATING IDENTITY IN ILLNESS SURVIVORSHIP

Ivy's experience with cancer began after a lifetime of various adversities. She discovered early in life that things can happen beyond a person's control, and throughout her experience with cancer, she struggled to figure out how the illness happened to her at a time when she was in control in her life and doing everything "right." Her physicians approached the illness as a simple process of surgery followed by taking medication the rest of her life: Taking pills every day would make her well. Ivy found herself becoming segmented, as the illness did not allow her to fulfill her role as a mother, a wife, and a friend. She dealt with people's blinders to her illness because they simply did not understand what was happening to her. Jack needed her to be a warrior and fight her illness, but there were times when she could not align herself with those expectations. Several members of the family came together with Ivy, Jack, and Brandon and she now sees the group as individual spokes on one wheel. Ivy needed reassurance that she was a whole person, not just an illness, and several individuals served as her guardian angels throughout extensive treatments by not being afraid of her. Ivy's scar is a badge of courage, and a reminder that the illness did not win.

Each person in this family had different things that contributed to his or her healing, but as a family, Ivy, Jack, and Brandon needed to heal as well. Leaning how to openly share information with one another was central to the family being able to heal as a cohesive unit. Brandon felt as though he could mask his feelings by censoring his conversations with his parents. Ivy thought she could control the amount of information given to Brandon so that she could maintain her motherly role and protect her child. Jack had to play the role of the positive, upbeat husband to help Ivy in her coping. By breaking down some of those barriers, the family opened up as a whole, and they were able to better communicate with one another, a trait they feel has improved even more since then.

We learn from these three narratives that supportive relationships are central to healing. Each person learned in whom he or she could confide, and once those ties were established, they became even stronger. This was evident for them going through the cancer journey, and also in recounting the experience through these narrative interviews. By telling the story again, all three family members were able to realize the key individuals they needed most throughout the experience. By this, we can return to the conversation about narratives being both a process and a product. Through the process of sharing their experiences, they discovered more about themselves as they retold the story. As a product, these stories may help others as they experience their own journeys with cancer and determine the supportive relationships central to their own healing processes.

Part of the healing process was rooted in positive thoughts about the future when Ivy's health was back to normal. Recovering from cancer meant that Ivy would be able to resume activities she enjoyed, or that she could anticipate beginning new endeavors. For example, Ivy's love for being outdoors and working in her garden was hindered by her illness. The thyroid cancer made her extremely tired and worn down, so gardening was impossible, but the anticipation of returning to her favorite hobby kept her hopes high. Communication about resuming pastimes gave Ivy the hope she needed to survive. We see this through Jack's and Brandon's factual, logical approach to thyroid cancer and treatment, through Ivy's need to be physically active again, and through Jack simply believing that his wife was going to survive. Goffman's (1963) discussion of stigma factors into this part of the healing process: Being sick precluded Ivy from engaging in her normal, daily activities, thus feeding the sick or spoiled identity that came along with her cancer diagnosis. All three family members, in their own ways, needed to focus on a positive future in order to heal. Maintaining the sick role (Parsons, 1978) was contrary to Ivy's way of dealing with her illness, and a positive approach to the illness journey helped all three family members heal from the impact of the experience.

Hearing all three stories emphasizes the concept that by letting our guards down and admitting that we need other people, we can find a place for healing. Much of the literature presented in this chapter advocates for sharing illness experiences as a means of catharsis and healing (e.g., Brody, 1987; Frank, 1991, 1993; Pennebaker & Beall, 1986; Pennebaker et al., 1988). Sharing the experience, in this case, was helpful for the entire family. Once they realized the importance of sharing experiences with one another and with others outside of the immediate family, they found it easier to communicate their feelings. Ivy, as she explained, needed to be nurtured and comforted. Brandon found that he needed his parents to be open with him about the details of Ivy's illness. Jack and Ivy both needed Brandon to share his feelings about Ivy's experience with them. All of these issues meant that they would have to break down the walls that inhibited this type of communication, and in doing so, they found that they needed each other much more than they previously realized. More importantly, they realized that needing other people is a good thing. Learning how to openly express this need for one another helped each one of them in their healing processes.

One of the most important implications we glean from these three narratives is the impact the experience had on this family's aging process. As we grow older, our likelihood for developing cancer increases. For example, according to the American Cancer Society, between age 45 and 50, the chances of women developing breast cancer nearly doubles. For Ivy and Jack, cancer was one reminder of their own aging processes. Although the vast amount of information told them that Ivy's type of thyroid cancer was completely curable, Ivy still believed there was a possibility that she could die. In confronting her own mortality, she felt it necessary to write out her last words to her husband and son. In doing so, she was able to grasp on to the control she so much wanted, and move forward with her surgery. For Brandon, the diagnosis came during a time when he was beginning his adult life. Seeing a rather young parent deal with a potentially fatal disease made him confront his own aging process (becoming an adult) as well as that of his parents. On learning of the diagnosis, and researching the illness, he knew that the chances of his mother dying were nearly zero. But, that did not prevent him from addressing this feeling when he learned more about the necessary treatment to cure her. Through these narratives, we are able to realize the profound changes that occurred in each family member's approach toward aging and death.

LEARNING THROUGH NARRATIVES: THEORETICAL IMPLICATIONS OF THIS RESEARCH

We can begin to theorize about communicating health in our lives and the lives of others through considering the personal complexities revealed in stories. Frank (1995) suggested that theory meets story when we think with a story rather than about it:

> To think about a story is to reduce it to content and then analyze the content. . . . To think with a story is to experience its affecting one's own life and to find in that effect a certain truth of one's own life. (p. 23)

Arthur Bochner (1997) echoed Frank's recommendation:

> We do not turn stories into data to test theoretical propositions. Rather, we link theory to story when we think with a story, trying to stay with the story, letting ourselves resonate with the moral dilemmas it may pose, understanding its ambiguities, examining its contradictions, feeling its nuances, letting ourselves become part of the story (Ellis, 1995). We think with a story from the framework of our own lives. We ask what kind of person we are becoming when we take the story in and consider how we can use it for our own purposes, what ethical directions it points us toward, and what moral commitments it calls out in us. (Coles, 1989, p. 436)

Focusing on narratives in the contexts of health, aging, illness, and providing care opens up opportunities for understanding and participating in our own health care with greater vigor and freedom. Each of us should consider how useful it is to compare our interpretations with others and to consider the personal, cultural, and political complexities of health care decisions. This is especially vital in health communication encounters that are tied to fateful moments (Giddens, 1991). Fateful health care moments, such as pregnancy, miscarriage, surgery, and diagnosis of a life-threatening disease are filled with uncertainty and may also have spiritual implications for the patient (Gonzalez, 1994). When such moments are treated as opportunities to interweave the voices of care providers, individuals, and their families, the potential exists for people to feel as if they have some sort of influence and impact on their courses of treatment, and are able to take control of their decision-making processes (O'Hair et al., 2003).

This research adds to the current dialogue in communication, aging, and cancer survivorship in several ways. The data and findings presented in this research parallel Kleinman's (1988) and Frank's (1991, 1995) argument that we can best learn about illness through narratives. Not only are narratives told and heard among families while coping with the illness, but also narratives are a primary means of learning about illness in the research process. This study yielded multivoiced texts, and included the voice of not just the survivor, but her family members as well. In order to see the communication that takes place during the illness, we must juxtaposition the voices of the family members. By eliciting and re-presenting narratives that are focused on families as a unit, we are able to learn how illness is a communicative phenomenon.

The narratives presented in this research also show that communicating in identity composition and recomposition is not unique to the ill individual, and it is through their interaction with family that they are able to develop survivor identities. Combining the stories of the individuals in this study showed that illness narratives are not just about the patient, and families recover along with the patient. Additionally, the discoveries made in the stories confirm the notion that renewal of the self comes through the shared experience of illness (Frank, 1991).

This research makes a theoretical argument that the identity and emotion literature would benefit from bridging the two disciplines. In other words, by addressing the emotional discoveries made in this study, the literature on identity roles would provide a better understanding of how those roles are composed as well as how communication of emotions is integral to the compositions. Communication literature can apply the conclusions from this study to expand the theoretical acumen concerning how individuals cope with the experience and expression of emotions present in life-threatening illness.

Some authors propose that identity can be categorized as victim identities (Lichter, 1987; Parsons, 1978; Verwoerdt, 1966), warrior identities (Doka, 1993; LeShan, 1977; Lorde, 1980), and survivor identities (Gotcher & Edwards, 1990; Rossman, 1989). This study contradicts the delineation of the three fixed identity roles, and broadens the approach that we should take in understanding these roles. We learn from this research that identity composition and recomposition is a continuous process that does not begin one day and end the next. The development of the survivor identity does not mark the end of the illness journey because a person can be a survivor one day, a victim the next, and a warrior in between. The communication that occurs on a daily basis affects how ill individuals perceive themselves, and through that communication they may assume any identity on any day.

Literature about survivorship suggests that illness provides the opportunity to change a life and illuminate new "truths" that illness brings into their lives (Ellis, 1996; Rossman, 1989). New truths that arise in survivorship may include the perception of a life-threatening illness as a "wake-up call" for the mind to attend to the needs of the body. A diagnosis of cancer can change the life of not only the person diagnosed, but for the family as well (Nussbaum, Baringer, & Kundrat, 2003). Those new truths may also include reappraisals of what is important in life.

Ivy's illness did spark a re-evaluation of her family's life and goals. Appraisal theories in communication suggest that reactions to situations and experiences result from a person's cognitive interpretation of those situations or experiences (see e.g., Smith, 1989). In other words, different environmental circumstances yield different interpretations of events even if the event is similar (Burleson & Goldsmith, 1998). For example, a man who has had prostate cancer cannot fully relate to and identify with the emotional experience of a woman who had breast cancer, or vice versa. Although both individuals experienced cancer, the varying environments, goals, and resources create different appraisals of the two situations that neither party can fully understand. Burleson and Goldsmith explained that "the only way a distressed emotional state can be altered is through an individual changing the appraisals that underlie and constitute the emotional distress" (p. 258). As such, the emotional turmoil experienced by cancer patients is only alleviated by the patient understanding the source of his or her distress, and making reappraisals of his or her environment, goals, and resources.

Appraisal theories are commonly found in emotion literature dealing with social support. During her illness, Ivy made cognitive assessments about her situation trying to determine where the illness would fit into the rest of her life. She knew that she was the only person who could completely understand her fears, uncertainty, and emotional distress. Supportive individuals (family, physicians, and support group members) were able to ask questions and console her, and those interactions were therapeutic. Comforting and supporting ill individuals simply means helping those individuals work through and generate emotional relief (Burleson & Goldsmith, 1998). In other words, the people dealing with the illness needed to make their own assessments and find their own paths to survivorship and recovery. From their own appraisals and reappraisals, illness survivors can adopt new truths about their relationships, communication, and family dynamics. "Well" individuals, however, cannot and should not provide the answers for ill individuals, as those answers may intensify resistance. This research reminds us that the only person who can come to terms with the illness is the person experiencing the illness him or herself, but through narratives, we are permitted to learn about those experiences so that we may better deal with them in future situations.

We constantly learn from stories of health and illness—the stories others tell, the stories we tell, and the stories we construct in conversation. Critical to learning from stories of health and illness is encouraging people to speak and tell their stories of being silenced, discredited, excluded, and stigmatized as well as to tell their stories of being heard, encouraged, and included. A sincere desire on all our parts to learn about, theorize from, and understand the personal complexities of our own and another's experience is vital to communicating health.

REFERENCES

Benjamin, H. H. (1987). *From victim to victor: The Wellness Community guide to fighting for recovery for cancer patients and their families*. New York: St. Martin's.

Bochner, A. (1997). It's about time: Narrative and the divided self. *Qualitative Inquiry, 3*, 418-438.

Brody, H. (1987). *Stories of sickness*. New Haven, CT: Yale University Press.

Bruner, J. (1987). Life as narrative. *Social Research, 54*, 11-32.

Burleson, B. R., & Goldsmith, D. J. (1998). How the comforting process works: Alleviating emotional distress through conversationally induced reappraisals. In P. A. Andersen & L. K. Guerrero (Eds.), *Handbook of communication and emotion: Research, theory, applications, and contexts* (pp. 245-280). San Diego: Academic Press.

Charmaz, K. (1983). Loss of self: A fundamental form of suffering in the chronically ill. *Sociology of Health and Illness, 5*, 168-195.

Charmaz, K. (1987). Struggling for a self: Identity levels of the chronically ill. In J. Roth & P. Conrad (Eds.), *Research in the sociology of health care: A research manual* (Vol. 6, pp. 249-281). Greenwich, CT: JAI Press.

Charmaz, K. (1991). *Good days, bad days: The self in chronic illness and time*. New Brunswick, NJ: Rutgers University Press.

Charmaz, K. (1994). Identity dilemmas of chronically ill men. *Sociological Quarterly, 35*, 269-288.

Charmaz, K. (1995). The body, identity, and self: Adapting to impairment. *Sociological Quarterly, 36*, 657-680.

Coles, R. (1989). *The call of stories: Teaching and the moral imagination*. Boston: Houghton-Mifflin.

Czarniawska, B. (1997). A four times told tale: Combining narrative and scientific knowledge in organization studies. *Organization, 4*, 7-30.

Denzin, N. K. (1997). *Interpretive ethnography: Ethnographic practices for the 21st century*. Thousand Oaks, CA: Sage.

Doka, K. J. (1993). *Living with life-threatening illness: A guide for patients, their families, and caregivers*. New York: Lexington.

Ellis, C. (1995). *Final negotiations: A story of love, loss, and chronic illness*. Philadelphia: Temple University Press.

Ellis, C. (1996). On the demands of truthfulness in writing personal loss narratives. *Journal of Personal and Interpersonal Loss, 1*, 157-177.

Ellis, C., & Bochner, A. (2000). Autoethnography, personal narrative, and reflexivity: Researcher as subject. In N. K. Denzin & Y. S. Lincoln (Eds.), *Handbook of qualitative research* (2nd ed., pp. 733-768). Thousand Oaks, CA: Sage.

Emerson, R. M., Fretz, R. I., & Shaw, L. L. (1995). *Writing ethnographic fieldnotes*. Chicago: University of Chicago Press.

Fisher, W. (1987). *Human communication as narration: Toward a philosophy of reason, value, and action*. Columbia: University of South Carolina Press.

Frank, A. W. (1991). *At the will of the body: Reflections on illness*. Boston: Houghton Mifflin.

Frank, A. W. (1993). The rhetoric of self change: Illness experience as narrative. *The Sociological Quarterly, 34*, 39-52.

Frank, A. W. (1995). *The wounded storyteller: Body, illness, and ethics*. Chicago: University of Chicago Press.

Geist, P., & Dreyer, J. (1993). Juxtapositioning accounts: Different versions of different stories in the health care context. In S. L. Herndon & G. L. Kreps (Eds.), *Qualitative research: Applications in organizational communication* (pp. 79-106). Cresskill, NJ: Hampton Press.

Geist-Martin, P., Ray, E. B., & Sharf, B. F. (2003). *Communicating health: Personal, cultural, and political complexities*. Belmont, CA: Wadsworth.

Gerhardt, U. (1989). *Ideas about illness: An intellectual and political history of medical sociology*. New York: New York University Press.

Giddens, A. (1991). *Modernity and self identity: Self and society in the late modern age*. Stanford: Stanford University Press.

Goffman, E. (1963). *Stigma: Notes on the management of spoiled identity*. Englewood Cliffs, NJ: Prentice Hall.

Gonzalez, M. C. (1994). An invitation to leap from a trinitarian ontology in health communication research to a spiritually inclusive quatrain. In S. A. Deetz (Ed.), *Communication yearbook* (Vol. 17, pp. 378-387). Thousand Oaks, CA: Sage.

Gotcher, J. M., & Edwards, R. (1990). Coping strategies of cancer patients: Actual communication and imagined interactions. *Health Communication, 2*, 255-266.

Hammersley, M., & Atkinson, P. (1995). *Ethnography: Principles in practice* (2nd ed.). New York: Routledge.

Hanne, M. (1994). *The power of the story: Fiction and political change*. Providence, RI: Berghahn Books.

Jackson, M. (1989). *Paths toward a clearing: Radical empiricism and ethnographic inquiry*. Bloomington: Indiana University Press.

Kleinman, A. (1988). *The illness narratives: Suffering, healing, and the human condition*. New York: Basic Books.

Leder, D. (1990). *The absent body*. Chicago: University of Chicago Press.

LeShan, L. (1977). *You can fight for your life: Emotional factors in the causation of cancer*. New York: M. Evans.

Lichter, I. (1987). *Communication in cancer care*. New York: Churchill Livingstone.

Lindlof, T. R. (1995). *Qualitative communication research methods*. Thousand Oaks, CA: Sage.

Lorde, A. (1980). *The cancer journals*. San Francisco: Sheba.

Mathieson, C. M., & Barrie, C. M. (1998). Probing the prime narrative: Illness, interviewing, and identity. *Qualitative Health Research, 8*, 581-601.

Mathieson, C. M., & Stam, H. J. (1995). Renegotiating identity: Cancer narratives. *Sociology of Health and Illness, 17*, 283-306.

Merleau-Ponty, M. (1962). *Phenomenology of perception* (C. Smith, Trans.). London: Routledge.

Metzger, D. (1992). *Tree and the woman who slept with men.* Berkeley, CA: Wingbow Press.

Nijhof, G. (1997). "Response work": Approaching answers to open interviews as readings. *Qualitative Inquiry, 3*, 169-187.

Nussbaum, J. F., Baringer, D., & Kundrat, A. (2003). Health, communication and aging: Cancer and older adults. *Health Communication, 15*, 185-192.

O'Hair, D., Villagran, M. M., Wittenberg, E., Brown, K., Ferguson, M., Hall, H. T., & Doty, T. (2003). Cancer survivorship and agency model: Implications for patient choice, decision making, and influence. *Health Communication, 15*, 193-202.

Ott, J. K. (1999). *Emotional experiences embraced: Communicating identity and illness survivorship.* Unpublished master's thesis, San Diego State University, San Diego, CA.

Parsons, T. (1978). *Action theory and the human condition.* New York: The Free Press.

Payer, L. (1989). *Medicine and culture.* New York: Penguin Books.

Pennebaker, J. W. (1992). Putting stress into words: Health, linguistic, and therapeutic implications. *Behavioral Research Therapy, 31*, 539-548.

Pennebaker, J. W., & Beall, S. K. (1986). Confronting a traumatic event: Toward and understanding of inhibition and disease. *Journal of Abnormal Psychology, 95*, 274-281.

Pennebaker, J. W., Kiecolt-Glaser, J. K., & Glaser, R. (1988). Disclosure of traumas and immune function: Health implications for psychotherapy. *Journal of Counseling and Clinical Psychology, 56*, 239-245.

Richardson, L. (1997). *Fields of play: Constructing an academic life.* New Brunswick, NJ: Rutgers University Press.

Ronan, R. (1982). *Narratives from America.* Port Townsend, WA: Dragon Gate.

Rossman, M. (1989). Illness as an opportunity for healing. In R. Carlson & B. Shield (Eds.), *Healers on healing* (pp. 78-81). Los Angeles: Jeremy P. Tarcher.

Smith, C. A. (1989). Dimensions of appraisal and physiological response in emotion. *Journal of Personality and Social Psychology, 56*, 339-353.

Sontag, S. (1989). *Illness as metaphor and AIDS and its metaphors.* New York: Doubleday.

Sparkes, A. C. (1996). The fatal flaw: A narrative of the fragile body-self. *Qualitative Inquiry, 2*, 463-494.

Sparkes, A. C. (1997). Reflections on the socially constructed physical self. In K. Fox (Ed.), *The physical self: From motivation to well-being* (pp. 83-110). Champaign, IL: Human Kinetics.

Sparkes, A. C. (1998). Athletic identity: An Achilles' heel to the survival of self. *Qualitative Health Research, 8*, 644-664.

Verwoerdt, A. (1966). *Communication with the fatally ill.* Springfield, IL: Charles C. Thomas.

White, H. (1981). The value of narrativity in the representation of reality. In W. J. T. Mitchell (Ed.), *On narrative* (pp. 1-23). Chicago: University of Chicago Press.

8

When Black Women Talk About Breast Cancer

How Health Care Workers Need To Learn To Listen

Margaret Chamberlain Wilmoth

Boyd Davis

L. Delores Sanders

University of North Carolina at Charlotte

> When women speak, how they mean and therefore how they say something is what they are talking about.
>
> —Morgan (2002, p. 110)

Key issues for health care educators and health care workers (HCWs) to consider when working with African American women diagnosed with breast cancer are the ways black women communicate about the diagnostic process and the subsequent impact of breast cancer on their lives. Increasing breast cancer incidence and survival rates make this a critical issue for the HCW. This chapter will link two areas of key communications study, that of intercultural or interethnic communication and patient-to-HCW communication, by identifying African American women's ways of speaking in focus groups about their breast cancer experience. Such an analysis will provide insights to HCWs who have been educated in the mainstream medical model.

LITERATURE REVIEW

The American Cancer Society (ACS) has estimated for 2007 that there will be 178,480 new breast cancer diagnoses in women; 159,470 in European American women and 19,010 in African American women (2007a). Numerous studies have shown that mortality from breast cancer is greater among African Americans than among Caucasians (American Cancer Society, 2007b; Gotay & Wilson, 1998). The anticipated mortality from breast cancer in European American women is 34,630 and 5,830 in African American women (ACS, 2007a, 2007b). Between 1990 and 1994, breast cancer mortality decreased approximately 6% among Caucasian women but only 1% among African American women (Phillips, Cohen, & Moses, 1999). In 2007, African American women continue this trend (ACS, 2007b).

Common beliefs about why African Americans have their cancer diagnosed at a later stage than other Americans include a lack of awareness of advances in health promotion strategies; financial concerns, including a lack of medical insurance; receipt of less than adequate health care and distrust of the healthcare system (Pierce, 1997). Other data also suggests that differences in stage at diagnosis between Caucasian American and African American women are linked to noneconomic access barriers (Bibb, 2000). These findings were based on data obtained from women in an equal-access system and indicated that barriers to access occurred at the individual level, not system level (Bibb, 2001). Bibb suggests that perception of appropriate care includes tending to cultural values, beliefs and practices, including the provision of culturally sensitive care and enhancement of intercultural communication.

The reasons for disparity in outcomes in breast cancer survival between Caucasian American and African American women are multi-faceted; McTavish et al. (2003) note the "conflicting findings" about differences in reaction to diagnosis as well as in coping skills (cf. Bourjolly 1998, 1999), adding that "African American women may bring different expectations and resources to the breast cancer experience" (McTavish et al., 2003, p. 104). However, one key component in reducing the higher mortality rates in African American women continues to be the availability of culturally appropriate and effective early detection in conjunction with health care workers who are conversant in the culture with which they are working.

Recent studies suggest that culturally appropriate health care within the African American community is keyed to that community's strong base in spirituality, is combined with social support that accepts and extends that spirituality, and establishes opportunity for people to story about their experience, recounting it in the ways they prefer (Lackey, Gates, & Brown, 2001; Newlin, Knafl, & Melkus, 2002; Taylor, 2001). Culturally appropriate care includes the ability to listen to communication patterns and nuances in order to identify cues that suggest the need for practitioner intervention. For example, McTavish et al. (2003) reviewed differences in how African American and Caucasian women use online information and discussion groups, commenting that "for women of color, the overwhelming topic of conversation is treatment, while it is a distant second for Caucasian women" (McTavish et al., 2003, p. 110). In this discussion, we will focus on the narrative styles used in face-to-face focus groups by African American women with breast cancer, looking particularly at how their narratives signal linkages between spirituality and self-efficacy in their discussions of living with the disease, and then provide suggestions for what practitioners need to listen for when caring for these women.

SPIRITUALITY

Spirituality has been defined as "a belief in non-causation . . . merely the force that resides in all beings, things, places/times and modalities" (Jones, 1991). There is growing support for accepting the influence that both religion and spirituality have on the experience of disease, health and well-being (Daaleman & Nease, 1994). Spirituality has been identified as a key variable that influences an individual's response to a cancer diagnosis and sense of identity as expressed in religious ritual practice (Haynes & Smedley, 1999; Lackey, Gates, & Brown, 2001). This is also true for women diagnosed with diseases other than cancer. Samuel-Hodge et al (2000) found that among women with diabetes, spirituality and religiosity were the most significant factors in gaining emotional support and coping with the disease. Several studies of illness and wellness in different segments of the larger African American community claim that many believe their degree of health or presence of illness to be God's will (Abrums 2000; Gregg & Curry, 1994). While this may be viewed as fatalism and contradicts HCW notions of self-efficacy, for many African American women their faith is a source of strength during adversity and what leads them to consider self-efficacy. The elements of spirituality, in the sense of reliance both on the church as an institution of support and on personal faith, are fundamental elements that African American women report as assisting them in coping with disease in the white-dominated healthcare system (Abrums, 2000; Henderson, Gore, Davis, & Condon, 2003).

Spirituality has also been found to be an effective component in cancer prevention and detection programs that reach into the African American community. Culturally relevant screening programs draw on the leadership of women recognized as spiritual leaders, natural healers, or survivors of breast and/or cervical cancer to encourage cancer screening in the African American community (Altpeter, Earp, Bishop, & Eng, 1999; Erwin, Spatz, & Turturro, 1992). These programs are also based on the construct of self-efficacy in that survivors are urged to tell their story so other women will have the confidence that they, too, can overcome and survive a diagnosis of breast cancer.

Self-Efficacy

A strong belief in God provides many African American women with strength and a positive outlook on life that allows them to get through difficult times (Lackey, Gates, & Brown, 2001). The confidence they obtain from their belief system is congruent with Self-Efficacy Theory as described by Bandura (1977, 1986). In 1986, Bandura outlined features of social cognitive theory which grounded his understanding of health behaviors. Bandura (1997) suggests that the principle of *reciprocal determinism* is the most important assumption of social cognitive theory, and that the interaction between interpersonal personal factors, behavior and the external environment can aid in the understanding of human behavior. Self-efficacy is a key cognitive personal factor that shapes behavior.

The importance of self-efficacy as a cognitive factor affecting health has been well documented in the literature (Bandura, 1977; Hickey, Owen, & Froman, 1992; O'Leary, 1985; Strecher, DeVellis, Becker, & Rosenstock, 1986; Newman, 1991, 1993, 1997), however its relationship to the storytelling used by African American women has not been fully explored. Self-efficacy includes the belief that one can carry out a behavior necessary to reach a desired goal or achieve an expected outcome (Bandura, 1997). As one example of the acceptance of the interrelationship between self-efficacy, social cognition, and health, the National Institute of Health program on Social Cognition and Aging includes this statement in its description of funding:

> Research suggests that complex cognitive functioning—involved in coping, everyday problem-solving and decision-making in health and social domains—depends not only on basic cognitive mechanisms, but also on socially-derived content and organization of existing knowledge structures as well as on socially-derived emotional and motivational influ-

> ences on performance. (Program PA-97-065: grants1.nih.gov/grants/guide/pa-files/PA-97-065.html, last accessed 8 July 2003)

In a review of health-related research generated by self-efficacy theory, O'Leary (1985) reported that research in such diverse areas as depression, motivation, career choice, weight control, smoking cessation, and childbirth "provide converging evidence of people's perception of efficacy significantly affect their level of motivation and psychosocial functioning" (p. 438). Clark and Dodge (1999) explored self-efficacy as a predictor of disease management behaviors in older women with heart disease. They noted that self-efficacy is relatively easy to measure and measuring a patient's baseline self-efficacy beliefs could provide an initial starting point for interventions focused on exercise, stress management, diet, and medication use.

Self-efficacy, or one's judgment about his or her ability to bring about "wished-for-results" (Clark & Dodge, 1999, p. 74), provides another link between health-promotion behaviors and spirituality. Concepts of spirituality and religious affiliation are fundamental to African-American women's worldview of health and disease process. These concepts provide a framework for coping with disease and the dominant health care system. They are interrelated with community and family support. One's ability to maintain strong and viable spiritual and religious ties within their chosen groups reflects self-efficacy. Research that examines the role of self-efficacy among ethnic groups should have the potential both to promote utilization of health care services and health-promotion behaviors within that group, and to move health care professionals toward a more inclusive and less dichotomized viewpoint about the group and its preferred ways of talking and storying about wellness and illness.

Story and Spirituality

Researchers note that African-American women typically do not talk about their breast cancer to HCWs, thus limiting their potential for obtaining support from HCWs while they cope with the disease and its treatment. This reticence also extends to talking about breast cancer among each other and was emphasized by all of the women in a set of three focus groups with low- and middle-income African-American women in an urban area (J. Phillips, 1999; J. Phillips, Cohen, & Moses, 1999).

Because African-American women draw on dialogue with others to discover new information and learn new ways of acting, storytelling is one effective way to share survival stories after a breast cancer diagnosis. Storytelling is one of the ways African-American women link interpersonal communication with their spirituality. Belief in God and use of prayer emerged as crucial components in one set of focus group discussions about storytelling and its use by African-American women. Researchers leading those discussions used a storytelling technique keyed to spirituality to teach breast health information to older African-American women (Williams-Brown, Baldwin, & Bakos, 2002).

Storytelling has been reported to provide four types of therapeutic benefits: cognitive, affective, interpersonal, and personal growth (Heiney, 1995). The cognitive benefits of storytelling can lead to improved learning and problem solving, whereas affective benefits include catharsis and hope. Interpersonal benefits are translated into social support and building of trust. Storytelling can provide insight and a sense of mastery over emotional distress that may be translated into improved self-confidence (Heiney, 1995). This is one effect of the healing that comes from participation in Alcoholics Anonymous. Storytelling, particularly when the stories are positive, can also provide models for one's own coping with a similar situation (S. Taylor, Aspinwall, Giuliano, Dakof, & Reardon, 1993).

Results from a series of focus group sessions and one-on-one interviews with older ($N = 31$) African-American women living with breast cancer suggest that they need social support from other women with the disease, but that their opportunities to find this support are limited (Sanders, Wilmoth, & Lowery, 2004; Wilmoth & Sanders, 2001). Participants commented that family members, spouses, and significant others were reticent in discussing their cancer because of the part of the anatomy involved. When support from family members and friends appeared lacking, those in focus groups indicated that participation in the group was important for coping with the disease. The focus group transcripts evidence the importance of spirituality and of the collaborative, participatory story these women offered to themselves and to each other as support.

Language and Style

Several important studies of African-American English (AAE) that analyzed women's style, both in the sense of what is talked about and of how women speak, have appeared since 2000. AAE is not a set of slang words and specific pronunciations spoken by urban teenage males. Morgan (2002) defined AAE as "the language, discourse and interactional styles and usage of those socialized in the speech community" (p. 65).

Although Morgan reviewed specific conversational strategies such as indirectness, or ways to joke, tease, or signify, that review is in the context of larger issues, such as the preservation of social "face," which she sees as the core of African-American language ideology that can perhaps best be seen in the contrast between being "cool" and being a "fool" (p. 43). This dichotomy is echoed in the discussion by Abrums (2000), who noted the emphasis by women in her study on wisdom, knowledge (as distinguished from education), and knowing and speaking that wisdom as rooted in spirituality. This distinction resonates with Houston's (2002a, 2002b) findings from a study of 134 African-American women's views about African-American women's talk. Their comments identify three dimensions characterizing this talk: wisdom, with themselves as authorities; fortitude, seen as being tough, strong, and assertive; and caring, seen as being warm, sensitive, context-sensitive, and confrontational—which is not necessarily negative, but is instead forthright. These dimensions contribute to understanding language style. Green's (2002) survey of AAE includes a discussion of women's styles in their narrative and conversational strategies, frequently citing African-American female scholars who are authorities on African-American women's speech such as folklorist, Zora Neale Hurston; rhetorician, Geneva Smitherman-Donaldson; anthropologist, Marcyliena Morgan, and sociolinguist, Sonja Lanehart.

Thus, it is important that HCWs have an understanding of the grounding of African-American women's talk in terms of their spirituality, how they talk about their breast cancer and begin to learn the social practice of their talk among themselves (Pope, 2003), and the cues that surround such talk. Learning these cues as well as the corresponding appropriate response can lead to better understanding and, hopefully, to improved health care outcomes.

METHOD

Sample

The sample narratives were derived from African-American women with breast cancer who were willing to talk at length about their experiences related to sexuality, intimacy, and living with breast cancer. One set of narratives analyzed for this chapter is from the second of two focus group interviews with African-American women with breast cancer, about the impact of the cancer on sexuality. A second set of eight narratives analyzed for this report was drawn from a study that conducted one-on-one interviews with breast cancer survivors to learn about the personal issues of African-American women with breast cancer. A convenience sample of women who participated in these two studies were recruited from churches, sororities, and service groups (Sanders, Wilmoth, & Lowery, 2004; Wilmoth & Sanders, 2001) and were willing to have their conversations audiotaped. All procedures for protection of human rights and privacy were followed in accordance with university protocol.

Sixteen women participated in two focus group discussions on the topic of personal issues and how they dealt with them after diagnosis (Wilmoth &

Sanders, 2001). These women were between the ages of 30 and 75, were middle to upper middle class, and all had private health insurance. They were 6-month to 5-7 year survivors of breast cancer. The focus group interviews were conducted by two researchers, one African American, the other Euro-American. Sixteen women who participated in the one-on-one interviews ranged in age from 37 to 80 (mean age: 59; Table 8.1). Nine were more than 5 years post-diagnosis, three were 3 to 5 years post-diagnosis, three were within 1 to 2 years of diagnosis, and one was within 1 year of diagnosis. Ten women had received mastectomy as their primary therapy and five lumpectomy. All had received some form of adjuvant therapy (Sanders, Wilmoth, & Lowery, 2004). All individual interviews were conducted by African-American researchers.

TABLE 8.1
Demographic Data: One-on-One Interviews

SUBJECT	AGE/ MARITAL STATUS	EDUCATIONAL LEVEL	TIME SINCE DIAGNOSIS	TREATMENT
1	49/Divorced	College graduate	5 years	Lumpectomy/ radiation therapy
2	55/Married	Technical school	15 years	Lumpectomy—then mastectomy both breasts with reconstruction/RT
3	47/Divorced	Technical school	5 years	Mastectomy with reconstruction/Tamoxifen
4	41/Married	Some college	8 years	Mastectomy/Tamoxifen
5	70/Widow	High school graduate	13 years	Mastectomy
6	64/Married	High school graduate	3 years	Lumpectomy/RT/ Tamoxifen
7	62/Single	High school graduate	19 years	Mastectomy
8	79/Widow	High school graduate	4 years	Lumpectomy/Tamoxifen

NOTE: RT, radiation therapy.

Data Analysis

The selected narratives were analyzed to identify patterns within the narratives using ethnographic and interactional approaches to discourse analysis as typified in studies of power, gender, and community by Ainsworth-Vaughn (1998), Foster (1995, 2001), and Tannen (1989; see also Johnstone, 2002, for an overview of specific techniques such as dividing narrative into stanza-like chunks or sections). Interactional sociolinguistics is focused on situated meaning, such as how participants in the communicative situation of a focus group collaboratively create that meaning; ethnographic analyses explore "the structures and functions of communicating that organize the use of language in speech situations, events, and acts" (Schiffrin, 1994, p. 185).

FINDINGS AND DISCUSSION

HCWs will profit from looking closely at the use of specific stylistic features of African-American oral narrative, and, in particular, women's discourse, to better learn to hear what the women are saying in the full focus group discussions and one-to-one interviews. How the women say is part of what they say; understanding their style is crucial. This was true of the narratives analyzed in this report.

Style is, as Rickford and McNair-Knox (1994) noted, a "resource and strategy . . . an interactive and dynamic process" that speakers can manipulate as they respond to changes in a situation or as they initiate such changes (p. 264). In her study of style in African-American sermon techniques, Wharry (2003) summarized a number of the discourse features shared by oral cultures. These features are collaborative in nature. Performance by the audience as well as by the primary speaker is expected, so that the audience and the performer are in dialogue with each other. Wharry added that distinct textual features such as rhyme, formulaic expression, exaggeration, or repetition characterize different kinds of language situations, or different stages or components of an interaction. The women participating in the breast cancer focus groups and interviews used many of these textual features, and a variety of strategies of involvement, including the following:

- "Side chats," which Gollop (1997) said are used by African-American women to individualize themselves in research interview settings. These surface in one-on-one follow-up interviews in our data, rather than in the full focus group, indicating that the focus groups were on task, and members adhered to their mission of responding to questions.

- Narrativizing, which is different from reportorial narrating. Smitherman (1997) noted that narrativizing "is a characteristic feature of general Black discursive strategies. Everyday conversational talk may be rendered as a 'story.' Narrativizing is a Black rhetorical strategy . . . to create word-pictures about general, abstract observations about life, love, and survival" (p. 12).
- Co-constructed meanings, where several people contribute to what listeners or a group can accept as being "cool" (as opposed to being an uninformed "fool": on the dichotomy, see Morgan, 2002, p. 39).
- Sermonizing adaptations from testifying and preaching, such as a display narrative in a round or sequence of narratives offered at times in unofficial competition (Foster, 2001), incorporating some degree of indirectness and signifying (Morgan, 1996) along with the use of sermonizing techniques. As Dance (2002) commented, "The Black sermon and the rhetorical practices growing out of it are characterized by the use of improvisation, popular formulaic lines, and familiar expressions . . . [with] insistence upon audience response [. . . and] the use of repetition and parallel structure . . ." (p. 250).

It would be highly surprising if the ways storytellers handle topic, story, and style were *not* culture-specific. Drawing on post-structuralist philosophers such as Foucault and Derrida, and on current feminist theories, nursing researchers D. Philips and Drevdahl (2003) explained that we are unconsciously shaped by cultural discourses: "language in the shape of written, verbal, and performed frameworks of knowledge" (pp. 23-24). They said whatever stands out, whatever seems unusual, is seen as different and often as inferior. Working only with identifying cultural and linguistic differences runs the danger of privileging one side or the other; as Houston (2002a) commented, communications researchers have without realizing it, centered the White by constantly comparing Black and White communications practices. Y. Taylor (1999) said that colonizing and stereotypic images of African-American women, such as the mammy (Aunt Jemima), the welfare mother, or the Jezebel temptress-figure are part of the cultural practices of labeling and denigrating. Such labels, said Taylor, contribute to how African-American women are viewed and treated (Y. Taylor, 1999; cf. Bogle, 1973). In the next section, we emphasize looking at the interviews and focus group conversations from the viewpoint of how speakers tell and retell stories using conversational and narrative strategies valued in and associated with African-American oral discourse.

Conversational and Narrative Strategies

Stories are often embedded in conversation, as was found in the narratives that were analyzed. In Ainsworth-Vaughn's (1998) study of power in doctor–patient talk, the cultural role of storytelling and story-sharing is emphasized:

> stories can invoke shared cultural background and thus establish a link between storyteller and audience. Stories are supposed to be told in such a way that listeners can understand the teller's evaluation of the events. Was the teller angered, saddened, made joyous? Other narrative forms, such as reports, do not have this esthetic dimension. . . . Evaluation is a way of representing ourselves; in evaluation, as its name implies, we most clearly express our values. (p. 128)

Evaluation, said O'Connor (2000), tells the listener the point of a story, and is often used to "cue the importance of moments" (p. 119). Speakers use a range of devices to signal where and how the listener can hear what is being emphasized, and the extent to which the listener is expected to become involved in the storytelling. Cultures will vary in the degree to which they invite involvement. To know—although not necessarily consciously—when and how to become involved in a story is to be competent in the discourse of the culture in which the story is embedded, either through the story, the storyteller, or the situation of telling (Tannen, 1989)

A story is a cultural discourse in the sense that D. Phillips and Drevdahl (2003) defined it previously: a performed, verbal framework of knowledge. What is particularly interesting about the stories we examined is that (a) they surfaced not in ordinary conversation, but in the constraints of a focus group and one-on-one health interviews, and (b) participants drew on their preferred and culturally sanctioned modes of public discourse to increase involvement of interviewer and interviewee alike in the stories being shared and co-constructed.

Involvement allows the hearer to participate in making meaning, said Tannen (1989). Involvement strategies can be keyed to the "sound and the music" of language, drawing in the listener through repetition and variation of individual sounds, words, or phrases, or keyed to different aspects of meaning, by varying amounts of dialogue, imagery and detail, or narrative structures.

Narrativizing: Madeline's Repetition and Reported Dialogue. All of the women in the focus groups and in the one-on-one interviews responded to the researchers' questions by narrativizing their experience into story, which they interweave with non-narrative accounts. In her story for the group, "Madeline Walker" uses two particular techniques: the repetition of key verbs and the presentation of reported dialogue. Both of these techniques enable her to highlight the drama of her diagnosis. We have used formatting cues to highlight different sections and rearranged the lines into idea groups (Chafe, 1980).

Madeline begins by differentiating her story of diagnosis from that of other women, by positioning herself in her professional identity: the nursing profession. Her self-representation is as a member of the medical community, with access to knowledge beyond that of the general public. Her repetition of the verb "check" is suggestive because this is a word that has semi-official status, as a popular and generally accepted term for self-diagnostic technique, breast self-examination. (Since the early 1990s, "check" has been the verb for the desired action suggested by national cancer, birth control, and similar organizations; see the spread across the country of Buddy Check programs sponsored by local media stations, such as WUSA, targeting particularly African-American women in Washington, DC.) Madeline's emphasis is on her own leadership and personal agency, first, in the finding of the lump; next, her insistence on a medical professional's immediate review; and then, on her ability to control the doctor's time.

Well, my experience was something different.
I'm in the nursing profession
and when I first found a lump,
I was **checking** myself like I tell all my patients
—how to check for breast cancer.
So I was **checking** the lump,
checking my breasts,
and I felt a lump.
I was home that day and I was off,
and I called my doctor and said, "Hey."
Cause he usually gets off on Wednesday afternoon.
I said, "I think I've got something here and I need it **checked** right now."
I said, "Don't leave the office, I'm on my way."
He didn't and he could feel it and we went from there.

She reiterates her control over the situation, which is to be taken as metonymic for her control of her own body and success with overcoming the cancer, with her use of reported dialogue to move listeners into the drama of her story. She calls her doctor with "Hey," and outlines the diagnostic sequence by reporting specific speech interactions: He spoke "very nonchalant"; everybody—presumably medical staff—"was afraid" to tell her the diagnosis behind the scenes; instead, she followed the protocol for patients, by requesting an appointment to be told.

> *He ordered* a mammogram.
> It did not show on the mammogram.
> *So he said*, "Well since you are 40, I think we need to do a biopsy."
> *Very nonchalant he said*, "Go have a biopsy."
> And when the report came back, it was just—
> *Everybody was afraid to come to me and say* "What is happening."
> *I had to make an appointment* to see him, go in the office,
> *and he told me.*

In the communal and collaborative focus group, Madeline reports dialogue that shows her control over the situation and summarizes events she could not control, adding a final editorial comment that echoes her initial statement of how her experience was different:

> So I took it fairly well, you know,
> but my husband and my family did not.
> I had surgery on Friday,
> and my husband had a heart attack on Monday. . . .
> We were upstairs in the bed,
> and someone else was running my house.
> *It's sort of been different.*

Retelling a story and Changing the Audience: Madeline's One-on-One Interview. Madeline's retelling of the story in a follow-up interview uses repetition and narrativization again, but for a different purpose. She has a single immediate hearer, even though she knows the interview is being recorded, and she is answering a specific question:

> INT: Were there any changes in terms of self, the way that your husband saw you, the way that you dressed, the way he touched or kissed, or any of this after the mastectomy?

"No," she says, "We have always talked"—but there is one time they were unable to talk, and that was right after the lumpectomy. In this retelling, Madeline uses *But* and *So* to signal the near-simultaneous hospitalization in two different towns:

> *Now* when I first had my lumpectomy—this is real funny—
> *Well*, it was not funny at the time—my husband had a heart attack.
> *So* he was out of town, in Tarboro, NC.
> I had the lumpectomy on that Friday,
>   and **I said**, *"Well 'Hank,' you can go to work."*
> Because my parents were here and he really didn't need to be home—not thinking about how he was feeling or whatever.
>   It had not dawned on me.
>   **He said**, *Yeah, he could go to work.*
> *But then* on Monday, he had a heart attack.
> *So, therefore,* he was in Tarboro, NC, and I was here at [the hospital].
> *So here* we had two children in high school and him there, and when he came from Tarboro—he was in Tarboro for about a week—they transferred him to [the hospital] .
> *So, therefore,* we didn't see each other for about 3 weeks, because I couldn't go see him and he couldn't come to see me.
> *Laughs*
> *So when* we got home, it was just—here we were upstairs in the bed.
> We couldn't do a thing.

In Madeline's one-on-one retelling, her emphasis is on their mutual inability to do anything for themselves, and her editorial commentary shifts to the spiritual, with the word *blessed*: Thanks to others, the house and children were cared for, and she and her husband could recuperate side-by-side, talking things through:

> We were **blessed**
> because they were old enough to take care of themselves,
> but somebody had to come in.
>   My mom and my neighborhood and my church members
>   just literally took over my house for about 2 weeks.
>   It was something, but we got over that.
> And, like I say, we are totally, totally **blessed**.
> We had a lot of time to talk,
> because we were in the bed together.

Sermonizing: Cassaundra's Contribution. A focus group is a more formal occasion than an everyday circle of chat. It has a convener, a recognized task, and unofficial and unspoken regulations as to the number of speakers who may have the floor at any one time: one. It is expected that the convener will ask questions and that participants in the group will each have the floor to answer the questions and, in this case, tell their stories. It is also typical to see short bursts of collaborative, emotion-filled conversation where everybody talks to her or his neighbor at once, usually in support of or in direct opposition to a speaker's point. The women in our focus group met these expectations. However, they added information using styles often used among women in the African American community, including sermonizing. Cassaundra's use of parallel structures and repetition of key words and phrases, particularly at points in the story that allow evaluation or editorial comment, is sufficiently sermon-like to evoke audience reaction. Notice how she uses verbal extenders, such as "that kind of thing," inviting her listeners to collaborate silently with her in finishing the meaning. In classical sermon technique, she elaborates a key concept or verbal picture, as if it were a text, in each stanza-like section of her personal testimony before the group. Cassaundra is doing more than revealing personal information, she is witnessing, testifying to her own travail and personal survival, suggesting emotional depth by tone of voice and repetition. (Key segments are italicized.)

I always want to deal with my own body,
even if, at the time, I felt that it betrayed me,
I always want to deal with my own body.
Immediately after hearing my diagnosis, I felt betrayed,
you know, the whole thing—
shaking my fist at God and *that kind of thing*,
but then after that, *you know*,
I wasn't depressed or *anything like that.*
There were certain things I didn't know like losing hair.
Well, you only relate that to your head.
You don't realize that you are going to be bald all over your body,
and I would stand and look in front of the mirror and just say
"Look there's nothing anywhere."
So I was glad when my lashes grew back *and that kind of thing.*
And keloids, also, you mentioned keloids.
I do have a keloid on the right side.
This was the breast I had mastectomized,
but I don't let any of that bother me.
I'm still the person I was before,
and once you get that diagnosis,
you're never the same after that,
but you gotta keep going.
You are still the person you were before,
probably even more.

Once Cassaundra finished showing that she has survived the loss and regrowth of hair, the development of scar tissue, and similar blows to surface, earthly beauty, and has extended the changes to self to her listeners, they join in the next part, cued by the phrase, "*once you get that diagnosis.*" Their collaborative voices underscore key points and help her turn the narrative just as she has turned a corner in her life: she doesn't want her old life back. She has a new one.

That's the thing I've learned, that once you get that diagnosis,
you really have a choice.
You can either give up—
Estelle: Exactly!
Or you can choose to deal with it and keep going.
The whole time I was in recovery,
I would say to my mother and my friends, all the time,
"I want my life back."
Marlena: Absolutely!
I want my life back!
I want this to stop.
I want my life back!
Regina: You've got to demand it!
But I don't want *that* life back.
I've got a different life now.
I've got a new life,
and I like this life better than the other one.
I'm glad I got rid of that life.
You need to weed your garden and get rid of the trash.
Cancer teaches you about living.
It teaches you to enjoy the wind on your face,
and you realize how green the grass and the trees are,
stuff that you just take for granted.
It's just amazing.

No one speaks for a moment as Cassaundra ends.

IMPLICATIONS: NARRATIVE IDENTITY AND CULTURE-SENSITIVE PRACTICES

Pierce (1997) suggested self-awareness, knowledge, and honing of skills in working with individuals of different cultures will have a positive impact on enhancing intercultural care and cultural sensitivity. We propose a fourth skill that is necessary to enhance effectiveness of HCWs; that is awareness of patterns of communication used by African-American women to enhance listening abilities of providers.

Analysis of taped conversations with African-American women living with breast cancer provides the following guidelines on what to listen for when seeking to learn how they are coping with this disease. The narratives from these samples of African-American women share several of the emphases reported by researchers as prevalent in discourse among African American women: that is, spirituality, wisdom, proud and strong individual identity, the roles of testimonial and witness as modes of cultural transmission, and beauty of the spirit as opposed to that of the body, with cautions against adopting White-given cultural stereotypes about hair and about the body (see Banks, 2000; Pereira, 2000). Sexuality is considered part of one's God-given, spiritually blessed life. Spirituality is what grounds notions of self-efficacy: in brief, one draws the strength for the achievement of self-efficacy from God.

African-American women diagnosed with breast cancer draw strength from their belief in God and include references to God when describing their symptoms. It is not uncommon for them to delay seeking diagnosis and treatment until they have "given it over" to God. HCWs need to understand this and encourage them to continue to draw strength from their spirituality during treatment rather than chastise them for what may be perceived as needless delay in seeking treatment. Offering opportunities for prayer and including references to their faith during treatment are ways HCWs can offer culturally sensitive care.

For example, narrativizing, or as HCWs term it, storytelling, often occurs in conjunction with references to spirituality. HCWs who want to be more effective and empathetic can listen for one or more of the stylistic techniques we have detailed, particularly around story and storytelling practices:

- Narrativizing: The HCW should be aware that many women will answer questions about symptoms, diagnosis, or current management of therapy and recovery with stories. These stories have two points: one is to transmit information in a deep, wise way; the other is to signal a depth of feeling. The storyteller expects signals from the HCW that they recognize she is giving important information in her own way; typically, nods, murmurs, and pauses in the HCW's part of the conversation, discussion, or interview will be seen as polite and involved:
- Repetition: The HCW must be aware that repetition of words or phrases, particularly phrases that sound like slogans, mottoes, or Bible verses, will not necessarily mean that the woman is fumbling for words; instead she may be emphasizing important issues and is unable to say them any more directly or thinks she is saying them directly. In her culture, the speaker is being direct. HCWs should practice active listening by offering verbal and nonverbal signals that they are listening.
- Sermonizing: HCWs need to be aware that the speaker may use religious references, not in an effort to convert the HCW, but as

> a frame of reference; if others have come with the primary speaker, they may reinforce her key points with interjections and comments.

Listening to the words used in narratives also provides strong cues as to the level of self-efficacy in the speaker. For example, Cassaundra exhibits a strong level of self-efficacy as she rejoices over her new life. She is confident in her ability to live life to its fullest, even after the diagnosis of cancer. Listening for the cues of wisdom, fortitude, and caring can also signal levels of self-efficacy. For example, each of these characteristics were evident in the talk collected in the focus group, with Madeleine's group talk showing the fortitude by reporting her confrontation and control, and her one-on-one interview exhibiting the caring. Listening carefully as women speak will enable the HCW to discern one of two emphases: a fatalistic avoidance of choices and a passive acceptance, which can get in the way of diagnosis, treatment, and recovery, or an emphasis on fortitude and self-control, which can actually lead to increased self-efficacy. The HCW can then formalize the perception by asking the woman to complete an appropriate self-efficacy measure and using the results to provide the appropriate degree and type of support and education.

African-American women, although having a lower incidence of breast cancer than Euro-American women, die more frequently from the disease. Survival rates of breast cancer in African-American women will only improve with a multipronged approach that is grounded in cultural appropriateness and improved intercultural communication abilities. Improving how HCWs hear what women say about how they found their lump, what the diagnosis means to them, and how they are coping with the diagnosis and treatment will, over time, improve both their quality of care, quality of life and, we hope, quantity of life. Knowing that HCWs *really hear* what they are saying will encourage women to tell their friends *not* to be afraid to seek health care. Increasing the possibility that they will be heard and thus seen and valued will lead to improved health care and survival for all.

REFERENCES

Abrums, M. (2000). "Jesus will fix it after awhile": Meanings and health. *Social Science & Medicine, 50,* 89-105.

Ainsworth-Vaughn, N. (1998). *Claiming power in doctor-patient talk.* Oxford: Oxford University Press.

Altpeter, M., Earp, J. A. L., Bishop, C., & Eng, E. (1999). Lay health advisor activity levels: Definitions from the field. *Health Education and Behavior, 26*, 495-512.

American Cancer Society. (2007a). *Cancer Facts & Figures 2007*. Atlanta: Author. Retrieved June 2007, from http://www.cancer.org/downloads/STT/CAFF2007PWSecured.pdf

American Cancer Society (2007b). *Cancer Facts & Figures for African Americans 2007-2008*. Atlanta: Author. Retrieved June 2007, from http://www.cancer.org/downloads/STT/CAFF2007AAacspdf2007.pdf

Bandura, A. (1977). *Social learning theory*. Englewood Cliffs, NJ: Prentice-Hall.

Bandura, A. (1986). *Social foundations of thought and action: A social cognitive theory*. Englewood Cliffs, NJ: Prentice-Hall.

Bandura, A. (1997). *Self-efficacy: The exercise of control*. New York: W. H. Freeman.

Banks, I. (2000). *Hair matters: Beauty, power, and Black women's consciousness*. New York: New York University Press

Bibb, S.C. (2000). Access and late-stage diagnosis of breast cancer in the military health system. *Military Medicine, 165*, 585-590.

Bibb, S.C.G. (2001). The relationship between access and stage at diagnosis of breast cancer in African American and Caucasian Women. *Oncology Nursing Forum, 28*(4), 711-719.

Bogle, D. (1973). *Toms, Coons, Mulattoes, Mammies and Bucks: An interpretive history of blacks in American films*. New York: Continuum.

Bourjolly, J. N. (1998). Differences in religiousness among black and white women with breast cancer. *Social Work Health Care, 28*(1), 21–39.

Bourjolly, J. N. (1999). A comparison of cognitive appraisal, coping, coping resources and social functioning among black and white women with breast cancer. *Social Work Health Care, 28*(3), 1–20.

Chafe, W. (1980). The deployment of consciousness in the production of a narrative. In W. Chafe (Ed.), *The pear stories: Cognitive, cultural, and linguistic aspects of narrative production* (pp. 9-50). Norwood, NJ: Ablex.

Clark, N., & Dodge, J. (1999). Exploring self-efficacy as a predictor of disease management. *Health Education & Behavior, 26*(1), 72-89.

Daaleman, T., & Nease, D. (1994). Patient attitudes regarding physician inquiry into spiritual and religious issues. *The Journal of Family Practice, 39*(6), 564-568.

Dance, D.C. (Ed.). (2002). *From my people: 400 years of African American folklore*. New York: Norton.

Erwin, D. O., Spatz, T. S., & Turturro, C. L. (1992). Development of an African-American role model intervention to increase breast self-examination and mammography. *Journal of Cancer Education, 7*, 311-319.

Foster, M. (1995). "Are you with me?" Power and solidarity in the discourse of African American women. In K. Hall & M. Bucholtz (Eds.), *Gender articulated: Language and the socially constructed self* (pp. 323–350). New York: Routledge.

Foster, M. (2001). Pay Leon, Pay Leon, Pay Leon Paleontologist: Using call-and-response to facilitate mastery and literacy acquisition among African American students. In S. Lanehart (Ed.), *Sociocultural and historical contexts of African American English* (pp. 281–298). Amsterdam: John Benjamins.

Gollop, C. (1997). Where have all the nice old ladies gone? Researching the health information-seeking behavior of older African American women. In K. Vaz (Ed.), *Oral narrative research with black women* (pp. 143–155). Thousand Oaks CA: Sage.

Gotay, C. C., & Wilson, M. E. (1998). Social support and cancer screening in African American, Hispanic, and Native American women. *Cancer Practice, 6,* 31-37.

Green, L. (2002). *African-American English: A linguistic introduction* Cambridge: Cambridge University Press.

Gregg, J., & Curry, R. H. (1994). Explanatory models for cancer among African-American women at two Atlanta neighborhood health centers: The implications for a cancer screening program. *Social Science & Medicine, 39*(4), 519-526.

Haynes, M. A., & Smedley, B. D. (1999). *The unequal burden of cancer*. Washington, DC: National Academy Press.

Heiney, S.P. (1995). The healing power of story. *Oncology Nursing Forum, 22*(6), 899-904.

Henderson, P.D., Gore, S.V., Davis, B.L., & Condon, E.H. (2003). African American women coping with breast cancer: A qualitative analysis. *Oncology Nursing Forum, 30*(4), 641-647.

Hickey, M. L., Owen, S.V., & Froman, R.D. (1992). Instrument development: Cardiac diet and exercise self-efficacy. *Nursing Research, 41(6),* 347-351.

Houston, M. (2002a). Multiple perspectives: African American women conceive their talk. *Women and Language, 23,* 11-17.

Houston, M. (2002b). Seeking difference: African Americans in interpersonal communications research, 1975-2000. *Howard Journal of Communication, 13*, 25-41.

Johnstone, B. (2002). *Discourse analysis: An introduction*. Oxford: Blackwell.

Jones, J. M. (1991). Racism: A cultural analysis of the problem. In R. L. Jones (Ed.), *Black psychology* (p. 626). Berkeley, CA: Cobb & Henry.

Lackey, N.R., Gates, M.F., & Brown, G. (2001). African American women's experiences with the initial discovery, diagnosis, and treatment of breast cancer. *Oncology Nursing Forum, 28*(3), 519-527.

McTavish, F., Pingree, S., Hawkings, R., & Gustafson, D. (2003). Cultural differences in use of discussion group. *Journal of Health Psychology, 8*, 103-116.

Morgan, M. (1996). Conversational signifying: Grammar and indirectness among African American women. In E. Ochs, E. Schegloff, & S. Thompson (Eds.), *Interaction and grammar* (pp. 405-434). Cambridge: Cambridge University Press.

Morgan, M. (2002). *Language, discourse and power in African American culture*. Cambridge: Cambridge University Press.

Newlin, K., Knafl, K., & Melus, G.D. (2002). African-American spirituality: A concept analysis. *Advances in Nursing Science, 25*(2), 57-70.

Newman, A. (1991). Effect of the arthritis self-help course on adaptation in people with arthritis. *Arthritis Care and Research, 4*(3), 26.

Newman, A. (1993). Effects of self-help course on adaptation in people with arthritis. In S. Funk, E. Tournquist, M. Champagne, & R. Weiss (Eds.), *Key aspects of caring for the chronically ill: Hospital and home* (pp. 150-157). New York: Springer.

Newman, A. (1997). Arthritis self-help in minorities: Preliminary results. *Arthritis Care and Research, 10,* 16.

O'Leary, A. (1985). Self-efficacy and health. *Behavior Therapy and Research, 23,* 437-451.

O'Connor, P. (2000). *Speaking of crime: Narratives of prisoners*. Omaha: University of Nebraska Press.

Pereira, M. (2000). *Embodying beauty: twentieth-century American women writers' aesthetics*. New York: Garland.

Phillips, D., & Drevdahl, D. (2003). "Race" and the difficulties of language. *Advances in Nursing Science, 2,* 17-29.

Phillips, J. M. (1999). Breast cancer and African American women: Moving beyond fear, fatalism, and silence. *Oncology Nursing Forum, 26,* 1001-1007.

Phillips, J. M., Cohen, M. Z., & Moses, G. (1999). Breast cancer screening and African American women: Fear, fatalism, and silence. *Oncology Nursing Forum, 26,* 561-571.

Pierce, R. L. (1997). African-American cancer patients and culturally competent practice. *Journal of Psychosocial Oncology, 15*(2), 1-17.

Pope, C. (2003, November). *Social practices in talk as sources of disparities for health literacy.* Presented at the annual meeting of the American Public Health Association, San Francisco, CA.

Rickford, J., & McNair-Knox, F. (1994). Addressee and topic-influenced style shift: A quantitative sociolinguistic study. In D. Biber & E. Finegan (Eds.), *Perspectives on register: Situating register variation within sociolinguistics* (pp. 235-276). Oxford: Oxford University Press.

Samuel-Hodge, C., Headen, S., Skelly, A., Ingram, A., Keyserling, T., Jackson, E., Ammerman, A., & Elasy, T. (2000). Influences on day-to-day self-management of type 2 diabetes among African-American women: Spirituality, the multi-caregiver role, and other social context factors. *Diabetes Care, 23*(7), 928-933.

Sanders, L. D., Wilmoth, M. C., & Lowery, B. (2004). Overcoming: Older African American women and breast cancer. *Journal of the Black Nurses Association, 15*(2), 32-39.

Schiffrin, D. (1994). *Approaches to discourse.* London: Blackwell

Smitherman, G. (1997). "The chain remain the same": Communicative practices in the hip hop nation. *Journal of Black Studies, 28,* 3-25.

Strecher, V., DeVellis, B., Becker, M., & Rosenstock, I. (1986, Spring). The role of self-efficacy in achieving behavior change. *Health Education Quarterly, 13*(1), 73-92.

Tannen, D. (1989). *Talking voices: Repetition, dialogue and imagery in conversational discourse*. Cambridge: Cambridge University Press.

Taylor, E. J. (2001). Spirituality, culture, and cancer care. *Seminars in Oncology Nursing, 17*(3), 197-205.

Taylor, J. Y. (1999). Colonizing images and diagnostic labels: Oppressive mechanisms for African American women's health. *Advances in Nursing Science, 21*(3), 32-45.

Taylor, S. E., Aspinwall, L. G., Giuliano, T. A., Dakof, G. A., & Reardon, K. K. (1993). Storytelling and coping with stressful events. *Journal of Applied Psychology, 23*(9), 703-733.

Wharry, C. (2003). Amen and hallelujah preaching: Discourse functions in African American sermons. *Language and Society, 32*, 203-225.

Williams-Brown, S., Baldwin, D.M., & Bakos, A. (2002). Storytelling as a method to teach African American women breast health information. *Journal of Cancer Education, 17*(4), 227-230.

Wilmoth, M.C., & Sanders, L.D. (2001). Accept me for myself: African American women's issues after breast cancer. *Oncology Nursing Forum*, *28*(5), 875-879.

9

Cancer and Older Adults

A Model of Technology and Social Support

James D. Robinson
University of Dayton

Jeanine Warisse Turner
Georgetown University

Teresa L. Thompson
University of Dayton

Although it is not clear if the increase in cancer pathology among older adults is a primary or a secondary characteristic of aging (Busse, 1969), it is clear that older adults are more susceptible than their younger adult counterparts to many types of cancer. In fact, Wallace (2001) argued that "Fundamentally, cancer is a disease of older people" (p. 146). More than 25% of all deaths in the United States are attributable to cancer (Wallace, 2001) and only cardiovascular disease accounts for more deaths in adults 65 years of age and older. Males over the age of 65 are most likely to fall victim to lung, prostate, colon, rectum, urinary system, and bladder cancers. Females of the same age cohort are most vulnerable to breast, colon, rectum, lung, and pancreatic cancers (Solomon, 1999).

The rate of cancer does not, however, increase monotonically across the lifespan. Between the ages of 65 and 74, 25% of all deaths are attributable to cancer. Between the ages of 74 and 84 approximately 20% of all deaths are caused by cancer. After the age of 85, the percentage of adults dying of cancer decreases to about 12% (Solomon, 1999).

Patients with cancer often need assistance as they battle the disease. Such assistance is often called *social support* in the health communication literature. Social support typically refers to those situations where one person provides help or services to others. Albrecht, Burleson, and Goldsmith (1994) pointed out that social support contains a communicative dimension. They defined *supportive communication* as "verbal and nonverbal behavior that influences how providers and recipients view themselves, their situations, the other, and their relationship and is the principal process through which individuals coordinate their actions in support-seeking and support-giving encounters" (p. 421).

Both social support and supportive communicative relationships have been shown to play an important role in mental and physical health. Social support has been linked to improved patient resistance to infection and disease, increased longevity, a reduction in patient mortality, increased feelings of self-efficacy, enhanced psychological adjustment to health, and social functioning (Albrecht & Adelman, 1987; Berkman & Syme, 1979; Bloom, 1982; Dimond, 1979; Jemmott & Magloire, 1988; Kasl, Evans, & Neiderman, 1979; Kurdek, 1988; Litwak & Messeri, 1989; Major et al., 1990).

Research into the provision of formal and informal social support indicates that older adults look first to their families for assistance (Shanas, 1979; Shanas & Maddox, 1985). Older adults typically live relatively close to at least one of their children (Hanson & Sauer, 1985), and most often one or two of the children provide the lion's share of the familial social support (Chappell & Havens, 1985). Chappell and Guse (1989) pointed out that most of the familial social support is provided by women. Wives, daughters, and daughters-in-law are the three most likely providers of social support. Social support provided by male caregivers is less common and generally only occurs when female caregivers are not available. It is interesting to note that when daughters provide social support, their husbands typically do not help. The spouses of sons providing social support to an older parent are much more likely to provide additional assistance to the parent (Chappell & Guse, 1989).

Discussions of social support all too often typically ignore the siblings of older adults. Chappell (1987) observed that siblings typically are the second most likely source of social support of older adults. Cicirelli (1985) argued that elderly people report feeling closer to their siblings than to any other relatives except their children and their spouses. Grandchildren and extended family members such as nieces, nephews, cousins, and inlaws are less likely to provide social support than are friends and neighbors (Chappell & Guse, 1989).

Friends of older adults are the third most common source of social support (Adams, 1986; Cantor, 1979; Hochschild, 1973; Litwak, 1985; Rosow, 1967; Shanas, 1962) and it is clear that friendships play an important role in the psychosocial well-being of the elderly (Adams, 1967, 1986; Arling, 1976; Larson, 1978; Lowenthal & Haven, 1968; Nussbaum, 1985; Roberto & Scott, 1986; Rosow, 1976; Wood & Robertson, 1978). It is interesting to note that the relationship between friendship and psychosocial well-being is stronger than the relationship between family activity and psychological well-being. In fact, the friendship variable is so important that the single strongest predictor of psychosocial well-being is the presence of a confidant or close friend (Connidis & Davies, 1990, 1992; Lowenthal & Haven, 1968; Rawlins, 1995). Although the family may play an important role in the provision of support, confidants or close friends who share in intimate communication and have a high level of involvement have a much more significant impact on the psychosocial well-being of elderly adults than do family members (Connidis & Davies, 1990, 1992; Lowenthal & Haven, 1968; Rawlins, 1995).

TYPES OF SOCIAL SUPPORT

Goodman (1984) also noted that the elderly are often provided some assistance by their neighbors. In his research on neighbors and social support, Goodman identified three general categories or types of neighborhood helpers: high helpers, mutual helpers, and neighborhood isolates. High helpers provide their neighbors with a great deal of very professional assistance and receive little or no help in return. Mutual helpers are those people who provide some assistance to others and also accept some help in return. Neighborhood isolates generally receive social support from people who do not live nearby. Immediate family, siblings, friends, and neighbors provide most of the social support received by older adults. Exactly what constitutes socials support is another complex question that has been examined by a number of researchers.

In an effort to better understand the concept of social support, Cutrona and Russell (1990) carefully reviewed the extant literature. They noticed that previous studies attempting to identify the dimensions of social support consistently uncovered six distinct types. The first type of social support is *emotional support,* which occurs when we communicate that we care about an individual who is going through a time of difficulty. Such interactions result in feelings of comfort and/or a sense of being cared for and about by others. Being empathetic, sympathetic, or compassionate are all examples of trying to provide emotional support to another individual.

The second type, *social integration,* occurs when an individual feels included by others in social or recreational activities by the members of a group. Typically, those group members have some common interests and/or concerns and the relationships are most commonly described as being casual friendships. Inviting someone to a ball game or lunch are examples of providing social integration support.

The third type of social support is *esteem support*, which occurs when one helps others feel that they are competent or capable of performing a task. Feedback indicating task competence can enhance feelings of self-efficacy and self-worth. Telling someone his or her yard looks great, while the person is gardening, or telling the person he or she is doing a great job of adjusting to the loss of a loved pet are both examples of efforts at providing esteem support to a neighbor.

The fourth type of support is what lay people often think of initially when asked about providing help to others. It is called *tangible support*. Tangible support occurs when someone provides concrete instrumental assistance such as helping wrap a package, providing a loan, or shoveling a driveway. Typically, the individual receiving the assistance cannot remedy the problem without the help and the circumstances are somewhat stressful.

The fifth type of support is *informational support*, which is provided to others when information is shared and advice or guidance is provided. Telling a neighbor when the bus will stop, or suggesting that someone can call the pharmacist to find out if a medication can be taken at night are both examples of informational support.

The sixth and final type of social support is described by Cutrona and Russell (1990) as the *support of others,* which occurs when an individual provides support to someone else. It is based on the belief that people have a need or a desire to be needed by others and feel useful. The act of providing social support to others helps individuals feel better about themselves and their abilities and can serve to improve their physical and mental well-being.

OPTIMAL MATCHING

In addition to identifying the six dimensions of social support just described. Cutrona and Russell (1990) also argued that successful socially supportive interactions occur when the type of support being provided by a caregiver is consistent with the type of social support needed or desired by the recipient. This consistency is described by Cutrona and Russell as optimal matching. Because Cutrona and Russell argue that there are six types of social support, it is easy to see how a social support provider may be trying very hard to help and at the same time be ineffectual because they are not providing the type of support desired by the individual in need. From the optimal matching perspective, receiving emotional social support will not be of much benefit to individuals in need of informational social support.

So far, social support has been discussed as a purely interpersonal phenomenon because much of the research examining it has focused on face-to-face interaction. Given the advent of the Internet and other new technologies, social support could also be provided through e-mail, chatrooms, and interactive web pages. In short, the Internet could be used as a functional alternative to face-to-face social support. Before further examination of the use of computer-mediated communication (CMC) as an avenue or vehicle for social support, a brief examination of older adult usage of personal computers is warranted.

Computer Use in Older Adults

The percentage of U.S. households with personal computers (PCs) has risen dramatically in recent years. In December 1998, approximately 42% of all homes contained one or more PCs (NTIA, 2000). By August 2000, the percentage of households with PCs had increased to 51% (NTIA, 2000). By 2001, that percentage had increased to 56.5% (U.S. Census Bureau, 2003) and projections for the year 2003 indicated that nearly 70% of all U.S. homes contained one or more PCs (Brunner, 2004). A 1998 survey of older computer users indicated that 60% of the respondents reported using their computers on a daily basis (Schwab, 1998).

Similarly, Internet access has also increased dramatically (see Table 9.1). In December 1998, 26% of all U.S. homes had Internet access (primarily through dial-up connections). By August 2000, that number had climbed 41.5% (NTIA, 2000) and by 2001, Internet access had increased to 50.5% (U.S. Census Bureau, 2003). It is interesting to note that, although the 55 years of age and older cohort is least likely to own a PC and the least likely to have Internet access in their homes, this segment of the population is expected to increase their computer activity significantly over the next decade (NTIA, 2000). Many computer users gained their experience with PCs and the Internet at school or in the workplace. As today's computer users grow older, the percentage of homes with computers and Internet access will undoubtedly increase dramatically. Evidence of this claim is in recent labor force statistics. Slightly more than 46% of adults aged 50 years, who were still working, reported using the Internet whereas only 16.6% of all unemployed adults over age 50 reported using the Internet (NTIA, 2000). This workforce effect is even more dramatic for older adults than younger adults. A little experience goes a long way in decreasing the digital divide.

TABLE 9.1
HOUSEHOLDS WITH COMPUTERS AND INTERNET ACCESS BY AGE: 2001

AGE OF HOME OWNER	HOMES WITH COMPUTERS	HOUSES WITH INTERNET ACCESS
	2001 (%)	2001 (%)
Less than 25 years of age	51.1	44.7
25–34 years of age	62.5	57.3
35–44 years of age	69.9	62.6
45–54 years of age	66.9	60.9
55+ years of age	39.1	33.9
All U.S. households	56.5	50.5

Note: Data: U.S. Census Bureau, Statistical Abstract of the US—2003.

As can be seen in Table 9.2, older adults are far less likely to have Internet access at home or at work and are less likely to have Internet access available to them anywhere (at home or work or from some other source such as a friend or the library) than their younger counterparts. The percentage of Internet users increased along with the increase in home access to the Internet. The percentage of people using the Internet rose from 32.7% in December 1998 to 44.4% in August 2000 (NTIA, 2000). By September 2001, 54% of the U.S. population was using the Internet (Brunner, 2004). For all the claims of providing Internet service at public libraries, unemployed indi-

TABLE 9.2
INTERNET ACCESS AND USAGE BY AGE: 2003

AGE OF HOMEOWNER (YEARS)	INTERNET ACCESS ANYWHERE (%)	HOME ACCESS (%)	WORK ACCESS (%)	USED THE INTERNET PAST 30 DAYS (%)
18–34	37.8	33.0	34.3	38.2
35–54	45.5	46.5	53.9	45.4
55+	16.7	20.5	11.8	16.4

Note: Data: U.S. Census Bureau, Statistical Abstract of the US—2003.

viduals are much more likely to access the Internet than are employed individuals. According to the NTIA (2000), in August 2000, 4% of unemployed individuals reported using the Internet from the public library compared to 2% of employed individuals.

Examination of Internet usage statistics suggests that the single most common use of the Internet is for sending and receiving e-mail (see Table 9.3). This finding holds true for all three age cohorts. An argument—consistent with engagement theory—could be made from this data that older adults use the Internet to stay engaged in society. Adults 55 years of age and older are most likely to report sending and receiving e-mail, to have sent an electronic postcard, to research products and services on the Internet, and to access daily news. Given the relative newness of Instant messaging to the older age cohorts (those older than 34 in this comparison), the percentage of older adults reporting usage of instant messaging is surprisingly high.

It is apparent that older adults are jumping the "digital divide" and using the Internet and other such technologies at an increasingly rapid rate. With Internet access increasingly available, it is no wonder that older adults are using it to gather information and to stay connected to the world around them. With the passage of time, the percentage of older adults who will have

TABLE 9.3
ONLINE ACTIVITIES BY AGE: 2002

ONLINE ACTIVITY	AGE 18–34 (%)	AGE 35–54 (%)	AGE 55+ (%)
Sent/received e-mail	92.2	93	95
Used a search engine	78	80	76
Gathered local information	61	61	55
Sent an electronic postcard	49	54	57
Researched products and services	59	65	68
Used instant messaging service	59	49	45
Accessed phone numbers and addresses	46	45	45
Chatted online	48	38	31
Accessed local, national, & international daily news	51	55	57
Gathered travel information	41	47	54

Note: Data: From Brunner (2004).

had experience with computers and the Internet will resemble their younger counterparts. At that time, older adults will be far more likely to have had and to maintain an online presence.

Desire for Medical Information

A growing body of research has demonstrated that patients—old and young alike—have a strong desire for medical information. Often, patients want more information about their disease and treatment options than their doctor provides. Furthermore, patients often report that they would like more written patient information or health care literature to supplement the information provided during the office consultation (Donovan & Blake, 1992) so they do not forget what they were told after they leave the office.

Evidence of this desire for medical information can be observed in the search behavior and chatroom activity of Internet subscribers. Lamberg (1997) and others noted that discussion groups and chatrooms are among the most widely visited Web sites on the Internet. In fact, research by Green and Himelstein (1998) suggests as many as 46% of all online users—or nearly 31 million people—use the Internet to learn about medical or personal problems. It should be no surprise, then, that older patients with cancer might use their computers to gain information about their illnesses and treatment options from others online. People who find themselves in need of information—particularly if other sources are unavailable—would seem likely to try to find alternative informational resources.

CMC AND SOCIAL SUPPORT

It is becoming clear that CMC can serve as a functional alternative to face-to-face social support (see Braithwaite, Waldron, & Finn, 1999; Brennan, Moore, & Smythe, 1992; Lamberg, 1997; Lieberman, 1992; Mickelson, 1998; Scheerhorn, Warisse, & McNeilis, 1995). Because older adults want information about their medical conditions and the treatment options available to them, it is not surprising that they turn to the Internet and Web sites like WebMD for information.

Turner, Grube, and Meyers (2001) argued that under conditions of dependency—that is to say when face-to-face social support opportunities were unavailable to them—people are more likely to go online for social support. In their research, Turner et al. supported this hypothesis, reporting that individuals were more inclined to turn to alternatives when they lacked such opportunities within their face-to-face relationships. This lack of opportunity could stem from a variety of different reasons, including not being mobile enough to have interaction with people face to face, not knowing others in their particular medical situation, or concern over being a burden to others.

Turner et al. (2001) also provided evidence of the need to extend the optimal matching hypothesis beyond face-to-face relationships into the computer mediated context. They found that people lacking social support regarding their illnesses and/or treatment options within their significant face-to-face interactions were indeed more likely to turn to online alternatives for social support. These individuals were drawn to the Internet for information and contact with similar others and found the most comfort and value in what similar others had to say.

Robinson and Turner (2003) suggested that the notion of optimal matching needs to be extended to include the type of relationship between the provider and recipient of social support. This argument stems from the fact that the relationship between communicants plays a critical role in the creation of meaning (see Watzlawick, Beavin, & Jackson, 1967). That relationship information provides much of the context information necessary for understanding the content of the message. Changing the context of a message changes the meaning of that message, so it is important to consider both the content of the message and nature of the relationship between the communicants to understand the effectiveness of social support.

In many ways, computer-mediated social support may be preferable to face-to-face social support because providing social support can be a burden for a friend or family member. In these virtual social support relationships, additional burdens are not being placed on loved ones, friends, and/or family members.

Additionally, the social support literature has demonstrated that recipients of social support prefer to get their support from nonfamilial sources. These relationships that exist outside the pressures and dynamics of close family relationships (Adelman, Parks, & Albrecht, 1987) are preferred because additional burdens are not being placed on loved ones or family members. These relationships are called *weak-tie relationships*. Some researchers argue that the support offered by *weak-ties* provide anonymity and objectivity not found in close personal relationships (Adelman et al., 1987; Walther & Boyd, 2002; Wellman & Gulia, 1999).

THE STRENGTH OF WEAK TIES

Weak-tie relationships exist outside the pressures and dynamics of close family relationships (Adelman et al., 1987). An individual typically goes to a specific place to receive weak-tie support. This place might be a church to talk to a priest or an online community to talk with other sufferers of a similar illness. Some researchers argue that the support offered by weak ties provides anonymity and objectivity not found in close personal relationships (Adelman et al., 1987; Walther & Boyd, 2002; Wellman & Gulia, 1999).

Mediated channels create many opportunities for support from weak-tie relationships. Wellman and Gulia (1999), Walther and Boyd (2002), and others suggest that online communication fosters development of weak-tie relationships because the discussions often concentrate on the topic most salient to the individual in need of social support. Additionally, because these weak-tie relationships can be established with a wide variety of different individuals, more expertise may be brought to bear on the problem. In cases where social support is being provided in the traditional face-to-face relationship with friends and family members, the support groups and/or individuals tend to be more homogeneous in their attitudes, experiences, and their knowledge about the situation.

What is interesting here is that the use of computer-mediated social support may at times be preferred over face-to-face support—even if face-to-face sources of social support are available. Support for this claim comes from Kogan and Shelton's (1962) work, which found that, even though young people thought that the elderly would find familial interactions to be the most rewarding, the elderly themselves expressed a strong desire to meet and interact with new people. Chappell and Guse (1989) said it succinctly when they wrote "most elderly live close to at least one child and the elderly prefer intimacy-at-a-distance" (p. 219). Thus, social support via the Internet may be preferred in those cases where one of the goals of the recipient is to make contact with new people.

EXTENDING THE OPTIMAL MATCHING HYPOTHESIS

It makes sense, then, to consider the possibility of extending the notion of optimal matching to include not only consistency in the type of social support being provided but in addition to consider the nature of the relationship between communicants. In the context of optimal matching, it may be important to consider the possibility that the type of relationship between social support providers and recipients affects the effectiveness and desirability of socially supportive behaviors. Certainly, it provides much of the context information necessary to interpret these social behaviors and interactions. Social support that is matched to the need of the recipient may not be well received depending on the nature of the relationship between the provider and the recipient.

The argument that the type or nature of the relationship between support providers and recipients plays an important role in the effectiveness and desirability can easily be supported by anecdotal evidence. One of the authors of this chapter is fortunate enough to have a couple of wonderful older neighbors living next door. The lessons learned from those neighbors could fill many book chapters, but the lesson in this case was learned on a cold snowy day about 15 years ago.

THE IMPORT OF THE RELATIONSHIP

Although it does not snow a great deal in Springfield, Ohio, there are a couple of days in a given year where timely snow removal can make the difference in being able to get in and out of the house easily. On those days, I augment the beauty of the silent white day with the staccato exhaust sounds of a two-cycle Snapper snow blower. After completing the removal of the snow from my driveway and sidewalk, I noted that none of my neighbors had dug out from the snow. My neighbor to the east was a 70-year-old woman I will call "Martha." Martha's husband had died several years before we moved next door and I thought it would be a nice neighborly gesture—not to mention tangible social support—to plow her driveway. I would not consider Martha a "friend" but we are friendly—waving and speaking about the weather if we meet going to the mailbox. Martha values her privacy a great deal and has no interest in our relationship escalating beyond being neighbors who wave.

For nearly 12 years I have removed all of the snow from Martha's driveway and the extent of our interaction remains short weather discussions at the mailbox and the occasional glance and wave out the window while I am running the snow blower. It is clear from her behavior, our relationship, and the small amount of social support I provide is plenty.

My neighbor on the west side of my house is a very hardworking man in his 80s named "Paul." Paul works in his yard every day and he works longer and harder in his yard than any three middle-aged lawn jockeys. Paul is the kind of guy who will spend 4 hours making a gasket for a lawnmower rather than pay $9 for a new gasket at K-mart. As I was dragging my snow blower back home from Martha's house I decided I would help Paul out and finish the snow-blowing "trifecta." About 5 minutes into the delicate snow-removal exercise, Paul came out of his house and assured me that he didn't need any help with snow removal. He was nice about it, but he was also adamant that I need not remove the snow from his drive.

Because it is his driveway, I didn't feel like I should remove the snow from it against his will—even though it clearly burst my snow-removal dreams and the opportunity to provide tangible assistance to my neighbor. Little did I realize that by tugging on the starter cord in Paul's driveway, I transformed the nature of my relationship with Paul.

It began simply enough that spring. If I mowed a couple of rows of Paul's grass in the front yard, Paul would "quid-pro-quo" me by mowing a few rows in the backyard or rake some of the leaves that technically were in my yard. Usually, we would do "favors" for each other while the other was not working in their yard. You would just come home and find something done that needed to be done and it was never spoken about. Occasionally, we would come home to find these favors "in progress," but the rule was to act as if you did not notice the raking or the mowing or the weeding. I noticed that Paul would always cut a few more rows or rake a few more leaves in my yard. And rather than escalate the process I decided I would remove his snow in the winter and call it even.

In the hope that Paul would think I was working on my driveway, when the first snow fell, I went out and cleared Paul's driveway first. Then I cleared mine and then I finished up at Martha's house. Paul never comes out or mentions it to me. But if we have had a lot of snow that year, I do notice Paul will cut some serious grass in my backyard and pick up a trashcan full of sticks if the wind picks up. It is clear to me that the nature of my relationship with Paul changed and that change allows me the opportunity to provide social support to Paul that I would not otherwise be allowed to do. Similarly, my relationship with Martha has to be just right, too. Martha has the money to schedule snow removal if she needs it, and it is clear that if our relationship becomes more than it is today that my days of snow removal are over.

As you can see from these stories, the same type of support was perceived differently depending on the nature of the relationship between providers and recipients. This suggests that social support may be more effective when the support comes from a provider who is involved in an appropriate type of relationship with the recipient. It is also clear from these stories that the nature of the relationship between the provider and recipient of the social support can change over time. In the case of Paul, the relationship can be characterized as a stronger tie, whereas the relationship with Martha necessarily remained a weak-tie relationship.

A MODEL

Recently Nahm (2004) proposed a model of the relationship between computer-mediated social network (CMSN), perceived social support from the CMSN, and psychological well-being of older adults. Using a convenience sample of 809 older adult SeniorNet members, Nahm used a web-based survey and structural equation modeling to test the model (see Fig. 9.1 for the model).

In the test of her model, Nahm (2004) found that the size of the SeniorNet members' CMSN was positively related to the time they spent using the Internet and e-mail and to SeniorNet members' knowledge about computers. The size of the CMSN was also positively related to their perceptions of the amount of social support gained through CMC interaction. She reported inverse relationships between the size of SeniorNet members' CMSN and age and physical barriers to computing. She also found that female SeniorNet members maintained larger computer-mediated social support networks than their male counterparts. Nahm (2004) also observed that levels of face-to-face social support were positively related to feelings of psychological well-being and feelings of psychological well-being were inversely related to the number and severity of physical barriers to computing reported by SeniorNet members.

The relationships described here were expected by Nahm (2004) and are supportive of the notion that people can and do receive social support in the computer mediated context. It is interesting to note that Nahm found no relationship between CMSN size and perceptions of psychological well-being. Additionally, she found that SeniorNet member perceptions of psychological well-being were unrelated to perceptions of social support received from the CMSN.

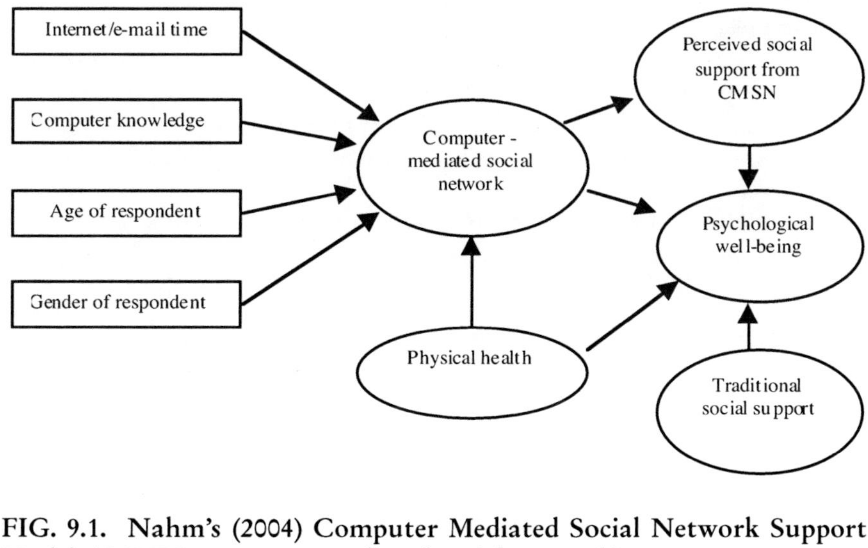

FIG. 9.1. Nahm's (2004) Computer Mediated Social Network Support Model. (CSMN, computer mediated social network)

Obviously, Nahm expected a relationship between CMSN size and perceptions of psychological well-being, and perceptions of psychological well-being to be related to CMSN size. Those relationships or lack of relationships may be attributable to measurement and/or conceptual issues. Using general measures of CMSN and perceived social support from the CMSN and a more specific measure of psychological well-being could be part of the problem. The persuasion literature is littered with small and nonsignificant correlations between variables measured at different logical levels (Davidson & Jaccard, 1979). Perhaps more importantly, however, it may well be that it is not the size of the computer-mediated social support network that matters but rather the relationship between the social support provider and recipient that matters. That would explain the fact that size of network is related to perceptions of social support but not psychological well-being. With more people in the network, there is more chance to have social support. But it is not necessarily the type of social support needed for feelings of psychological well-being. One optimally matched interaction, here used to mean that the type of social support is consistent between provider and recipient and relationally matched (that is to say the support comes from someone who is in the appropriate type of relationship with the recipient) may well be effective in either the face-to-face or computer-mediated context. Future examination of this very important model should examine specific types of social support (as identified by Cutrona & Russell, 1990) and types of relationships (as suggested by Robinson & Turner, 2003).

What has not been discussed here in any detail is what exactly constitutes "types of relationships." A good place to start would be the weak ties–strong ties dichotomy discussed in the social support literature. At the most basic level this would allow researchers to see if these two types of relationships are equally effective in general, and it would allow researchers to determine if particular types of relationships are more effective for specific types of social support. Furthermore, this simple dichotomy can be used to compare face-to-face weak-tie relationships with computer-mediated weak-tie relationships. Again, such a comparison may help us better understand not only the weak-tie relationship but in addition the differences between face-to-face and computer-mediated social support.

AND A META-MODEL

Underlying the notion that older adults with cancer adapt to their illnesses through socially supportive communicative relationships is a meta-model of adaptation developed by Baltes and Baltes (1990). This model—the Selective Optimization with Compensation (SOC) Model—attempts to explain adaptation to aging across the life span (see the Appendix for a more detailed explanation of the model). Baltes and Baltes suggested that adaptation to the losses associated with aging can be explained by examining the processes of selection, compensation, and optimization. The SOC model is based on the principles of Social Exchange Theory (see Thibaut & Kelly, 1959) and suggests that people select their behavior based on the goals they have selected (selection), the resources and opportunities available to them (optimization), and their perceptions of their abilities to enact behaviors that will help them attain those goals (compensation). Although the individual may not be able to perform a particular task as in the past, often times nominal performance is more than adequate for goal attainment. Through the selection, optimization, and compensation process, older adults are able to maintain satisfying, successful, and efficacious lives by selecting behaviors that will help them fulfill their needs at a reasonable cost. Furthermore, those behaviors that are too difficult, impossible, or simply too costly in a social exchange sense are less likely or not at all likely to be selected from their behavioral repertoire.

The SOC model is important to this discussion of social support because it explains the principles underlying how adaptation occurs in a general sense and provides a framework for understanding the middle-range theories employed above to generate specific hypotheses. Specifically, the SOC provides a rationale for what constitutes an optimal match in terms of a good or desirable relationship. From the social exchange perspective that underlies the SOC model, a good relationship is one where the rewards of the relationship exceed the costs of the relationship relative to the available relational alternatives. Those relational alternatives, in this case, can be found in the face-to-face context or in a computer-mediated context. CMC, then, may be perceived as desirable because relationships that are impersonal can be established at a low cost or at a relatively low rate of exchange. Given the value of CMC in finding others with similar experiences, illnesses, and/or treatments as well as similar demographic characteristics—few social opportunities offer so much for so little. Similarly, with a large potential audience of communicative partners, the opportunities for older adult cancer victims to fulfill their need to provide social support for others is precariously close to limitless.

APPENDIX: SELECTIVE OPTIMIZATION WITH COMPENSATION MODEL (Baltes & Baltes, 1990)

Selection. As we get older, some physical and cognitive abilities decline. As a consequence of these new limitations or restrictions, older adults adapt by selecting from among the potential goals those that are most likely to be successfully accomplished and those that will most contribute to their physical and psychological well-being. Some of these goals may be the same across the life span and others may be adapted or revised as the actual or anticipated changes associated with aging occur. Selection, then, can be viewed as adaptation through limiting the number of goals the individual may pursue.

Optimization. In an effort to attain the selected goals, older adults may hone or refine their skills, acquire new skills, focus their efforts, and/or expend their energies in a particular life domain. For example, a writer who finds he or she has trouble concentrating may organize his or her life such that he or she sleeps several hours and then gets up and writes for an hour or makes sure he or she write before expending efforts on other tasks that are less important. That same author may write in the morning and edit what was written later in the day when he or she is too tired to continue writing effectively. Optimization can be viewed as the marshalling of skills and resources within a limited goal or life domain to remain effective.

Compensation. Although selection refers to the choosing among the assortment of goals an individual may have, compensation is used to describe the individual's response to a loss in behavioral capacity. Many of the losses or restrictions that occur to older adults do not significantly impact their abilities to function because the losses tend to occur near the limits of their latent reserves. Because many of the skills and abilities we have far exceed the requirements of completing a task, we have a latent reserve of skills and abilities that we have but are not using in the completion of a task. Because our skills often exceed the tasks, a slight loss in a skill or ability as a consequence of aging may not present much of a problem because the losses tend to occur in those skill or ability areas that are not typically used.

REFERENCES

Albrecht, T. L, & Adelman, M. B. (Eds.). (1987). *Communicating social support*. Newbury Park, CA: Sage.

Albrecht, T., Burleson, B., & Goldsmith, D. (1994). Supportive communication. In M. Knapp & G. Miller (Eds.), *Handbook of interpersonal communication* (pp. 419-459). Thousand Oaks, CA: Sage.

Adelman, M. B., Parks, M. R., & Albrecht, T. L. (1987). Beyond close relationships: Support in weak ties. In T. L. Albrecht & M. B. Adelman (Eds.), *Communicating social support* (pp. 126-147). Newbury Park, CA: Sage.

Adams, B. (1967). Interaction theory and the social network. *Sociometry, 30*, 64-78.

Adams, B. N. (1986). *The family: A sociological interpretation* (4th ed.). New York: Harcourt Brace, & Jovanovich.

Arling, G. (1976). The elderly widow and her family, neighbours, and friends. *Journal of Marriage and the Family, 38*, 757-768.

Baltes, P. B., & Baltes, M. M. (1990). Psychological perspectives on successful aging: The model of selective optimization with compensation. In P. B. Baltes & M. M. Baltes (Eds.), *Successful aging: Perspectives from the behavioral sciences*. New York: Cambridge University Press.

Berkman, L. F., & Syme, S. L. (1979). Social networks, host resistance, and mortality: A nine-year follow up of Alameda County residents. *American Journal of Epidemiology, 109*, 186-204.

Bloom, J. (1982). Social support, accommodation to stress and adjustment to breast cancer. *Social Science and Medicine, 16*, 1329-1338.

Braithwaite, D. O., Waldron, V. R., & Finn, J. (1999). Communication of social support in computer-mediated groups for persons with disabilities. *Health Communication, 11*, 123-151.

Brennan, P. F., Moore, S.M., & Smythe, K.A. (1992). ComputerLink: Electronic support for the home caregiver. *Advances in Nursing Science, 13* 14-27.

Brunner, B. (2004). *Time Almanac, 2004*. Boston: Information Please.

Busse, E. (1969). Theories of aging. In E. Busse & E. Pfeiffer (Eds.), *Behavior and adaptation in later life* (pp. 11-32). Boston: Little, Brown.

Cantor, M. H. (1979). Neighbours and friends: An overlooked resource in the informal support system. *Research on Aging, 1*, 434-463.

Chappell, N.L. (1987). *Intergenerational helping patterns*. Paper presented at the annual meeting of the Canadian Sociology and Anthropology Association, Hamilton, Ontario.

Chappell, N. L., & Guse, L. W. (1989). Linkages between informal and formal support (1989). In K. Markides & C. Cooper (Eds.), *Aging, stress, and health* (pp. 217–237). New York: Wiley.

Chappell, N. L., & Havens, B. (1985). Who helps the elderly person: Discussion of informal and formal care. In W. Peterson & J. Quadagno (Eds.), *Social bonds in later life* (pp. 211-227). Beverly Hills, CA: Sage.

Cicirelli, V. G. (1985). The role of siblings as family caregivers. In W. J. Sauer & R. T. Coward (Eds.), *Social support networks and the care of the elderly* (pp. 93–107). New York: Springer.

Connidis, I. A., & Davies, L. (1990). Confidants and companions in later life: The place of family and friends. *Journal of Gerontology, 45*, S141-S149.

Connidis, I. A., & Davies, L. (1992). Confidants and companions: Choices in later life. *Journal of Gerontology, 47*, S115-S122.

Cutrona, C., & Russell, D. (1990). Type of social support and specific stress: Toward a theory of optimal matching. In B. Sarason, I. Sarason, & G. Pierce (Eds.), *Social support: An interactional view* (pp. 319-366). New York: Wiley.

Davidson, A., & Jaccard, J. (1979). Variables that moderate the attitude-behavior relation: Results of a longitudinal survey. *Journal of Personality and Social Psychology, 37*, 1364-1376.

Dimond, M. (1979). Social support and adaptation to chronic illness: The case of maintenance hemodialysis. *Research in Nursing and Health, 2*, 101-108.

Donovan, J., & Blake, D. (1992). Patient compliance: Deviance or reasoned decision making? *Social Science Medicine, 34*, 507-513.

Green, H., & Himelstein, L. (1998, October 19). A cyber revolt in health care. *Business Week*, p. 154.

Goodman, C. (1984). Natural helping among older adults. *The Gerontologist, 24*, 138-143.

Hanson, S. M., & Sauer, W. J. (1985). Children and their elderly parents. In W. J. Sauer & R. T. Coward (Eds.), *Social support networks and the care of the elderly* (pp. 41–66). New York: Springer.

Hochschild, A. R. (1973). *The unexpected community*. Englewood Cliffs, NJ: Prentice-Hall.

Jemmott, J. B., & Magloire, K. (1988). Academic stress, social support, and secretory immunoglobulin A. *Journal of Personality and Social Psychology, 55*, 803-810.

Kasl, S. V., Evans, A. S., & Neiderman, J. C. (1979). Psychosocial risk factors in the development of infectious mononucleosis. *Psychosomatic Medicine, 41*, 445-466.

Kogan, N., & Shelton, F. C. (1962). Differential cue value of age and occupation in impression formation. *Psychological Reports, 7*, 203-216.

Kurdek, L. A. (1988). Perceived social support in gays and lesbians in cohabiting relationships. *Journal of Personality and Social Psychology, 54*, 504-509.

Lamberg, L. (1997). Online support group helps patients live with, learn more about the rare skin cancer CTCL-MF. *Journal of the American Medical Association, 277*, 1422-1423.

Larson, R. (1978). Thirty years of research on the subjective well-being of older Americans. *Journal of Gerontology, 33*, 109-125.

Lieberman, D. (1992). The computer's potential role in health education. *Health Communication, 4*, 211-225.

Litwak, E. (1985). *Helping the elderly.* New York: Guilford Press.

Litwak, E., & Messeri, P. (1989). Organizational theory, social supports, and mortality rates: A theoretical convergence. *American Sociological Review, 54*, 49-66.

Lowenthal, M.F., & Haven, C. (1968). Interaction and adaptation: Intimacy as a critical variable. *American Sociological Review, 33*, 20–30.

Major, B., Cozzarelli, C., Sciaccitano, A. M., Cooper, M. L., Testa, M., & Mueller, P. M. (1990). *Journal of Personality and Social Psychology, 59*, 452-463.

Mickelson, K. (1998). Seeking social support: Parents in electronic support groups. In S. Kiesler (Ed.), *Culture of the Internet* (pp. 157-178). Mahwah, NJ: Erlbaum.

Nahm, E. (2004). *Exploring internet use among older adults*. June 2002. [Online]. SeniorNet. Available: http://www.seniornet.org.

NTIA. (2000). *Falling through the net: Toward digital inclusion*. [Online]. Washington, DC: U.S. Commerce Department. Available: http://www.ntia.doc.gov/ntiahome/fttn00/contents00.html

Nussbaum, J. F. (1985). Successful aging: A communicative model. *Communication Quarterly, 33*, 262-269.

Rawlins, W. K. (1995). Friendships in later life. In J. F. Nussbaum & J. Coupland (Eds.), *Handbook of communication and aging research* (pp. 227-257). Mahwah, NJ: Erlbaum.

Roberto, K. A., & Scott, I. P. (1986). Equity consideration in the friendships of older adults. *Journal of Gerontology, 41*, 241-247.

Robinson, J.D., & Turner, J W. (2003). Impersonal, interpersonal, and hyperpersonal social support: Cancer and older adults. *Health Communication, 15*(2), 231-239.

Rosow, I. (1967). *Social integration of the aged.* New York: The Free Press

Rosow, I. (1976). Status and role change through the life span. In R. Binstock & E. Shanas (Eds.), *Handbook of aging and the social sciences* (pp. 457-482). New York: Van Nostrand Reinhold.

Scheerhorn, D., Warisse, J., & McNeilis, K. (1995). Computer-based telecommunication among an illness-related community: Design, delivery, early use, and the functions of the HIGHnet. *Health Communication, 7*, 301-325.

Schwab, C. (1998). *Research on senior's computer and internet usage: A report of a national survey.* [Online]. Available: http://www.seniornet.org

Shanas, E. (1962). *The health of older people: A social survey.* Cambridge, MA: Harvard University Press.

Shanas, E. (1979). The family as a support system in old age. *The Gerontologist, 19*, 169-174.

Shanas, E., & Maddox, G. (1985). Health, health resources, and the utilization of care. In R. Binstock & E. Shanas (Eds.), *Handbook of aging and the social sciences* (pp. 697–726), New York: Van Nostrand Reinhold.

Solomon, D. H. (1999). The role of aging processes in aging-dependent diseases. In V. L. Bengsten & K. W. Schaie (Eds.), *Handbook of theories of aging* (pp. 133-150). New York: Springer.

Thibaut, J.W., & H.H. Kelly (1959). *The social psychology of groups.* New York: Wiley.

Turner, J. W., Grube, J., & Meyers, J. (2001). Developing an optimal match within online communities: An exploration of CMC support communities & traditional support. *Journal of Communication, 51*(2), 231-251.

U.S. Census Bureau. (2003). *Statistical Abstract of the United States: 2003.* Washington DC: US Government Printing Office.

Wallace, R. B. (2001). Prevention of cancer in the elderly. In E. Swanson, T. Tripp-Reimer, & K. Buckwalter (Eds.), *Health promotion and disease prevention in the older adult: Interventions and recommendations* (pp. 146–155). New York: Springer.

Walther, J.B., & Boyd, S. (2002). Attraction to computer-mediates social support. In C. A. Lin & D. Atkin (Eds.), *Communication technology and society: Audience adoption and uses* (pp. 153–188). Cresskill, NJ: Hampton Press.

Watzlawick, P., Beavin, J. H., & Jackson, D. (1967). *Pragmatics of human communication: A study of interactional patterns, pathologies, and paradoxes.* New York: Norton.

Wood, Y., & Robertson, J. F. (1978). Friendship and kinship interaction: Differential effect on morale of the elderly. *Journal of Marriage and the Family, 40*, 367-375.

Wellman, B., & Gulia, M. (1999). Net surfers don't ride alone: Virtual communities as communities. In M. A. Smith & P. Kollock (Eds.), *Communities in cyberspace* (pp. 167-194). London: Routledge.

10

Online Support Groups Among Older Adults With Cancer and Their Lay Caregivers

Jim L. Query, Jr.
University of Houston

Kevin B. Wright
University of Oklahoma

This chapter explores the potential of online support groups for older adults with cancer and their lay caregivers in terms of providing health benefits. It begins by reviewing literature on computer-mediated support groups for older adults, individuals with cancer, and caregivers. Next, the authors present a model of online support group participation based on communication competence, social support, and coping theory, social network theory, and theories of computer-mediated communication. The implications of this model for individuals with cancer and their lay caregivers are discussed.

As individuals become older, they often become more susceptible to certain types of cancers, such as breast, colon, lung, and prostate cancers (American Cancer Society [ACS], 2001; Hewitt, Rowland, & Yancik, 2003). Although the 5-year average survival rate for all cancers is increasing and currently resides at 62% (ACS, 2001), the ACS recently reported that approximately 548,000 individuals or 1,500 per day per year would die from cancer.

Further exacerbating this health crisis is the decreasing social networks many older individuals confront (Query & James, 1989; Query & Kreps, 1996), and the higher likelihood of experiencing a symbolic crisis that often forges new and undesirable self- and relational identities (Query & Flint, 1996; see also Flint, Query, & Parrish, 2005). As Query and associates reported, this type of crisis is three-dimensional and blocks informed understanding and decision making; thereby often worsening the impacts of particular diagnoses. An example is a male cancer patient who refuses treatment primarily because he mistakenly believes that it would be futile in slowing or curing the disease (Kreps, 1988). Past research has demonstrated that individuals combating such life stressors can help protect themselves based, in part, on their communication competence, social support network size, and satisfaction, as well as coping skills (Query & James, 1989; Query & Kreps, 1996; Query & Wright, 2003; Wright & Query, 2004). Burleson, Albrecht, Goldsmith, and Sarason (1994) captured the inescapable link between social support processes and health outcomes when they stated, "The presence of caring relationships and the experience of social support indisputably contribute to the quality of a person's life" (p. xi).

More than 9 million Americans are currently living with some form of cancer, with about 1 million new cases diagnosed each year (ACS, 2001). Older adults currently account for 61% of all new cancer cases and 70% of all cancer deaths (Lewis et al., 2003). Although advances in cancer diagnosis and treatment have led to a growing number of long-term cancer survivors (Kreps, 2003), there have been relatively few studies of the communication processes and practices that may help individuals cope with living with cancer, including communication-based studies of support groups for individuals with cancer or their caregivers (for a review, see Kreps & Chapelsky Massimilla, 2002). Today, cancer survivors and caregivers have many choices in terms of sources of social support, including traditional support networks, such as family and friends, as well as other face-to-face and computer-mediated sources of social support.

In recent years, there has been tremendous growth in computer-mediated communication (CMC) as a result of the increased availability of computers, user-friendly Web browsers, and the popularity of the Internet in our culture. These technologies allow for the maintenance and expansion of social networks because of their ability to transcend geographical and temporal barriers by allowing individuals to conveniently and cheaply communicate with family and friends and by providing opportunities to meet new people with similar interests in online communities. A common stereotype of older individuals is that they do not use the Internet or have an interest in using this technology for relationships. Several studies have found, however, that increasing numbers of older individuals are using the Internet than previously and the number of older users is projected to climb in the coming decade (Fox, Giles, Orbe, & Bourhis, 2001; National Telecommunications and Information Administration, 2002; Wright, 2000a). Additionally, these studies have found that older individuals enjoy using the Internet as a means for maintaining relationships formed in the face-to-face world and meeting new acquaintances.

One type of online community that has become important for individuals with health concerns, including cancer, in our society is the online support group. Davison, Pennebaker, and Dickerson (2000), in a study of online health-related support groups, found that cancer groups were the most frequent type of support group on the Internet. Hundreds of cancer support groups have been identified on the Internet (Alexander, Peterson, & Hollingshead, 2003), and organizations such as the National Cancer Institute (NCI) and the ACS provide links to many online support groups for virtually all types of cancer. The use of online support groups has rapidly increased during the past decade, gaining the attention of communication scholars (Alexander et al., 2003; Braithwaite, Waldron, & Finn, 1999; Query & Wright, 2003; Sharf, 1997; Sullivan, 2003; Wright, 2002; Wright & Bell, 2003).

These groups have the potential for providing access to a larger support network for older individuals with cancer and their family members, and the features of these groups may be very helpful for those who have a limited number of people in their traditional support network, and/or problems receiving adequate support from current members. Online support groups, however, may not be helpful for all older people with cancer or their caregivers, especially those who have strong traditional support networks. They also may not be beneficial for individuals who lack access to the Internet, or the ability to participate effectively in these groups because of a variety of reasons such as low communication competence levels, income, education, and/or disabilities. Although the digital divide has become smaller in recent years, older adults who use the Internet are disproportionately more affluent and better educated than those who do not use it (see Wright & Query, 2004).

This chapter explores the potential of online support groups for older adults with cancer and their lay caregivers in terms of providing health benefits. Toward that end, we begin by reviewing literature on computer-mediated support groups for older adults, individuals with cancer, and caregivers. A model of online support group participation featuring communication competence, social support, and coping theory, as well as social network theory, and theories of CMC is then advanced.

STUDIES OF ONLINE SUPPORT GROUPS FOR OLDER ADULTS AND INDIVIDUALS WITH CANCER

There have been relatively few studies of online support groups for individuals with cancer, their lay caregivers, or peers, but there is some evidence that suggests these groups may provide health benefits. In a recent study by the authors, 76 older adults, recruited from 50 cancer-related e-mail list-serves and online communities, who were either cancer survivors or caregivers for a family member with cancer participated in a survey about how they used the Internet for social support. Employing quantitative and qualitative measures this study tested Kreps' (1988) Relational Health Communication Model by examining relationships among social support, communication competence, and perceived stress in a study of well elders, elderly individuals with cancer, and their lay caregivers. The authors also examined participant narratives focusing on positive and negative expressions of social support. The results indicated partial support for Kreps' (1988) Relational Health Communication Model. In particular, participants who were more communicatively competent were found to have lower levels of perceived stress, and they were more satisfied with the support offered by members of their support network. Additionally, the critical incidents revealed that participants received significantly more emotional/esteem support from their network than other social support types. This finding is in concert with the widespread view that emotional support, of all the support types, is most closely associated with health outcomes (Broadhead et al., 1983; Wills & Fegan, 2001).

In a study of an online cancer support group (with one-third of the sample being older adults), Wright (2002) found a modest significant correlation between perceptions of emotional support obtained within the online group and perceived life stress. Both individuals with cancer and their caregivers had similar perceived stress scores and similar motives for using the groups in that they were more interested in interpersonal relationships as opposed to obtaining information. Wright (2002) also found that caregivers for individuals with cancer enjoyed the same benefits of online support groups as individuals with cancer. Caregivers often experience frustration with caregiving duties and have difficulties talking about caregiving issues with friends and family. The Internet provides access to other caregivers who understand these frustrations, and participating in online cancer caregiver support groups can provide many caregivers with opportunities to find increased empathy and specialized information about caregiving that may be difficult to access in the face-to-face world. The findings of this study also indicated that individuals who perceived the online support group to be problematic in terms of the ability to assess the nonverbal cues of other participants had significantly lower emotional support scores.

Sullivan (2003) found that female users of online cancer support groups differed from male users in terms of the types of support they sought and provided others within the group. Although both men and women reported the groups to be beneficial in terms of coping with the cancer experience, women with cancer in this study were more likely to share their feelings, talk about pain and frustrations, and to be more emotionally expressive than male participants. Male participants tended to seek and provide information as opposed to sharing feelings and bonding emotionally with other men. Specifically, male participants tended to suggest helpful sources online that discussed relevant cancer research, talk about case histories and risk factors, and pose questions to the group and clarify information. However, male cancer patients did find the informational support they received online to be helpful and even empowering.

Although Sullivan's work was consistent with traditional male and female stereotypes, in one of the few experimental studies of gender effects and social support, Derlega, Barbee, and Winstead (1994) reported that "Even for relationship problems, females were not found to be superior to males as support providers in the laboratory situation" (p. 147). Additional investigations should assess the potential influences of gender.

Although there have been relatively few studies of online support groups for older individuals with cancer or their caregivers (or for individuals with cancer in general), there have been a number of studies in recent years that have examined other types of online support groups for people with health concerns. These studies have provided scholars with some insights into the unique nature of these groups and possible reasons why individuals use them. As Query and Wright (2004) reported in an earlier work, notwithstanding their growing popularity, to date, there has been no systematic attempt to catalogue and evaluate online support groups, and in particular, online cancer support groups.

Proceeding further, we noted that there has been no sustained inquiry that has attempted to measure the relationship between cancer support members' online communication competencies and health outcomes such as perceived coping and treatment choices. And although a variety of extant measures exist to assess face-to-face interaction, to the best of our knowledge, no similar measures are available for evaluating the efficacy of virtual cancer support group interaction. To help address the preceding gap, the following section presents a model of online support group participation based on previous work in this area.

A MODEL OF ONLINE SUPPORT GROUP PARTICIPATION

There are many reasons why individuals might be attracted to online support groups that have been identified in recent studies. Researchers have found that (a) participants feel these groups are more convenient than face-to-face groups because of their ability to transcend time and distance (Braithwaite et al., 1999; Sullivan, 2003; Wright, 2002); (b) the anonymity of the groups provide a safe environment for disclosing feelings and for minimizing judgments from others based on the stigma of illness, ethnicity, gender, and age (Braithwaite et al., 1999; Scott, 1999; Wright & Bell, 2003); (c) participants feel they have more time and control when constructing supportive messages (Braithwaite et al., 1999; Sullivan, 2003; Wright & Bell, 2003); (d) the perception exists that writing about one's health within these groups has therapeutic value (Binik, Cantor, Ochs, & Meana, 1997); and (e) users feel they can obtain multiple viewpoints and increased empathy from others facing similar health concerns (Preece & Ghozati, 2001; Wright & Bell, 2003).

Although these studies have helped provide a better understanding of online support groups for individuals with health concerns, they have not attempted to link empirical findings to a larger theoretical framework. Although there are many theories and models that have been used to explain certain aspects of online support groups in this body of research, a more encompassing theoretical framework is needed to explain the reasons why individuals may use online support groups over traditional support networks. Ideally, such a theoretical framework can also help undergird the measurement of key variables that are associated with selected health outcomes. In the following sections, we present a model of online support group participation based on previous work (see Wright & Bell, 2003; Wright & Query, 2004).

The model of online support group participation (Fig. 10.1) draws upon theoretical perspectives from extant research in communication competence, social support, and coping, as well as sociological inquiry, and the CMC literature. Specifically, it combines aspects of Communication Competence Theory (Kreps & Query, 1990; Spitzberg & Cupach, 1984; Wiemann, 1977), Weak Tie Support Network Theory (Adelman, Parks, & Albrecht, 1987; Granovetter, 1973, 1982), Social Network Analysis (Berkowitz, 1982; Wasserman & Faust, 1993; Wellman, 1997), and Social Information-Processing Theory (Walther, 1996; Walther & Boyd, 2002). The specific components of the model are discussed here.

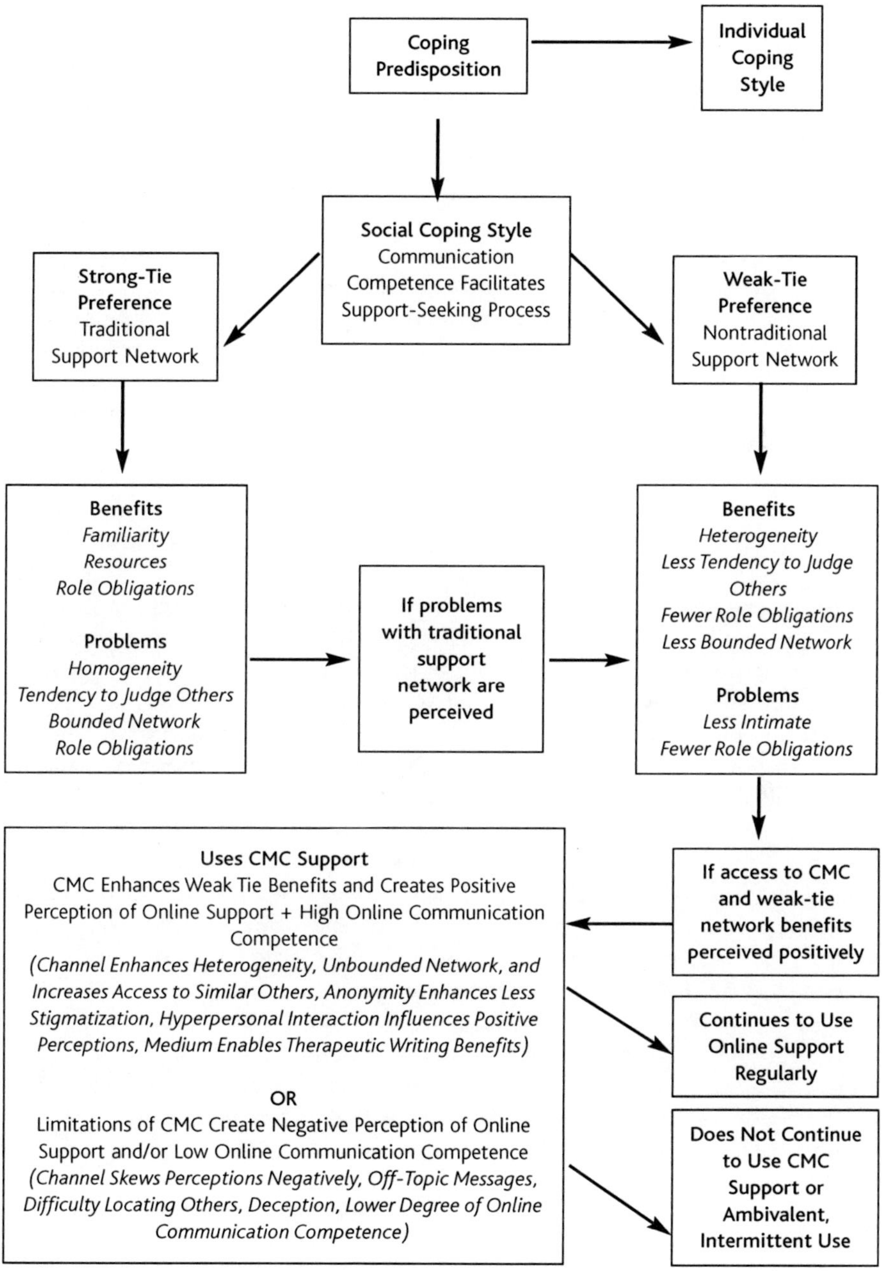

FIG. 10-1. Model of online support group participation.

Communication Competence and Moving Toward Online Conceptualizations

In a state-of-the-art review, Kreps and Query (1990) stated that, "Central to health communication inquiry is the assumption that effectiveness of health care depends largely on the communication skills and competencies of health care providers and consumers" (p. 294). Two years earlier, Kreps (1988) developed a model of relational health communication that posited that communication competence shaped a variety of health care outcomes, and that individuals' communication competence level should increase as the difficulty of negotiating the terrain (i.e., relevant context, such as cancer) increased. Query and associates confirmed key parts of the preceding model (see Query & James, 1989; Query & Kreps, 1996; Query, Parry, & Flint, 1992; Query & Wright, 2003) which cover a wide range of research participants including elders residing in retirement communities, caregivers for individuals with Alzheimer's disease, nontraditional students, and online support group and lists on members experiencing or providing care across cancer contexts. In those investigations, Wiemann's (1977) competence instrument, as altered by Brunner (1979), was used and yielded sound reliability levels.

Both scales used a five-point Likert scale where participants indicated the extent to which they agreed or disagreed with 36 statements describing their interaction with others. Sample items included, "I am easy to talk to"; "I am interested in what my partner has to say"; I am sensitive to others' needs of the moment." Based in part on the preceding foundation, it is reasonable to posit that communication competence should influence variables such as social coping style preference, ability to use strong or weak tie networks, and ability to use computer mediated communication (CMC).

As indicated earlier, to the best of our knowledge, no measure of online communication competence has been developed to help gauge online support group efficacy in general, and in particular, online cancer support groups. To begin to bridge this theoretical and methodological abyss, we (Query & Wright, 2004) anticipated seeking external funding to compile a census of online cancer support groups; create a measure of online communication competence with construct and face validity, as well as reliability levels; and develop an online clearinghouse to better coordinate information dissemination as well as social support provision and reception. The specific aims of this project follow:

1. Develop a census of online cancer support groups. During this process, key information would be sought and ultimately reported, such as sponsoring agency or organization, type of cancer and stage data if available, group member size, focus and history

of the group, background and training of facilitator(s), frequency of participation, satisfaction with participation, types of support, and satisfaction based on using other channels such as phone, e-mail, and/or face-face interaction; as well as frequency and types of social support, and satisfaction with social support available as members migrate with each other to distinct channels facilitating more real-time interaction (e.g., phone and/or face-to-face meetings).

2. Create a measure of online communication competency and health outcomes. Ideally, such a measure could help individuals living with cancer, their caregivers, and support group members better assess key benefits and disadvantages of cancer support group participation.

Addressing the proposed methodology, we would first conduct an extensive online search using a variety of search engines and other means to create a census of online cancer support groups. Second, we would facilitate five to six focus groups, with sizes ranging from five to nine members each. Prospective participants would be current and former online cancer support group members. To help develop the online communication competence measure, the Critical Incident Technique (CIT; Flanagan, 1954) would be used during the focus groups to generate recurring themes that would lead to the scale's construction (Query, Kreps, Arneson, & Caso, 2001; see Query & Wright, 2004, for detailed reviews of the CIT). Once the scale had been developed, it would be pilot tested over a 6-month period and factor analyzed.

Coping Predispositions

A cancer diagnosis is one of the most taxing life events a person can face, and communication often plays an essential role in the process of coping with a variety of stressful events and anxiety associated with living with cancer. According to Kreps (2003):

> Cancer survivors have unique communication needs to help them cope with the many uncertainties of living with cancer. For example, survivors typically have to cope with the fear of their cancer recurring. Survivors also need access to social support and relevant information to help them live with side effects of cancer treatments. Peer support from others who adapted to living with cancer can often help cancer survivors overcome both physical and psychosocial challenges and enable them to readjust to their everyday lives. (p. 165)

Individuals often vary considerably in terms of the coping strategies they use when faced with life-threatening diseases such as cancer. There is some debate in the coping literature whether coping predispositions are based on traits, or learned from prior stressful situations; however, both trait and state coping predispositions are thought to be important. Depending on their circumstances, individuals may decide to use avoidance-focused coping strategies, such as diverting their attention away from the stressful situation by engaging in activities; problem-focused coping, such as gathering information about the problem or mobilizing resources; or emotional-focused coping, such as venting frustrations (Kohn, 1996). In general, researchers have found that individuals who use problem-focused coping tend to adapt to stressful situations better than those who employ avoidance or emotional-focused strategies (Folkman, Lazarus, Gruen, & DeLongis, 1986; Kohn, 1996).

Additionally, some people choose individually based strategies for coping with stressful events, whereas other individuals are more socially oriented in terms of coping with stressful situations, and they seek various types of social support (Kohn, 1996; Pierce, Sarason, & Sarason, 1996). For example, studies have found that individuals who are facing illness often perceive emotional support as being more helpful than informational support, thereby often triggering a higher occurrence of emotional support than any other type of social support (Martin, Davis, Baron, Suls, & Blanchard, 1994; Query & Wright, 2003). These individuals may be more likely to cope with stress by seeking emotional support through their social network than by using more individually based coping strategies (e.g., obtaining information about cancer from a book).

The process of seeking the support of others, however, as a means for coping with a stressful situation can be highly complex. Albrecht and Goldsmith (2003) contended that support researchers need to recognize" the importance of relational coordination in achieving satisfactory support outcomes" (p. 272). When approaching one's social network(s) to obtain support, individuals are often faced with a surprising array of challenges in terms of meeting their support and coping needs while balancing their relational needs. According to Albrecht and Goldsmith (2003):

> Several researchers have called for a revised conceptualization of support in close relationships. This new framing of support casts it as a more complex dyadic phenomenon, in which partners must not only cope with a stressor but also cope with the relational strains created by the stressor and the need to coordinate their individual coping attempts. (p. 272)

Thus, the process of seeking support within relationships can be difficult for many individuals who must coordinate meeting their needs while simultaneously attempting to manage relational concerns. For example, many individuals find it difficult to obtain appropriate support from friends and family because they may not feel comfortable discussing their problems for a variety of reasons. An alternative to family and friends, when seeking support, is the use of weak-tie support networks, which may include online support groups, as well as non-human entities such as a higher power, pets, favorite music or readings, and/or deceased loved ones (see Query et al., 1992, for a discussion of "inanimate ties").

Weak-Tie Network Theory and Preferences for Weak-Tie Support

Granovetter (1973) originally developed weak-tie support network theory, which has been found useful for explaining various aspects of support groups in the face-to-face world and on the Internet (Walther & Boyd, 2002; Wright & Bell, 2003; Wright & Query, 2004). Weak-tie relationships typically occur between individuals who communicate on a relatively frequent basis, but who do not consider each other to be members of their close personal network (e.g., close friends, family). Prior to the Internet, weak-tie networks for most individuals consisted of neighbors, service providers, and other individuals to whom a person could turn during times of stress when closer ties were unavailable. Individuals facing stressful situations, such as life-threatening diseases, often find that weak-tie networks offer certain advantages in terms of social support. These advantages are explicated here.

One reason why some individuals may decide to seek support through weak-tie networks, instead of within their strong-tie network, is that weak tie networks often provide access to diverse points of view and information that may not be available within more intimate relationships (Adelman et al., 1987). Typically, many individuals form close relationships with others who are similar to them in terms of demographics, attitudes, and backgrounds. This homogeneous preference can limit the diversity of information and viewpoints obtained about topics, including health concerns.

Access to more diverse viewpoints about health problems can provide individuals with more varied informational support about health issues, and interacting with varied types of people increases the number of social comparisons a person can make about his or her health condition vis-à-vis others (Adelman et al., 1987). The opportunity for more social comparisons has been found to be an integral component of support groups (Helgeson & Gottlieb, 2000), and they often help individuals reduce uncertainty about their health condition. For example, a person who has been recently diagnosed with cancer will probably not find many people within his or her traditional support network who also have cancer. Therefore, their network members may only have a limited perspective about how to cope with the disease. By moving outside of one's traditional support network and using weak-tie networks, such as support groups, the individual can obtain more information about cancer from someone who also has the disease and who is likely to share similar feelings about it (even if he or she is dissimilar in terms of demographics, attitudes, and background). Furthermore, by interacting with multiple individuals with cancer in a support group, assessments about how one is coping with the disease compared to others can be made. This process can help people reduce uncertainty. For example, individuals who are in earlier stages of cancer can interact with others who are in the later stages and learn about possible trajectories of the disease, and/or glean firsthand information about the efficacy of treatment options.

Communicating About Illness in Weak-tie versus Close-Tie Networks. Close-tie support networks are sometimes perceived to be inadequate in terms of providing satisfactory support for a variety of reasons, and this notion may influence a person's decision to use weak-tie support networks as an alternative. Life-threatening illnesses are difficult topics for most people to discuss, especially when they are affecting a close loved one. In terms of talking about cancer, researchers have found that family members and friends often minimize the concerns of persons with cancer, avoid interacting with the individual, and/or steer conversational topics away from emotional talk about the disease, or refrain from any discussion of cancer (Dakof & Taylor, 1990; Dunkel-Schetter & Wortman, 1982; Helgeson, Cohen, Shultz, & Yasko, 2000; Wortman & Dunkel-Schetter, 1979).

Even when they wish to do so, many individuals with the disease often find it problematical to discuss cancer with family and close friends, primarily because of their desire not to burden anyone with problems caused by the disease (DiMatteo & Hays, 1981; Gotcher & Edwards, 1990). When they feel discomfort surrounding the discussion of cancer and have no firsthand experience with the disease, friends and family may find it difficult to provide appropriate support, and individuals with cancer often perceive support from loved ones negatively. For example, Dunkel-Schetter and Wortman (1982) found that patients with early-stage cancer did not appreciate being told "they would be okay," and they did not like being given directional advice or material assistance from loved ones.

Additionally, studies have found that role obligations in close ties and reciprocity issues can lead to problems with the provision of social support. Support from close ties for a loved one who is ill can lead to increased conflict or negative feelings toward the person because of role obligations (Albrecht & Goldsmith, 2003; Chesler & Barbarin, 1984; LaGaipa, 1990; Pitula & Daugherty, 1995). Although one may care deeply for those who are close to him or her, they can feel overburdened when a loved one becomes ill and needs a great amount of support (particularly when family members become caregivers), and the stress experienced can lead to conflict. Many individuals with cancer who receive support from family members and friends may also feel uncomfortable when they do not have the ability to reciprocate (Chesler & Barbarin, 1984). This discomfort is based on a sense of inequity that may lead a person with cancer to feel overbenefitted if he or she cannot help his or her friends in a similar manner. According to LaGaipa (1990), "social obligations may override the positive effect of companionship and social support. Such constraints may have a negative effect on mental well-being that may not make up for the beneficial aspects of personal relationships" (p. 126).

By comparison, certain members of weak-tie networks may be more willing to talk about cancer because they tend to be less emotionally attached to the person with cancer. For example, within face-to-face and online cancer support groups, members of the group frequently allow other members to share their concerns and feelings about living with the disease. Because the other group members are also contending with cancer, the similarity between the members increases understanding of the other members' situation and fosters opportunities for increased empathy and other types of emotional support (e.g., validation). Additionally, weak-tie network members are often able to provide more objective feedback about a problem because they are less emotionally attached to a person with cancer than family and friends. According to La Gaipa (1990), "confidants are not likely to provide an accurate reflection of what a person is worth. Rather, one must turn to less intimate friends for more accurate feedback" (p. 126). The combination of increased similarity within these groups, being less emotionally attached to members than members of one's close-tie network, and the tendency to have fewer stringent role obligations in this context, allows support group members to discuss difficult issues related to diseases like cancer with a greater sense of freedom than is often found when discussing the same issues among closer ties.

Moreover, the combination of similarity of problems and the tendency of people in weak-tie networks to be somewhat removed from a person's primary social network has been found to facilitate the discussion of more risky topics. Because members of weak-tie networks do not typically share an intimate relational history with each other, they are less likely to be judgmental (Adelman et al., 1987). Cancer, like many other diseases and medical conditions, has been found to carry a social stigma (Mathieson, Logan-Smith, Phillips, MacPhee, & Attia, 1996; Sullivan & Reardon, 1985), and this dehumanizing process can negatively affect the provision of social support (Bloom & Spiegel, 1984).

For example, support group members often report feeling a greater sense of freedom communicating about their problems with other members who do not know them particularly well; yet, they understand their situation because they are experiencing similar issues, and therefore are less likely to pass judgment on what is said within the group (Cline, 1999). Weak-tie networks may also be helpful for caregivers, as well as individuals facing cancer. Wright (2000a) found that caregivers enjoyed talking to other caregivers in online support groups because they could complain about the difficulties associated with caregiving without being judged by others. In contrast, they often felt judged by family members and friends when they complained about their caregiving duties.

Members of online support groups are often separated by great distances and less likely to interact with one another than face-to-face weak-tie network members, and these features may facilitate the self-disclosure of intense feelings and concerns about cancer without fear of judgment from others. Additionally, the text-based communication within these groups can provide members with a greater sense of anonymity than in face-to-face support group contexts, which may further facilitate the discussion of interpersonally risky topics (Walther & Boyd, 2002; Wright & Bell, 2003).

Social Network Theory and Computer-Mediated Groups

Social Network Theory (Berkowitz, 1982; Wasserman & Faust, 1993) is a helpful framework for understanding differences between face-to-face and computer-mediated social networks. Wellman (1997) described computer networks as "unbounded networks," and relationships within this type of network "are usually better connected to other, more diverse social circles, and hence apt to be sources of new information" (p. 189). Essentially, face-to-face networks tend to be bounded, indicating that the interrelationships between network members are somewhat limited to contextual boundaries. Although social networks in the face-to-face world certainly have permeable boundaries to some extent, most relationships among network members typically stay within a contextually specific population (e.g., a workplace, neighborhoods, organizations).

According to Wellman (1997), although computer networks support bounded networks and unbounded networks, they facilitate the creation of unbounded networks in ways that would be very difficult in the face-to-face world, or through other media. As Wellman (1997) argued:

> Many computer networks support unbounded social networks because both private e-mail and computerized conferences make it easy and inexpensive to maintain connections with distant acquaintances and form new ties with strangers. Such "weak ties" are usually better connected to other, more diverse social circles, and hence are more apt to be sources of new information. (p. 189)

Wellman (1997) elaborated by stating that the low social presence of e-mail and other popular text-based forms of CMC makes it easier for many individuals to engage in conversations with online strangers with less concern about rude intrusions or interpersonal risks. In terms of social support, computer networks (including the Internet) often blur boundaries between people from different backgrounds, organizations, communities, and other social network contexts. Subsequently, relationships that would likely never develop because of contextual boundaries in the face-to-face world, flourish on the Internet because Internet relationships tend to be based on shared interests, as opposed to demographic similarity. Unlike other contexts, physical proximity is not necessary to build trust and consensus among communicators. Wellman (1997) mentioned that computer networks "help people to maintain a stockpile of potentially useful contacts outside of their work group, organization, or community that can provide information, instrumental aid, and emotional support" (p. 189).

Additionally, the Internet has the capacity to extend the range of social networks, or how large and diverse a population is within a particular contextual boundary. Because physical presence is not required to form and maintain relationships online, Internet users are able to maintain more relationships than is possible in the face-to-face world. Wellman (1997) contended, "the resulting expansion of the size and proximity of one's online 'communication audience' can increase the diversity of people encountered" (p. 191). This view is in contrast to traditional face-to-face social networks where individuals tend to interact with a finite set of individuals as opposed to sparse networks. Wellman (1997) argued that in the face-to-face world, "because of the difficulty of coordinating sparse networks, interactions are more apt to be one-on-one, and much information tends to be privately held with a dyad or selectively shared with sparsely knit sets of similar minded people" (p. 193).

Given these characteristics of the medium, the Internet has the potential to extend the support network of older individuals facing cancer. Older adults with cancer, who choose to use the Internet for social support, have the option of communicating messages privately using e-mail or they can obtain diverse viewpoints from others by posting their messages at the community level.

Computer-Mediated Communication Influences

Social Information-Processing Theory (Ramirez, Walther, Burgoon, & Sunnafrank, 2002; Walther, 1996) asserts that in CMC, message senders portray themselves in a socially favorable manner to draw the attention of message receivers and foster anticipation of future interaction. Message receivers, in turn, tend to idealize the image of the sender due to overvaluing minimal, text-based cues. Additionally, the asynchronous format of most computer-mediated interaction (and to some extent in synchronous formats, such as chatrooms) gives the sender and the receiver more time to edit their communication, making computer-mediated interactions more controllable and less stressful compared to the immediate feedback loop inherent in face-to-face interactions. Idealized perceptions and optimal self-presentation in the CMC process tend to intensify in the feedback loop, and this emphasis often leads to what Walther termed *hyperpersonal interaction*, or a more intimate and socially desirable exchange than face-to-face interactions. According to Walther (1996), the hyperpersonal nature of CMC is enhanced when long-term future interaction is anticipated and when no face-to-face relationship exists, so that users construct impressions and present themselves "without the interference of environmental reality" (p. 33).

Hyperpersonal interaction has been found to skew perceptions of relational partners in positive ways, and in some cases, computer-mediated relationships may exceed face-to-face interactions in terms of intensity (King & Moreggi, 1998; Ramirez et al., 2002; Walther, 1996; Wright & Bell, 2003). There is some evidence that relationships within computer-mediated support groups may be affected by hyperpersonal interaction (Walther & Boyd, 2002). For example, in a qualitative study of an online community for older adults, Wright (2002a) found that a relatively large number of caregivers reported that people in their online support network were perceived as being closer than even members of their own immediate family. Participants mentioned that the people they turned to for online support understood their problems better than non-Internet supporters, despite the fact that they had never met members of their online support network in the face-to-face world.

COMPUTER-MEDIATED SUPPORT GROUPS AS A FUNCTIONAL ALTERNATIVE TO FULFILLING UNMET SUPPORT NEEDS IN THE FACE-TO-FACE WORLD.

Ferguson and Perse (2000) provided a comprehensive explanation of when a specific medium can be a "functional alternative" to another medium (including the use of face-to-face social networks). According to these authors, most individuals select media they believe will help them achieve their goals or meet their needs; they make choices among functional alternatives, or communication channels that can fulfill similar goals or needs. Papacharissi and Rubin (2000) concluded that individuals use CMC as a "functional alternative" when face-to-face communication is perceived as difficult or not preferred. For example, individuals who were "less satisfied and who felt less valued in their face-to-face communication used the Internet as a functional alternative to interpersonal communication" (p. 192). In the case of online support, there is some evidence that computer-mediated support groups may be perceived as a functional alternative to face-to-face support, especially when face-to-face support networks are not perceived as helpful in terms of meeting goals/needs.

Some researchers have argued that electronic social support helps to satisfy unmet needs in face-to-face relationships (Egdorf & Rahoi, 1994; Walther & Boyd, 2002). For example, Finn and Lavitt (1994) found that the anonymity of an online support group of sexual abuse survivors decreased the level of anxiety members experienced about sharing shameful experiences in face-to-face relationships. Alexander et al. (2003) found that members of an online cancer support group were satisfied with the amount and quality of the information they received and "some members even stated that they used the group as a source of information because they mistrusted doctors and other members of the medical community" (p. 326). Moreover, computer-mediated support groups have been found to be an alternative source of information to that which is obtained from a professional such as a physician or therapist. According to Preece (1999), "Physicians can provide the facts, but other patients can tell you what it really feels like and what to expect next, in a way that only someone with personal experience can" (p. 63). That is, some individuals often need to identify with the feelings of a person who is experiencing a health issue first-hand, and this type of information is unlikely to be met by traditional providers (who tend to offer only information about diseases such as cancer).

Additionally, Walther and Boyd (2002) contended that users of online self-help groups tend to be less concerned about being judged negatively by fellow members of their virtual online group than they would be when discussing these matters with off-line friends and family. King and Moreggi (1998) argued that the increased opportunities for self-disclosure and intimacy with similar others in online support groups may lead participants to become actively engaged in their online relationships to the exclusion of all others.

Other Perceived Advantages of Computer-Mediated Support Groups. Weinberg, Schmale, Liken, and Wesse (1995) posited that the therapeutic value of writing down problems in text-based computer-mediated support groups may allow for more distance from others and reflection without worrying about the immediate responses from others. Diamond (2000) claimed that writing messages down seemed to create some distance between individuals and their dilemmas helping people connect with the larger culture. Braithwaite et al. (1999), in a study of online support groups for individuals with disabilities, mentioned that the lack of pressure for an immediate response when composing messages to online support group members created opportunities for more thoughtful comments, and that "this feature may be an especially salient advantage for those with communication-related disabilities who find the computer liberates them from the difficulties they encounter with oral speech" (p. 143).

Computer-mediated support groups can offer a forum for those who feel stigmatized by their health conditions thereby encouraging the disclosure of personal information with a sense of safety. This sense of safety is due, in part, to the anonymity (or at least pseudonymity) of online communication, which gives people an opportunity to talk about their problems with others coping with the same issues, without all the complications of face-to-face relationships (Wallace, 1999). Conversely, one's physical presence in face-to-face support groups, even those that strive to maintain the anonymity of their members, can undermine a person's sense of safety when communicating about health conditions that carry a social stigma, including cancer. According to Galagher, Sproull, and Kiesler (1998):

> Confidentiality regarding the (face-to-face) group's proceedings may be expected, but one's physical presence and the possibility of encountering others in one's community create a risk of unwanted public exposure. Furthermore, these groups often exert social pressure on members to participate actively and to disclose their thoughts and feelings. Small size, local geography, and social pressure make these groups less private, less anonymous, and more conformist than are electronic social support groups. (p. 497).

Perceived Disadvantages of Computer-Mediated Support Groups. Although online support groups may offer a number of advantages to participants, it is certainly possible for individuals to view features of these groups and aspects of CMC in ambivalent or negative ways. These ambivalent or negative perceptions, if perceived by individuals as outweighing positive aspects of the groups, are likely to curtail use of online support groups. Several researchers have identified negative aspects of online support groups. Wright (2000b) found that one of the most frequently reported disadvantages of asynchronous online support groups is the inability to find a particular person online at a specific time. This obstacle may have an adverse effect on the timing of support and the immediacy of communication between support providers and recipients. The inability of the medium to enable individuals to give and receive various types of touch has also been reported to be especially problematic for online support group members confronting health issues (Braithwaite et al., 1999; Wright, 2000b).

Additionally, studies have found other sources of dissatisfaction when using online support groups (Galinski, Schopler, & Abell, 1997; King & Moreggi, 1998; Preece, 1998; Preece & Ghozati, 2001; Walther & Boyd, 2002; Wright, 2000b). Participants often find the lack of immediacy when communicating with others frustrating; difficulty when expressing and interpreting emotions due to reduced nonverbal cues; dissatisfaction with the inability to touch others; frustration with unwanted messages from unsolicited parties participating in the group (including spam messages); and increased opportunities for some individuals to misrepresent themselves to the group.

Summary of Model and Implications for Older Adults With Cancer and Their Caregivers

The model of online support group participation posits that there are a number of factors that may influence individuals with health concerns, such as individuals with cancer or their caregivers, to use a computer-mediated support group. First, a person's coping predisposition when faced with a disease like cancer and level of communication competence may lead them toward individually oriented or socially oriented coping strategies. Although individuals can certainly engage in both individual and social coping strategies, previous research suggests that people can be somewhat trait-like in their choice of coping strategies (Kohn, 1996), with some individuals preferring more individually oriented strategies and others gravitating toward more socially oriented strategies. For those individuals who prefer to interact with others when coping with stressful situations associated with health conditions like cancer, they have two broad choices in terms of social support network types: strong ties or weak ties.

Strong-tie and weak-tie support networks have their relative advantages and disadvantages. In general, most people, including cancer patients, gravitate toward strong-tie support networks during times of stress (Albrecht & Goldsmith, 2003), but although this type of network has many advantages, there are a number of problems with them as well in terms of their ability to provide satisfactory support. Some individuals may choose weak-tie support networks initially, especially if there are few people to whom they can turn in their close-tie support network; or if they feel it would be difficult to obtain information or empathy from their existing close-tie network, or they simply may not want to burden family members and friends with problems associated with the stress of coping with a life-threatening illness.

Yet, most individuals tend to choose weak-tie networks when they feel that there are deficiencies in the type of support they are receiving from close-tie network members, or if their support needs are not being met by members of this network. In such cases, these individuals may be more likely to try using a weak-tie support network, including traditional weak ties in face-to-face daily interaction (e.g., chatting with a bus driver as one rides to work about some health condition) or face-to-face support networks in an attempt to benefit from the supportive advantages that this type of network can offer.

If individuals are cognizant of the advantages of using weak-tie networks for support, have access to the Internet, are aware of online support groups and view them positively, and have the ability to use them, then the model posits that they may be more likely to use these groups. If the features of the online support groups are seen as advantageous and perceived positively and individuals possess online communication competence, then participation in these groups should intensify the advantages of weak tie network support, and participation in these groups is more likely to continue. If there is ambivalence or it is perceived that disadvantages of using these groups outweigh the advantages, and/or there is low online communication competence, then participation in them is less likely to continue.

Implications of Model for Older Adults With Cancer and Their Lay Caregivers. For older individuals with cancer or their lay caregivers, this model may help to explain why some individuals are attracted to computer-mediated support groups whereas others are not. Additionally, it may help researchers identify potential barriers to using online supports, and the model may provide a theoretical framework for designing interventions for older individuals with cancer or their caregivers. The proposed model is not without limitations. It would also be presumptuous to suggest that it is all encompassing in terms of including all of the key variables that may predict online support group participation. The model needs to be tested empirically in future research to assess its validity, and as a series of empirical studies unfold, it is likely its initial form will be altered. In the interim, the embryonic model should help provide a heuristic framework for future inquiry in the area of online support group participation: particularly for individuals with cancer and their lay caregivers.

REFERENCES

Adelman, M. B., Parks, M. R., & Albrecht, T. L. (1987). Beyond close relationships: Support in weak ties. In T. L. Albrecht & M. B. Adelman (Eds.), *Communicating social support* (pp. 126-147). Newbury Park, CA: Sage.

Albrecht, T. L., & Goldsmith, D. J. (2003). Social support, social networks, and health. In T. L. Thompson, A. M. Dorsey, K. I. Miller, & R. Parrott (Eds.), *Handbook of health communication* (pp. 263-284). Mahwah, NJ: Erlbaum.

Alexander, S. C., Peterson, J. L., & Hollingshead, A. B. (2003). Help is at your keyboard: Support groups on the Internet. In L. R. Frey (Ed.), *Group communication in context: Studies of bona fide groups* (2nd ed., pp. 309-334). Mahwah, NJ: Erlbaum.

American Cancer Society. (2001). *Cancer statistics.* Retrieved November 1, 2002, from http://www.cancer.org/cancerinfo/

Berkowitz, S. D. (1982). *An introduction to structural analysis: The network approach to social research.* Toronto: Butterworth.

Binik, Y. M., Cantor, J., Ochs, E., & Meana, M. (1997). From the couch to the keyboard: Psychotherapy in cyberspace. In S. Kiesler (Ed.), *Culture of the Internet* (pp. 71-100). Mahwah, NJ: Erlbaum.

Bloom, J. R., & Spiegel, D. (1984). The relationship of two dimensions of social support to the psychological well-being and social functioning of women with advanced breast cancer. *Social Science Medicine, 19,* 831-837.

Braithwaite, D. O., Waldron, V. R., & Finn, J. (1999). Communication of social support in computer-mediated groups for people with disabilities. *Health Communication, 11,* 123-151.

Broadhead, W. E., Kaplan, B. H., James, S. A., Wagner, E. H., Schoenbach, V. J., Grimson, R., Heyden, S., Tibblin, G., & Gehlbach, S. H. (1983). The epidemiologic evidence for a relationship between social support and health. *American Journal of Epidemiology, 117,* 521-537.

Brunner, C. C. (1979). *An examination of the relationship between interpersonal communication competence and androgyny.* Unpublished master's thesis, Miami University, Oxford, OH.

Burleson, B. R., Albrecht, T. L., Goldsmith, D. J., & Sarason, I. G. (1994). Introduction: The communication of social support. In B. R. Burleson, T. L. Albrecht, & I. G. Sarason (Eds.), *Communication of social support: Messages, interactions, relationships, and community* (pp. xi-xxx). Thousand Oaks, CA: Sage.

Chesler, M. A., & Barbarin, O. A. (1984). Difficulties of providing help in a crisis: Relationships between parents of children with cancer and their friends. *Journal of Social Issues, 40,* 113-134.

Cline, R. J. (1999). Communication within social support groups. In L. R. Frey, D. S. Gouran, & M. S. Poole (Eds.), *Handbook of group communication theory and research* (pp. 516-538). Thousand Oaks, CA: Sage.

Dakof, G. A., & Taylor, S. E. (1990). Victim's perceptions of social support: What is helpful from whom? *Journal of Personality and Social Psychology, 58,* 80-89.

Davison, K. P., Pennebaker, J. W., & Dickerson, S. S. (2000). Who talks? The social psychology of illness support groups. *American Psychologist, 55,* 205-217.

Derlega, V. J., Barbee, A. P., & Winstead, B. A. (1994). Friendship, gender, and social support: Laboratory studies of supportive interactions. In B. R. Burleson, T. L. Albrecht, & I. G. Sarason (Eds.), *Communication of social support: Messages, interactions, relationships, and community* (pp. 136-151). Thousand Oaks, CA: Sage.

Diamond, J. (2000). *Narrative means to sober ends: Treating addiction and its aftermath.* New York: Guilford.

DiMatteo, M., & Hays, R. (1981). Social support and serious illness. In B. Gottlieb (Ed.), *Social networks and social support* (pp. 117-148). Beverly Hills, CA: Sage.

Dunkel-Schetter, C., & Wortman, C. D. (1982). The interpersonal dynamics of cancer: Problems in social relationships and their impact on the patient. In H. S. Friedman & M. R. DiMatteo (Eds.), *Interpersonal issues in health care* (pp. 69-100). New York: Academic Press.

Egdorf, K., & Rahoi, R. L. (1994, November). *Finding a place where "we all want to hear it": E-mail as a source of social support*. Paper presented at the annual meeting of the Speech Communication Association, New Orleans, LA.

Ferguson, D. A., & Perse, E. M. (2000). The World Wide Web as a functional alternative to television. *Journal of Broadcasting & Electronic Media, 44*, 155-174.

Finn, J., & Lavitt, M. (1994). Computer-based self-help/mutual aid groups for sexual abuse survivors. *Social Work with Groups, 17*, 21-46.

Flanagan, J. C. (1954). The critical incident technique. *Psychological Bulletin, 51*, 327-357.

Flint, L. J., Query, J. L., & Parrish, A. (2005). Negotiating communication obstacles while experiencing Alzheimer's disease: The case of one family. In E. B. Ray (Ed.), *Case studies in health communication* (2nd ed., pp. 223-232). Mahwah, NJ: Erlbaum.

Folkman, S., Lazarus, R. S., Gruen, R. J., & DeLongis, A. (1986). Appraisal, coping, health status, and psychological symptoms. *Journal of Personality and Social Psychology, 50*, 571-579.

Fox, S. A., Giles, H., Orbe, M. P., & Bourhis, R. Y. (200). Interability communication: Theoretical perspectives. In D. O. Braithwaite & T. L. Thompson (Eds.), *Handbook of communication and people with disabilities: Research and application* (pp. 193-222). Mahwah, NJ: Erlbaum.

Galagher, J., Sproull, L., & Kiesler, S. (1998). Legitimacy, authority, and community in electronic support groups. *Written Communication, 15*, 493-530.

Galinski, M. J., Schopler, J. H., & Abell, M. D. (1997). Connecting group members through telephone and computer groups. *Health and Social Work, 22*, 181-189.

Gotcher, J. M., & Edwards, R. (1990). Coping strategies of cancer patients: Actual communication and imagined interactions. *Health Communication*, 2, 255-266.

Granovetter, M. S. (1973). The strength of weak ties. *American Journal of Sociology, 78*, 1360-1380.

Granovetter, M. S. (1982). The strength of weak ties: A network theory revisited. In P. V. Marsden & N. Lin (Eds.), *Social structure and network analysis* (pp. 105-130). Newbury Park, CA: Sage.

Helgeson, V. S., Cohen, S., Schultz, R., & Yasko, J. (2000). Group support interventions for women with breast cancer: Who benefits from what? *Health Psychology, 19*, 107-114.

Helgeson, V. S., & Gottlieb, B. H. (2000). Support groups. In S. Cohen, L. G. Underwood, & B. H. Gottlieb (Eds.), *Social support measurement and intervention* (pp. 221-245). New York: Oxford University Press.

Hewitt, M., Rowland, J., & Yancik, R. (2003). Cancer survivors in the United States: Age, health, and disability. *The Journals of Gerontology, Series A*, *58*(1), 82-92.

King, S. A., & Moreggi, D. (1998). Internet therapy and self help groups—the pros and cons. In J. Gackenbach (Ed.), *Psychology and the Internet: Intrapersonal, interpersonal and transpersonal implications* (pp. 77-109). San Diego, CA: Academic Press.

Kohn, P. M. (1996). On coping adaptively with daily hassles. In M. Zeidner & N. S. Endler (Eds.), *Handbook of coping* (pp. 181-201). New York: Wiley.

Kreps, G. L. (1988). Relational communication in health care. *Southern Speech Communication Journal, 53*, 344-359.

Kreps, G. L. (2003). The impact of communication on cancer risk, incidence, morbidity, mortality, and quality of life. *Health Communication*, *15*, 161-169.

Kreps , G. L., & Chapelsky Massimilla, D. (2002). Cancer communications research and health outcomes: Review and challenge. *Communication Studies, 53*(4), 318-336.

Kreps, G. L., & Query, J. L. (1990). Health communication and interpersonal competence. In G. M. Phillips and J. T. Wood (Eds.), *Speech communication: Essays to celebrate the 75th anniversary of the Speech Communication Association* (pp. 293-323). Carbondale: Southern Illinois University Press.

LaGaipa, J. L. (1990). The negative effects of informal support systems. In S. Duck & R. C. Silver (Eds.), *Personal relationships and social support* (pp. 122-139). Newbury Park, CA: Sage.

Lewis, J., Ng, K., Hung, K. E., Bilker, W.B., Berlin, J. A., Brensinger, C., & Rustgi, A. K. (2003). Detection of proximal adenomatous polyps with screening sigmoidoscopy: A systematic review and meta-analysis of screening colonoscopy. *Archives of Internal Medicine*, *163*(4), 413-421.

Mathieson, C. M., Logan-Smith, L. L., Phillips, J., MacPhee, M., & Attia, M. L. (1996). Caring for head and neck oncology patients: Does social support lead to better quality of life? *Canadian Family Physician*, *42*, 1712-1720.

Martin, R., Davis, G. M., Baron, R. S., Suls, J., & Blanchard, E. B. (1994). Specificity in social support: Perceptions of helpful and unhelpful provider behaviors among irritable bowel syndrome, headache, and cancer patients. *Health Psychology*, *13*, 432-439.

National Telecommunications and Information Administration. (2002). *Falling through the Net: Toward digital inclusion* [Online]. Washington, DC: United States Commerce Department. Available: http://www.search.ntia.doc.gov/pdf/fttn00.pdf

Papacharissi, Z., & Rubin, A. M. (2000). Predictors of internet use. *Journal of Broadcasting Electronic Media*, *44*, 175-196.

Pierce, G. R., Sarason, I. G., & Sarason, B. R. (1996). Coping and social support. In M. Zeidner and N. S. Endler (Eds.), *Handbook of coping* (pp. 434-451). New York: Wiley.

Pitula, C. R., & Daugherty, S. R. (1995). Sources of social support and conflict in hospitalized depressed women. *Nursing and Health, 18*, 325-332.

Preece, J. (1998). Empathetic communities: Reaching out across the web. *Interactions, 2*, 32-43.

Preece, J. (1999). Empathetic communities: Balancing emotional and factual communication. *Interacting with Computers: The Interdisciplinary Journal of Human-Computer Interaction, 12*, 63-77.

Preece, J. J., & Ghozati, K. (2001). Experiencing empathy on-line. In R. E. Rice & J. E. Katz (Eds.), *The Internet and health communication: Experiences and expectations* (pp. 237-260). Thousand Oaks, CA: Sage.

Query, J. L., & Flint, L. J. (1996). The caregiving relationship. In N. Vanzetti & S. Duck (Eds.), *A lifetime of relationships* (pp. 455-483). Pacific Grove, CA: Brooks/Cole.

Query, J. L., & James, A. C. (1989). The relationship between interpersonal communication competence and social support among elderly support groups in retirement communities. *Health Communication, 1*(3), 165-184.

Query, J. L., & Kreps, G. L. (1996). Testing a health communication model among caregivers for individuals with Alzheimer's disease. *Journal of Health Psychology, 1*(3), 335-351.

Query, J. L., Kreps, G. L., Arneson, P. A., & Caso, N. S. (2001). Towards helping organizations manage interaction: The theoretical and pragmatic merits of the critical incident technique. In S. L. Herndon & G. L. Kreps (Eds.),*Qualitative research: Applications in organizational life* (2nd ed., pp. 91-119). Cresskill, NJ: Hampton Press.

Query, J. L., Parry, D., & Flint, L. J. (1992). The relationship among social support, communication competence, and cognitive depression for non-traditional students. *Journal of Applied Communication Research, 20*(1), 78-94.

Query, J. L., Jr., & Wright, K. B. (2003). Assessing communication competence in an online study: Toward informing subsequent interventions among older adults with cancer, their lay caregivers, and peers. *Health Communication, 15*(2), 205-219.

Query, J. L., & Wright, K. B. (2004, April). *Profiling and assessing online cancer support group efficacy and online communication competence.* Abbreviated NIH grant abstract presented at the annual conference of the Central States Communication Association, Cleveland, OH.

Ramirez, A., Jr., Walther, J. B., Burgoon, J. K., & Sunnafrank, M. (2002). Information-seeking strategies, uncertainty, and computer-mediated communication: Toward a conceptual model. *Human Communication Research, 28*, 213-228.

Scott, C. R. (1999). The impact of physical and discursive anonymity on group members' multiple identifications during computer supported decision making. *Western Journal of Communication, 63*, 456-487.

Sharf, B. F. (1997). Communicating breast cancer on-line: Support and empowerment on the Internet. *Women & Health, 26*, 65-84.

Spitzberg, B. H., & Cupach, W. R. (1984). *Interpersonal communication competence.* Beverly Hills, CA: Sage.

Sullivan, C. F. (2003). Gendered cybersupport: A thematic analysis of two on-line cancer support groups. *Journal of Health Psychology, 8*, 83-103.

Sullivan, C. F., & Reardon, K. K. (1985). Social support satisfaction and health locus of control: Discriminators of breast cancer patients' style of coping. In M. L. McLaughlin (Ed.), *Communication yearbook* (Vol. 9, pp. 707-722). Beverly Hills, CA: Sage.

Wallace, P. (1999). *The psychology of the internet.* Cambridge, UK: Cambridge University Press.

Walther, J. B. (1996). Computer-mediated communication: Impersonal, interpersonal, and hyperpersonal interaction. *Communication Research, 23*, 3-43.

Walther, J. B., & Boyd, S. (2002). Attraction to computer-mediated social support. In C. A. Lin & D. Atkin (Eds.), *Communication technology and society: Audience adoption and uses* (pp. 153-188). Cresskill, NJ: Hampton Press.

Wasserman, S., & Faust, K. (1993). *Social network analysis: Methods and applications.* Cambridge, UK: Cambridge University Press.

Weinberg, N., Schmale, J. D., Uken, J., & Wessel, K. (1995). Computer-mediated support groups. *Social Work with Groups, 17*, 43-55.

Wellman, B. (1997). An electronic group is virtually a social network. In S. Kiesler (Ed.), *Culture of the Internet* (pp. 179–205). Mahwah, NJ: Erlbaum.

Wiemann, J. M. (1977). Explication and test of a model of communicative competence. *Human Communication Research, 3*, 195-213.

Wills, T. A., & Fegan, M. F. (2001). Social networks and social support. In A. Baum, T. Revenson, & J. E. Singer (Eds.), *Handbook of health psychology* (pp. 209-234). Mahwah, NJ: Erlbaum.

Wortman, C. B., & Dunkel-Schetter, C. (1979). Interpersonal relationships and cancer: A theoretical analysis. *Journal of Social Issues, 35*, 120-155.

Wright, K. B. (2000a). The communication of social support within an on-line community for older adults: A qualitative analysis of the SeniorNet community. *Qualitative Research Reports in Communication, 1*, 33-43.

Wright, K. B. (2000b). Perceptions of on-line support providers: An examination of perceived homophily, source credibility, communication and social support within on-line support groups. *Communication Quarterly, 48*, 44-59.

Wright, K. B. (2002). Social support within an on-line cancer community: An assessment of emotional support, perceptions of advantages and disadvantages, and motives for using the community. *Journal of Applied Communication Research, 3*, 195-209.

Wright, K. B., & Bell, S. B. (2003). Health-related support groups on the Internet: Linking empirical findings to social support and computer-mediated communication theory. *Journal of Health Psychology, 8*, 39-54.

Wright, K. B., & Query, J. L., Jr. (2004). Online support and older adults: A theoretical examination of benefits and limitations of computer-mediated support networks for older adults and possible health outcomes. In J. F. Nussbaum & J. Coupland (Eds.), *Handbook of communication and aging research* (2nd ed., pp. 499-519). Mahwah, NJ: Erlbaum.

11

When the Parent Has Cancer

A Life-Span Developmental Approach to Adult Child Perceptions of Communication Competency, Humor Orientation, and Relational Satisfaction in the Older Adult Parent–Adult Child Relationship

Elizabeth Harzold

George Mason University

Lisa Sparks

Chapman University

REVIEW OF LITERATURE

When a parent is diagnosed with cancer, the entire family is affected. The ability for a parent to effectively communicate with his or her adult child during this period is one essential component for helping the adult child cope with the complexities of a cancer diagnosis. To maintain a satisfying relationship between the parent and adult child, coping tactics must be employed by both parties. Humor is one possible coping method. This chapter takes a life-span developmental communicative approach to evaluating the relationships between communication competency, humor orientation, and relational satisfaction based on adult children's perceptions of their cancer-diagnosed parent's communication with them.

COMMUNICATION ACROSS THE LIFE SPAN

Life-span communication is not just about communication by, with, and about older adults. Life-span communication, rather, is about the developmental processes related to the aging process also known as getting older, despite the age period examined in a particular study. Nussbaum, Pecchioni, Robinson, and Thompson (2000) stated that our communicative behaviors and functions change across the life span as we adapt to age-related diagnoses such as cancer. Close relationships that are defined, maintained, negotiated, and renegotiated by communication across the life span are not stagnant in nature because individuals change as their relationships age. The relationships we maintain with our children, parents, and grandparents; spouses; and our friendship relationships are in a steady state of fluctuation as we negotiate and adapt to age-related biological, economic, psychological, and social circumstances (Nussbaum, Baringer, Fisher, & Kundrat, Chapter 4, this volume). Furthermore, at various times throughout the life span, the intimacy as well as power elements of the parent–child relationship appear to govern our lives, whereas at other points in the life span, our marital and friendship relationships take over with a much diminished role for our parents and siblings.

The diagnosis of cancer simultaneously changes an individual's life course with the disease and the life and relational courses of adult children as well as the spouse, grandchildren, siblings, and friends (Nussbaum et al., Chapter 4, this volume). The caring and psychosocial adaptations that must transpire to ensure a reliable quality of life for the older cancer patient depend to a great extent on those family and friends who have shared meaningful life moments and support throughout life (Nussbaum et al., 2000). However, the caring burden for adult children can be overwhelming and quite difficult.

CANCER COMMUNICATION

Cancer communication offers relevant health information at the interpersonal and family level with the goal of enhancing quality of life (Sparks, 2003). As a result of the broad range of different cancer conditions and issues, it is important to address the "psychological and socioemotional issues surrounding different individuals' experiences with cancer" (Kreps, 2003, p. 163). Once diagnosed, the patient with cancer is bombarded with a new environment characterized by intense emotions often including anger and fear. The cancer diagnosis reshapes social constructions of reality and the relationships with other healthy individuals, including their families (Sparks, 2003). How families learn to cope with cancer is important for improving their quality of life. Communication competency and humor orientation are traits that may aid patients and their families in this process.

Parents who can competently communicate their cancer diagnosis and treatment plans may offer their children a better understanding of the disease. Query and Kreps (1996) suggested that communication competence influences health outcomes. With increased competency, cancer patients can enact skills that include empathic listening and verbal and nonverbal messages that are encoded and decoded to manage the situation with sensitivity. Whether a child feels his or her parent is effectively conveying information and responding appropriately may affect the relational satisfaction of the parent–child dyad.

One type of communication that can be utilized skillfully is humor. Humor is an integral part of human existence. Occurring in the initiation, maintenance, and termination of relationships, humor is employed in a variety of communicative situations (Wanzer, Booth-Butterfield, & Booth-Butterfield, 1995). Weisberg and Haberman (1992) stated that humor and laughter may diffuse the anxiety associated with uncertainty, fear, and anger—all emotions felt during the initial stages of cancer. In the health field, humor is a comfortable way to share personal and often sensitive information (Sparks-Bethea, Travis, & Pecchioni, 2000). Recognized as one highly effective coping strategy among patients and health care professionals, humor enables individuals to manage face-threatening situations (Sparks-Bethea et al., 2000).

Prior research has shown the usefulness of humor in health care settings, but humor is also important in the family setting (Pasquali, 1991). Laughter can revitalize family caregivers both physically and psychologically, thus improving their quality of life. The integration of humor can offer a new perspective on a situation while helping to prevent burnout of the primary caregiver. When dealing with a serious illness such as cancer, a patient's sense of humor may affect the entire families' outlook on the experience. Because adult children are often caregivers to their sick parents, the parent's use of humorous tactics may affect the relational satisfaction of the parent–child dyad.

Cancer and the Family

The family dynamic is changed when one of its members is diagnosed with cancer. The psychological uncertainty associated with cancer alters traditional family relations, sometimes causing avoidance with a patient for fear of saying or doing something "wrong" (Gotcher, 1993). This avoidance often stunts the patients' ability to adjust to their illness. Those patients who report the most effective adjustment to the cancer experience also reported the highest quality of patient–family communication (Gotcher, 1993). There is a strong need for interaction with loving and caring family members. The communicative tactics patients and family members use will characterize these interactions. Furthermore, it is highly likely that the primary caregiver for the older cancer patient with cancer will be a spouse or a daughter (Cicirelli, 1992; Prohaska & Glasser, 1996). Thus, an understanding of the functions of competency, humor orientation, and relational satisfaction in the parent–adult child relationship is an important link to understand.

Communication Competency and the Cancer Context

Spitzberg and Cupach (1984) asserted that communication competence is integral to quality of life. Although the importance of communication competence is generally agreed on by scholars, the nature of competence in communicating remains elusive (Query & Kreps, 1996; Spitzberg & Cupach, 1984). Wiemann (1977) postulated five dimensions of communication competence that include affiliation/support, social relaxation, empathy, behavioral flexibility, and interaction management. Derived from Wiemann's ideas, communication competence is best conceptualized for this study using Query and Kreps' (1996) definition for health contexts. They described the concept as "the perceived tendency to seek out meaningful interaction with others, render support, be relaxed, appreciate others' plight and turn-take appropriately" (p. 339). During the cancer treatment period, it may be the parent's responsibility to communicate effectively with his or her child, particularly for younger children.

Although Query and Kreps (1996) discussed a relational model for communication competence, there is not much prior research on communication competency between the child and parent during the cancer experience. The cancer experience is a complex series of events that can possibly involve screening, diagnosis, treatment, recovery, and end-of-life care. How competently a parent communicates with his or her child during these different situations and throughout the cancer experience may greatly impact the nature of the parent–child relationship. Therefore, the first research question was put forth:

> RQ1: How does communication function in the older parent–adult child dyad throughout discussions during the parent's cancer experience?

Humor and Humor Orientation in the Health Context

Booth-Butterfield and Booth-Butterfield (1991) defined humor enactments as "intentional verbal and nonverbal messages which elicit laughter, chuckling, and other forms of spontaneous behavior taken to mean pleasure, delight, and/or surprise in the targeted receiver" (p. 206). Humor is commonly used throughout everyday interactions. In the health communication context, humor has positive benefits for patients.

Humor might improve a patient's overall health (Wrench & Booth-Butterfield, 2003). A predictive relationship exists between a patient's sense of humor and the patient's perceived health and morale. Medically speaking, the use of humor causes us to laugh, physiologically increasing endorphins, which are associated with decreased anxiety levels. Humor helps to revitalize people physically and improve quality of life. Pasquali (1991) stated that by stimulating the cardiovascular and respiratory systems and stimulating the production of T- lymphocytes, laughter strengthens the immune system. Humor reduces stress by allowing individuals to view the event in a different context (Davidhizar & Shearer, 1996). Thus, it appears that when humor and laughter are present, the patient is often healthier and stress is reduced for the family.

Aside from the physical benefits of humor, there are also psychological benefits. The use of humor allows individuals to save face when discussing uncomfortable topics (Wanzer, Frymier, & Sparks, 1995). This is best exemplified by the Arousal-Relief theory. When asked to describe their role reversal with aged parents and their inability to care for themselves, adult children will enact humorous messages, which function as relief or coping strategies (Sparks-Bethea et al., 2000). Treating cancer often involves situations where face is threatened or a perceived loss of dignity is present. Some patients may need to rely on their children to aid them in simple everyday functions of life. Humor can diffuse the tension built up by these situations and help patients preserve their face when dealing with their children. A study on health care providers by Wanzer, Booth-Butterfield, and Booth-Butterfield (2005) found that higher humor orientation (HO) was associated with greater self-perceived coping efficacy and claimed that humor is a useful coping strategy for patient's family members. The Arousal-Relief theory is supported by Wanzer, Frymier, and Sparks (2005), who found that high humor-oriented individuals gained a great deal of psychological relief by incorporating humorous coping communication in difficult situations.

Although humor can be a positive coping mechanism in interactions, misinterpretation of humor can enact negative effects. Sparks-Bethea et al. (2000) found that humor used by caregivers can be subdivided into either positive or painful relief functions. Humor must be selected wisely and take the form of "laughing with" and not "laughing at" in order to decrease stress and promote psychological and physical health (Davidhizar & Shearer, 1996). Family members often fear putting patients in an uncomfortable position, and patients must also be aware of the possible negative effects their use of humor might have on their family. Humor may have multiple functions throughout the communication of the cancer experience within the family, which leads to the next research question:

> RQ2: How does humor function both positively and negatively in the older parent–adult child dyad when communicating during a parent's cancer experience?

Humor Orientation

The awareness of proper use of humor is a skill. Just as people differ at enacting different levels of expertise in argumentativeness, assertiveness, or producing persuasive messages, individuals have differing levels of expertise in choosing, producing, and timing humor (Booth-Butterfield & Booth-Butterfield, 1991). Because people regularly enact humor in interactions, the humor orientation (HO) measure is a means of understanding humor usage. HO is a communication-based personality variable that enables some individuals to more skillfully produce humorous messages on a regular basis (Booth-Butterfield & Booth Butterfield, 1991). Individuals with high HO have a wider repertoire of humorous behaviors and require less planning to effectively generate humorous messages. People with high HO are more aware of the proper use of humor and therefore encounter fewer problems enacting humor (Wrench & Booth-Butterfield, 2003). Those predisposed to use humor perceive more situations as appropriate for humor use and fewer situations as inappropriate for humor (Booth-Butterfield & Booth-Butterfield, 1991). Additionally, Wanzer, Booth-Butterfield, and Booth-Butterfield (1995) stated that individuals with high HO report a strong need for creating a positive impression and attempt to elicit those images by entertaining and causing others to laugh and smile. The authors also found that low humor-oriented individuals do not try to make others laugh during interaction and avoid initiating humor attempts.

Whether individuals are high or low humor-oriented will likely affect whether they will enact humor tactics in interactions with others when dealing with their cancer diagnosis and treatment. Based on prior research on humor and communication, high HO patients are more likely to perceive their cancer experience as an appropriate situation to use humor than low HO patients and would also use humor more effectively. Because the use of humor may help in coping with illness, reducing stress, and improving quality of life, the patient/parents' interactions with their children is an important interaction to evaluate for humor usage.

Humor Orientation and Communication Competency

Booth-Butterfield and Booth-Butterfield (1991) stated that higher humor oriented individuals have the ability to effectively construct an appropriate humorous message. This ability to construct appropriate humor messages may be related to their skill as competent communicators. Both HO and communication competency require the skilled communicator to take into account the situation, relationship, and context before producing a message for their intended recipient. In a study operationalizing communication competence with social management, communication competency was correlated to HO (Wanzer et al., 1995). Furthermore, Wanzer, Frymier, and Sparks (2005) stated that humor-oriented individuals tend to be more communicatively competent and incorporate emotions more when making communication decisions. Wanzer, Booth-Butterfield, and Booth-Butterfield (2005) found that higher HO was associated with higher emotional expressivity. The relationship between HO and communication competency may exist in the cancer-diagnosed parent. Thus, the first hypothesis is put forth:

> H1: Adult children who perceive their cancer-diagnosed parent as high in HO will also perceive their parent high in communication competency.

Communication Competency and Satisfaction

Communication competency may be important for satisfaction within the parent–child dyad. In their review of previous literature, Spitzberg and Cupach (1984) found overwhelming evidence that there is a strong connection between competency in communication and marital satisfaction. Although prospective social support providers (the parent) must be able to interpret their recipient's situation before satisfactory support can be given, the social support recipient (the child) must be able to influence interactions with the provider (Query & Kreps, 1996). This concept of dyadic satisfaction related to communication competency may also apply to the parent–child dyad, specifically when offering communicative support during the cancer treatment period. Query and Kreps (1996) asserted the notion that the perceived competency is often more important than actual competency. Therefore, the child's perception of parent's interactions with them is possibly connected to satisfaction.

H2: Adult children who perceive their cancer-diagnosed parent as high in communication competency will report higher relational satisfaction than children who perceive their parent as low in communication competency.

Humor Orientation and Satisfaction

HO is positively associated with satisfaction (Wanzer et al., 1995). In a study examining teacher's use of HO and outside classroom communication, Aylor and Oppliger (2003) found increased student satisfaction with higher HO instructors. Wanzer, Booth-Butterfield, and Booth-Butterfield (1996) examined HO and popularity and determined high HO individuals experienced less loneliness. HO can positively affect an individual's happiness and overall satisfaction in certain interactions.

The use of humor in medical situations is both positive and satisfying for patients and their caregivers (Wrench & Booth-Butterfield, 2003). Wrench and Booth-Butterfield (2003) examined the relationship between physician HO and patient satisfaction. They found that although it is not the primary variable, a physician's humor orientation accounts for some of the variation in a patient's satisfaction. The stronger physicians' HO, the more likely patients reported cognitive satisfaction. HO also accounted for variation in physician credibility based on competence, caring/goodwill, and trustworthiness (Wrench & Booth-Butterfield, 2003). In health contexts, humor can be used appropriately to improve patient satisfaction.

Humor Orientation and Relational Satisfaction in the Cancer Context

Relational satisfaction is based on interactions with family members. Family communication standards that are positively associated with satisfaction include openness, expression of affection, emotional/instrumental support, and regular routine interaction (Caughlin, 2003). The use of humor and its positive relationship to satisfaction is dependent on the communication style of the individual family. Caughlin found that humor and sarcasm were appropriate communicative standards for satisfaction in some families. He also noted a possible relationship among humor, family satisfaction, and topic avoidance. Families reported an inverse connection between topic avoidance and satisfaction characterized by a higher endorsement of the standard of expressing affection and lower endorsement of the standard of humor/sarcasm. However, those families that associated humor/sarcasm with relational satisfaction were relatively untroubled by topic avoidance. The importance of humor use affects its desirability for relational satisfaction. If a parent is high in HO, humor is more likely important in the family's interactions, and therefore important to the relational satisfaction.

Emotional support is an important aspect in the cancer experience. In general, adult children report greater satisfaction with parents who communicate support (Golish, 2000). Similarly, emotional support was the most important factor in adjustment to cancer diagnosis and treatment (Gotcher, 1993). Booth-Butterfield and Booth-Butterfield (1991) stated that humor can be used to generate support. Humor, therefore, might be effective in the adjustment to the cancer experience and the overall satisfaction in the parent–child relationship.

Humor is useful to the parent–child relationship during the cancer experience in a number of ways. By reducing stress, improving health and quality of life, and offering support, the use of humor can alleviate many of the problems often associated with cancer adjustment and treatment. Individuals higher in HO are better equipped to use humor in a variety of situations and high HO parents would be more likely to use humor. Children of these individuals may feel more satisfaction with their relationship because of the benefits of humor. Thus, Hypothesis 3 predicts:

> H3: Adult children who perceive their cancer-diagnosed parent as high in HO will report higher relational satisfaction than children who perceive their parent as low in HO.

METHODOLOGY

Participants

Participants in this study were 46 adults recruited in a snowball sample from the pool of undergraduate students enrolled in the basic communication courses. Participants, who were at least 18 years old, had a parent who was currently diagnosed with cancer or treated for cancer within the previous 2 years. Respondents completed a variety of scales and open-ended questions on their own time through an online survey system, www.surveymonkey .com. The sample consisted of 17 males and 29 females. Most participants were under age 30 (65.2%), followed by ages 30 to 44 (23.9%), and 45 to 60 (10.9%). A majority were White (71.7%) and Asian/Pacific Islander (15.6%). The remaining participants were Black (6.7%), Hispanic (2.2%), or other (2.2%), with one participant not reporting ethnicity.

Also collected was demographic information about the parent to which respondents referred throughout the questionnaire, and information about the type and stage of cancer. There were 17 male parents and 29 females.

Most parents were between ages 45 and 60 (43.5%), followed closely by older than age 60 (41.3%), with a smaller percentage between ages 30 and 44 (15.2%). The race of the parent was also predominantly White (73.9%) and Asian/Pacific Islander (15.2%). The remainder of the participants were Black (6.5%), Native American (2.2%), or Hispanic (2.2%). Most parents had Stage II cancer (39.1%), which is localized cancer limited to the organ in which it began, without evidence of spread. This was followed by Stage III (30.4%), which is regional cancer that has spread beyond the original (primary) site to nearby lymph nodes or organs and tissues. Next, a few participants reported that their parent had Stage I (21.7%), which is early cancer present only in the layer of cells in which it began, followed by Stage IV (8.7%), known as distant cancer, which has spread from the primary site to distant organs or distant lymph nodes. A little less than one-third (29.5%) of participants reported that their parent was diagnosed with breast cancer. This was followed by lung (11.4%), melanoma (11.4%), colon (6.5%), and prostate (6.5%).

Measures

Participants completed an online survey and were asked to answer a variety of demographic questions about their own sex, ethnicity, and age, and the sex, ethnicity, and age of their cancer-diagnosed parent. The type of cancer and stage of cancer were also asked. Next, participants completed three scales and four open-ended questions. The scales included the Communicative Competence Scale (CCS Wiemann, 1977), Humor Orientation Scale (HO; Booth-Butterfield & Booth-Butterfield, 1991), and a modified version of the Marital Opinion Questionnaire (Huston, McHale, & Crouter, 1986). The open-ended questions asked participants to describe a satisfying and dissatisfying conversation with their parent about their parent's cancer and an effective and ineffective use of humor in reference to the cancer experience.

Communication Competence. The 36-item CCS measures attributes connected to an individual's ability to communicate effectively in a variety of social situations (Wiemann, 1977). Respondents use a Likert-type response format ranging from *strongly disagree* to *strongly agree.* The self-report scale has been modified to read "my parent" instead of "subject." High reliability (.96 coefficient was found with this scale (Wiemann, 1977). In the present study, the CCS had a $M = 139.63$, $SD = 28.36$, and $\alpha = .977$.

Humor Orientation. Booth-Butterfield and Booth-Butterfield (1991) developed the HO Scale to measure a person's sense of humor, or variations in what is perceived, appreciated, or labeled as funny. This self-report scale generates a list of 17 statements that directly reference the communicative use of humor in a variety of interpersonal situations. Respondents use a Likert-type response format ranging from *strongly disagree* to *strongly agree*. Scores for the HO range from 17 to 85. The scale has shown good reliability (Cronbach's $\alpha = .92$) and face validity (Wanzer, Booth-Butterfield, & Booth-Butterfield, 1995). For the purposes of this study, the scale was modified for children to answer the questionnaire about their parent. In the present study, the HO scale had a $M = 65.22$, $SD = 13.08$, and $\alpha = .945$.

Relational Satisfaction. A version of Huston et al.'s (1986) Marital Opinion Questionnaire was used to measure the overall satisfaction of the parent–child relationship. Vangelisti and Caughlin (1997) modified this instrument to evaluate the parent–child relational satisfaction and the scale was successfully used in several family relationship investigations (Caughlin, 2003; Caughlin & Golish, 2002; Golish, 2000). As Vangelisti and Caughlin described, the instrument was reworded to read "parent" instead of "marriage." The scale includes eight items measured with a 7-point semantic differential in a format ranging from opposites such as *miserable-enjoyable* or *worthwhile-useless* as well as one global indicator that ranges from *completely dissatisfied* to *completely satisfied*. This scale has high reliability (Cronbach's α =.91 and .94; Caughlin, 2003; Caughlin & Golish, 2002). In the present study, the Marital Opinion Questionnaire had a $M = 5.097$, $SD = 1.04$, and $\alpha = .834$.

Coding Open-Ended Data

Answers to the open-ended data necessitated the development of a category coding system. Using the model of content analysis set forth by Kaid and Wadsworth (1989), the responses were evaluated to determine possible content themes and humor usage. A detailed category system was developed to examine topic themes for all responses. Using Sparks-Bethea et al. (2000) as a model, humor anecdotes were also coded to categorize the type of humor usage. For the purposes of calculating intercoder reliability, each person was counted as one unit with four possible responses. Reliability for that unit was then calculated based on the agreement of the coders' analysis of the four responses giving a possible reliability score of .00, .25, .50, .75, or 1.00 for each unit. During the preliminary session, coders evaluated 10% of the data set and achieved a reliability of .550. Further descriptions of categories were added to the coding dictionary and discussion about the categories, types of responses that would fit in each, and coding procedures ensued. Both coders then evaluated the full data set and achieved a reliability score of .831.

RESULTS

Research Questions

The first research question addressed the function of communication between the parent and child during the parent's cancer experience. Respondents ($n = 36$) first described a satisfying conversation they had with their parents. The categories and percent of use were as follows: initial disclosure of diagnosis (22.2%), initial disclosure of treatment plans (13.9%), discussion of treatment procedures (27.5%), discussion of parent's feelings (50%), discussion of the outcome of cancer (13.9%), withholding information from the child (8.3%), discussion of side effects (0%), and no topic categories present (13.9%).

Respondents ($n = 34$) then were asked to describe a dissatisfying conversation with their parent. The categories and percent of use were as follows: initial disclosure of diagnosis (15.6%), initial disclosure of treatment plans (6.3%), discussion of treatment procedures (6.3%), discussion of parent's feelings (46.9%), discussion of the outcome of cancer (21.9%), withholding information from the child (34.4 %), discussion of side effects (0%), and no topic categories present (5.9%).

The second research question addressed how humor functioned in the dyad. Respondents ($n = 24$) were first asked to describe an appropriate use of humor by their parents. The categories and percent of use included initial disclosure of diagnosis (4.4%), initial disclosure of treatment plans (8.3%), discussion of treatment procedures (16.7%), discussion of parent's feelings (16.7%), discussion of the outcome of cancer (4.2%), withholding information from the child (0 %), discussion of side effects (70.8%), and no topic categories present (8.3%). The side effects were divided further into types: loss of hair (47.1%), loss of weight (11.8%), loss of breast (11.8%), other (29.4%).

Finally, respondents ($n = 13$) gave an example of inappropriate humor used by their parent. The breakdown included initial disclosure of diagnosis (15.4%), initial disclosure of treatment plans (0%), discussion of treatment procedures (15.4%), discussion of parent's feelings (23.1%), discussion of the outcome of cancer (23.1%), withholding information from the child (7.7%), discussion of side effects (15.4%), and no topic categories present (7.7%).

The responses about appropriate and inappropriate humor use were evaluated and assigned into categories described by Sparks-Bethea et al. (2000). Appropriate humor responses were categorized according to the following usages: relief (34.8%), which is characterized by the anecdote indicating closure and the respondent achieving a sense of pleasure from conveying the story; pain (2.3%), which is characterized by the anecdote indicating humor relief associated with some residual discomfort or pain; coping (39.1%), which is characterized by the anecdote being somewhat open-ended, and both listener and respondent are left with an inability to enjoy or lack of satisfaction from the story; and other or unsure (21.7%). Inappropriate humor responses were categorizes as relief (0%), pain (50.0%), coping (25.0%), and other or unsure (25.0%).

Tests of Hypotheses

The three hypotheses were tested using a Pearson correlation. The first hypothesis predicted that children who perceive their parent as high in HO will also perceive their parent high in communication competency. HO was positively correlated with communication competency ($r = .644, p < .0005$), providing significant support for the first hypothesis.

The second hypothesis predicted that children who perceive their cancer-diagnosed parent as high in communication competency will report higher relational satisfaction than children who perceive their parent as low in communication competency. Communication competency was positively correlated with relational satisfaction ($r = .346, p < .05$), providing significant support for the second hypothesis.

The third hypothesis predicted that children who perceive their cancer-diagnosed parent as high in HO will report higher relational satisfaction than children who perceive their parent as low in HO. HO was not significantly correlated with relational satisfaction ($r = .231, p = .123$). Thus, the third hypothesis was rejected.

DISCUSSION AND ANALYSIS OF ADULT–CHILD DIFFERENTIAL ACCOUNTS

Results overall indicate that communication competency, HO, and relational satisfaction work in complex ways for the cancer-diagnosed parent–child dyad. Content analysis was used to examine the child's report of discussions and humor use that took place during the cancer experience. This study also examined the relationships between communication competency and HO, communication competency and relational satisfaction, and HO and relational satisfaction.

The first research question sought to identify what areas of the cancer experience would produce satisfying and dissatisfying messages. Popular topics for the satisfying conversation included the initial disclosure of the cancer diagnosis (22.2%) and discussion of the treatment plan and procedures (27.5%). One respondent wrote, "I was satisfied with the way my mother would tell everyone the detail of her diagnosis and what the process was supposed to be." Respondents indicated that it was important to feel informed and included in their parent's cancer experience. Dissatisfying conversations often included discussions of the outcome of cancer (21.9%; e.g., "She talks about how life is short and she's going to die.") and the parent withholding information (34.4%). Caughlin (2003) found that family communication standards will affect whether a child will be accepting of topic avoidance. Although some families are relatively untroubled by topic avoidance or withholding information, this was not the case for many of the respondents. Perhaps the seriousness of a cancer diagnosis affects the level of acceptance of topic avoidance. One respondent wrote:

> My mom did not tell us that she had been diagnosed with chronic lymphocytic leukemia for about 4 months. I was angry at the fact that she had known about it for so long and did not tell us . . . at the time, I felt like I had been left out of an important loop that I wanted to be a part of. I felt like I had been betrayed because my mom did not trust me enough to tell me something of this magnitude . . . the fact that I wasn't made aware of everything made me feel powerless and less in control of the situation.

The parents who chose to withhold information were not competently communicating according to their child's standards.

Interestingly, 50% considered the discussion of their parents' feelings a satisfying conversation, whereas 46.9% found the parents' management of conversation of their feelings dissatisfying. The dissatisfying conversation of feelings also included a lack of willingness to discuss feelings. One adult child wrote, "He's hopeful. He talks about getting through the treatment, going into remission. . . . He's also straightforward about the fact it's hard for him," whereas another wrote, "The most dissatisfying thing my mother did was hide her feelings. She tried so hard to make sure everyone else was okay with her being sick that she rarely told us how she felt." The discussion of feelings with the child during the cancer experience appears to be an important topic element for most respondents. The fact that almost half of respondents discussed this topic in a negative way is troublesome. Emotional support is an important factor in adjustment to the cancer diagnosis and treatment, and in parent–child relational satisfaction (Golish, 2000; Gotcher, 1993). Additionally, the ability to express emotion and integrate emotions into messages is related to communication competency (Spitzberg & Cupach, 1984). Although many parents are doing an adequate job in relating feelings during the cancer experience, many others are not. This may affect adjustment and satisfaction for the child or parent.

The second research question sought to evaluate how humor functions in the parent–child dyad within the cancer context. The most interesting finding was that 70.8% of appropriate humor usage included topic elements about the side effects of cancer treatment. In a further breakdown of this result, almost half (47.1%) involved humor about hair loss, whereas some other side effects mentioned were loss of weight (11.8%) or of a breast (11.8%). One child wrote, "We talked about his hair falling out again and he said this time he would try a wig for looks instead of being Telly again," whereas another wrote, "She made a joke about how she would have less hair then my dad." Applying Sparks-Bethea et al.'s (2000) subdivisions of positive relief, painful relief, and coping uses of humor, the appropriate humor responses were mostly coping (39.1%) or positive relief (34.8%) anecdotes. This idea of coping humor often has an open-ended feeling of "just having to deal" and leaves the respondent unable to fully feel the relief effect of the anecdote. For example, one respondent wrote, "When my mother was talking about getting her surgery to remove her cancer, she would jokingly say that, 'at least now I can't have any more kids!'" Humor in sensitive situations such as the cancer context must take the form of "laughing with" and not "laughing at" (Davidhizar & Shearer, 1996). It is important to note that most of the appropriate humor anecdotes discussed by respondents took this form where both the parent and child appreciated the joke as either relief or coping.

Contrasting with the relief and coping anecdotes, the inappropriate humor responses discussed contained different topic elements including jokes about feelings (23.1%) and the outcome of cancer (23.1%). These anecdotes were usually made about inappropriate topics such as "I heard him say to my mom she needed to go out without him to get used to it" or "When my dad has trouble communicating he tries to laugh it off but once he made a joke concerning the hole in his throat. It made me uncomfortable and upset that he would joke about something that serious." No inappropriate anecdotes were considered a positive relief function of humor, but rather 50% were considered painful relief humor usage and 25% were considered coping. Individuals with lower levels of HO will be less likely to produce appropriate jokes that take into account the emotional needs of the recipient (Booth-Butterfield & Booth-Butterfield, 1991). The anecdotes described as inappropriate in this study may enact negative effects on the adjustment to cancer or emotional support needs during the cancer treatment period. The difference in topic preference for appropriate and inappropriate humor may indicate that humor that is appropriate is concentrated on more trivial or physical appearance topics such as hair loss or weight loss, while inappropriate jokes were topically serious such as fear of the death of the parent.

Humor can be used as a coping mechanism and is positively correlated with coping efficacy (Wanzer, Booth-Butterfield, & Booth-Butterfield, 2005). Many of the anecdotes discussed as both appropriate and inappropriate functioned as a coping tactic. However, it is important to note that not all coping humor attempts were viewed as positive. Therefore, humor as a coping tactic may work in more complex ways. Despite this, it is important to examine humor as an active coping tactic parents use with their children throughout the cancer experience.

The first hypothesis predicted that respondents who perceived their cancer-diagnosed parent as high in HO would also perceive them as high in communication competency. Not surprisingly, the children's reports of parents' HO were significantly and positively associated with communication competency. Consistent with studies that examined other population's HO and communication competency levels, the findings in this study once again support that individuals who are high in HO are also competent communicators (Wanzer et al., 1995). Individuals who can successfully formulate appropriate humor messages are also successful at other forms of competent communication.

The second hypothesis predicted that children who perceived their cancer-diagnosed parent as high in communication competency would be more satisfied with their relationship with the parent. The hypothesis was supported as communication competency was positively correlated with relational satisfaction. This finding supports previous research that found the ability to competently communicate a trait related to relational satisfaction (Spitzberg & Cupach, 1984). During the cancer experience, the ability for a parent to gauge the situational appropriateness and relational needs of the child when producing messages about the disease is important to how satisfied a child is with the relationship.

The third hypothesis predicted that HO was positively correlated with relational satisfaction. This hypothesis was not supported. Higher humor-oriented individuals did not report higher levels of relational satisfaction. This finding is similar to that of Wanzer, Frymier, and Sparks (2005), who did not find higher humor-orientated individuals reporting greater life satisfaction. Although not related directly to satisfaction, findings in this study and others have linked HO to communication competency, emotional support, decreased levels of loneliness, and coping efficacy, which are all related to satisfaction (Booth-Butterfield & Booth-Butterfield, 1991; Wanzer, Frymier, & Sparks, 2005; Wanzer et al., 1996; Wrench & Booth-Butterfield, 2003). Humor, therefore, might act in more complex ways with relational satisfaction. Wanzer, Frymier, and Sparks (2005) explained their findings, stating that although high HO individuals did not report greater life satisfaction, they did report greater coping efficacy and are therefore probably more satisfied with their lives. Because HO is significantly related to many factors that do positively correlate to relational satisfaction, it may be that HO acts as a secondary characteristic. Although the primary trait that correlates positively to satisfaction would be communication competency or coping efficacy, the secondary characteristic of humor might contribute to the execution of the primary trait. Therefore although not directly affecting satisfaction, HO may act as a part of another trait that does act as a catalyst for satisfaction.

Limitations

This study contains certain limitations. The sample used was one of convenience, does not vary much in cultural or ethnic diversity, and was limited in size. The sample's type of cancer was also well representative of patients with breast cancer and lacking in many other types. Another limitation to the qualitative data was the lack of completion by many respondents. Whether it was due to lack of motivation to complete the questionnaire or inability to recall situations that fit the criteria for the question is not certain. Data collection using an online survey Web Site may have produced compliance issues or a skewed demographic sample because of online computer access limitations. As a result of the limited sample size and composition, the findings of this study may only be considered as preliminary.

Future Research

This study was limited in population and therefore the results should be considered preliminary. Future research needs to include a population diverse in gender, age, and ethnicities to determine if these results are upheld. Demographic variance should also be studied to determine the differences in humor usage in the cancer context between different genders, age groups, or ethnicities.

Future research should examine HO as a possible secondary trait associated to other traits that positively correlate to relational satisfaction such as competency or coping efficacy. Studies need to ascertain the complexities of humor and its different uses and how humor functions within the primary traits such as communication competency and coping efficacy.

Finally, more qualitative research needs to be conducted to take an in-depth analysis of the use of humor. For instance, this study revealed an interesting topic preference of discussing the side effects of cancer treatment with humor that needs further evaluation. Qualitative research asking for the best and worst use of humor might be studied using a critical incident perspective or narrative analysis.

Practical Applications

Applications in these data may aid individuals working with patients and their families, researchers and practitioners creating message design, education, as well as theoretical considerations that translate research into practice.

Implications for Health Care Providers. The data presented here is useful for informal and formal health care providers who are faced with the challenges that come with communicating about and dealing with a cancer diagnosis. By understanding the functions of the communication variables that have been examined in this study, family members will have better communicative strategies in dealing with such a difficult transitional time as they negotiate their way through the disease as well as their newly defined relationship. These communicative strategies are aimed at understanding such complexities from a life-span developmental approach. Both informal and formal providers can read the real-life accounts of older adult–adult child interactions within this study and adapt their communication strategies in ways that fit their family culture.

Implications for Message Design and Education. Learning how to effectively communicate with a family member diagnosed with cancer is an extremely delicate endeavor. Family members are in the dark when it comes to dealing with these complex communicative issues. Present provider–patient communication research needs to be employed into applicable course content for family members of those diagnosed with cancer. Currently, the only exposure to provider–patient interaction that individuals have access to is medical students who take a course on bedside manners (Vandekieft, 2001; Yedidia, Gillespie, Kachur, Schwartz, Ockene et al., 2003). Informal and formal providers need to be taught the significance of communication strategies when such difficult bad news is delivered and through the entire cancer diagnosis, treatment, and recovery process. Training programs need to be created and implemented for such family providers and existing practitioners.

Implications for Theory. There are a few additional theoretical frameworks that further inform the older adult patient–adult child cancer context including Dialectical Theory (Baxter, 1986), Social Exchange Theory (Duck, 1976), Social Identity Theory (Harwood & Sparks, 2003; Robinson, 1996; Tajfel & Turner, 1986), and communication accommodation theory (see e.g., Barker, Giles, & Harwood, 2004; Giles, Coupland, & Coupland, 1991). Additional research to test such theoretical applications would be fruitful. There is an absence of a communication theory that informs informal and formal caregiver/provider negative interactions as a result of a cancer diagnosis. Within medical research, there are many findings on how to deliver bad news, such as a cancer diagnosis, however these findings are not organized in a cohesive communication framework that is user-friendly for providers.

CONCLUSION

This study sought to evaluate the communicative impact of an older parent diagnosed with cancer by utilizing a life-span developmental approach to investigate perceptions of communication competency, HO, and relational satisfaction from the adult child's perspective. Overall, communication competency was positively associated with HO and relational satisfaction. Although HO was not related directly to satisfaction, this line of research suggests that humor might act in more complicated ways. Qualitative data was also used to triangulate the data and understand what topics are discussed within this cancer context. This study supports the notion that the age-related diagnosis of cancer can greatly impact family communicative functions and behaviors across the life span as the family adapts to and renegotiates the many changes that take place (see Nussbaum et al., 2000). Thus, not only do such family relationships get redefined, maintained, negotiated, and renegotiated via the aging process, but also through various health issues that arise from the aging process. As Nussbaum et al. (Chapter 4, this volume) stated, the relationships maintained with adult children and other close relationships are constantly fluctuating as family members and friends negotiate and adapt to age-related biological, economic, psychological, and social circumstances. Although this study offers only preliminary data for the exploration of this specialized population, it is a necessary step in research in an effort to better understand and aid the parent–adult child dyad dealing with the difficulties surrounding a cancer diagnosis.

REFERENCES

Aylor, B., & Oppliger, P. (2003). Out-of-class communication and student perceptions of instructor humor orientation and socio-communicative style. *Communication Education*, *52*, 122-135.

Barker, V., Giles, H., & Harwood., J. (2004). Inter- and intragroup perspectives on intergenerational communication. In J. F. Nussbaum & J. Coupland (Eds.), *Handbook of communication and aging research* (2nd ed., pp. 139-166). Mahwah, NJ: Erlbaum.

Baxter, L. A. (1986). Gender differences in the heterosexual relationship rules embedded in break-up accounts. *Journal of Social and Personal Relationships*, *3*, 289-306.

Booth-Butterfield, S., & Booth-Butterfield, M. (1991). Individual differences in the communication of humorous messages. *The Southern Communication Journal*, *56*, 205-218.

Caughlin, J. P. (2003). Family communication standards: What counts as excellent family communication and how are such standards associated with family satisfaction? *Human Communication Research*, *29*, 5-40.

Caughlin, J. P., & Golish, T. D. (2002). An analysis of the association between topic avoidance and dissatisfaction: Comparing perceptual and interpersonal explanations. *Communication Monographs*, *69*, 275-295.

Cicirelli, V.G. (1992). *Family caregiving: Autonomous and paternalistic decision making*. Newbury Park, CA: Sage.

Davidhizar, R. E., & Shearer, R. (1996). Using humor to cope with stress in home care. *Home Healthcare Nurse*, *14*(10), 825-830.

Duck, S. (1976). Interpersonal communication in developing acquittance. In G. R. Miller (ed.) *Exploration in interpersonal Communication*. Beverly Hills, CA: Sage.

Giles, H., Coupland, J., & Coupland, N. (1991). Accommodation theory: Communication, context, and consequence. In H. Giles, J. Coupland, & N. Coupland (Eds.), *Contexts of accommodation: Developments in applied sociolinguistics* (pp. 1-68). Cambridge, UK: Cambridge University Press.

Golish, T. D. (2000). Is openness always better?: Exploring the role of topic avoidance, satisfaction, and parenting styles of stepparents. *Communication Quarterly*, *48*, 137-159.

Gotcher, J. M. (1993). The effects of family communication on psychosocial adjustment of cancer patients. *Journal of Applied Communication Research*, *21*, 176-188.

Harwood, J., & Sparks, L. (2003). Social identity and health: An intergroup communication approach to cancer. *Health Communication, 15,* 145-170.

Harwood, J. & Sparks, L. (2008). Social identity and health: An intergroup communication approach to cancer. In L. Sparks, H. D. O'Hair, & G. L. Kreps (Eds.), *Cancer, communication, and aging* (pp. 77-96). Cresskill, NJ: Hampton Press.

Huston, T. L., McHale, S. M., & Crouter, A. C. (1986). When the honeymoon is over: Changes in the marital relationship over the first year. In R. Gilmour & S. Duck (Eds.), *The emerging field of close relationships*. Hillsdale, NJ: Erlbaum.

Kaid, L. L., & Wadsworth, A. J. (1989). Content analysis. In P. Emmert & L. Barker (Eds.), *Measurement of communication behavior* (pp. 197-217). New York: Longman.

Kreps, G. (2003). The impact of communication on cancer risk, incidence, morbidity, mortality, and quality of life. *Health Communication*, *15*, 161-169.

Nussbaum, J. F., Baringer, D., Fisher, C. L., & Kundrat, A. L. (2008). Connecting health, communication, and aging: Cancer communication and older adults. In L. Sparks, H. D. O'Hair, & G. L. Kreps (Eds.), *Cancer, communication, and aging* (pp. 67-76). Cresskill, NJ: Hampton Press.

Nussbaum, J. F., Pecchioni, L. L., Robinson, J. D., & Thompson, T. L. (2000). *Communication and aging*. Mahwah, NJ: Erlbaum.

Query, J. L. Jr., & Kreps, G. L. (1996). Testing a relational model for health communication competence among caregivers for individuals with Alzheimer's Disease. *Journal of Health Psychology*, *1*, 335-351.

Pasquali, E. A. (1991). Humor: Preventative therapy for family caregivers. *Home Healthcare Nurse*, *9*(3), 13-17.

Prohaska, T. R., & Glasser, M. (1996). Patient's views of family involvement in medical care decisions and encounters. *Research on Aging, 18,* 52–69.

Robinson, W. P. (Ed.). (1996). *Social groups and identities: Developing the legacy of Henri Tajfel.* Boston: Butterworth Heinemann.

Sparks, L. (2003). An introduction to cancer communication and aging: Theoretical and research insights. *Health Communication, 15*, 123-131.

Sparks-Bethea, L. S., Travis, S. S., & Pecchioni, L. (2000). Family caregivers' use of humor in conveying information about caring for dependent older adults. *Health Communication, 12*, 361-376.

Spitzberg, B. H., & Cupach, W. R. (1984). *Interpersonal communication competence.* Beverly Hills, CA: Sage.

Spitzberg, B. H., & Cupach, W. R. (1989). *Handbook of interpersonal competence research.* New York: Springer-Verlag.

Tajfel, H., & Turner, J.C. (1986). The social identity theory of intergroup behavior. In S. Worschel & W. Austin (Eds.), The *social psychology of intergroup relations* (2nd ed., pp. 7-24). Chicago: Nelson-Hall.

Vandekieft, G. K. (2001). Breaking bad news. *American Family Physician, 64,* 1975-1978.

Vangelisti, A. L., & Caughlin, J. R. (1997). Revealing family secrets: The influence of topic, function, and relationships. *Journal of Social and Personal Relationships, 14*, 679-705.

Wanzer, M. B., Booth-Butterfield, M., & Booth-Butterfield, S. (1995). The funny people: A source-orientation to the communication of humor. *Communication Quarterly, 43*, 142-154.

Wanzer, M. B., Booth-Butterfield, M., & Booth-Butterfield, S. (1996). Are funny people popular?: An examination of humor orientation, loneliness, and social attraction. *Communication Quarterly, 44*, 42-52.

Wanzer, M. B., Booth-Butterfield, M., & Booth-Butterfield, S. (2005). "If we didn't use humor, we'd cry": Humorous coping communication in health care settings. *Journal of Health Communication, 10*, 105-125.

Wanzer, M., Frymier, A. B., & Sparks, L. (2005). *An exploration of the relationship between humor, coping efficacy, and life satisfaction for older adults.* Paper presented to the Interpersonal Division of the National Communication Association, Boston, MA.

Weisberg, J., & Haberman, M. R. (1992). Drama, humor, and music to reduce family anxiety in a nursing home. *Geriatric Nursing, 13*, 22-24.

Wiemann, J. M. (1977). Explication and test of a model of communicative competence. *Human Communication Research, 3*, 195-213.

Wrench, J. S., & Booth-Butterfield, M. (2003). Increasing patient satisfaction and compliance: An examination of physician humor orientation, compliance-gaining strategies, and perceived credibility. *Communication Quarterly, 51*, 482-503.

Yedidia, M. J., Gillespie, C. C., Kachur, E., Schwartz, M. D., Ockene, J., Chepaitis, A. E., Snyder, C. W., Lazare, A., & Lipkin, M. (2003). Effect of communications training on medical student performance. *Journal of the American Medical Association, 290*(9), 1157-1165.

PART III

COMMUNICATING ABOUT CANCER CONTEXTS AND AGING

Issues of Cultural Values, Spirituality, and End of Life

12

Investigating Cancer and Aging From a Cultural Perspective

Loretta L. Pecchioni
Louisiana State University

Janice L. Raup Krieger
Ohio State University

Lisa Sparks
Chapman University

Margaret J. Pitts
Old Dominion University

Hiroshi Ota
Aichi Shukutoku University, Japan

Cancer is an international public health problem that affects both developing and industrialized nations (Pisani, Bray, & Parkin, 2002). The global nature of the disease makes it increasingly important to understand the role of culture in shaping how cancer is experienced. Culture influences the most fundamental aspects of our existence, such as our assumptions about human nature, the nature of reality, and our relationships to one another and the environment (Gudykunst, 1998; Hofstede, 1984; Schein, 1985). Communication is central to this process because language is defined by, reflects, and transmits culture. The purpose of this chapter is to examine the ways in which culture influences the social context of cancer among older adults. A focus on older adults is warranted because they bear the largest burden of cancer, with 50% to nearly 66% of all cancer cases diagnosed in the United States occurring among those aged 65 and older (Hutchins, Unger, Crowley, Coltman, & Albain, 1999; Yancik, 1997). We begin this chapter with a discussion of the role of culture in social life. Then, we investigate intersections of communication and aging with a focus on Eastern and Western cultural perspectives. Next, we use the context of cancer clinical trials as an example to illustrate how culture shapes the experience of aging and cancer. We conclude the chapter with suggestions for future research and practical applications.

CULTURE IN SOCIAL LIFE

Culture is the collective way in which a group of people share and interpret their experiences of the world (Hecht, Jackson, & Pitts, 2005). It defines our socially expected roles (see Stryker, 1987; Thois, 1991), how to competently perform those roles, and the meanings attached to them (Ting-Toomey, 1999). As a result, there is social pressure to conform to the expectations of a social group. Moreover, culture is intergenerationally transmitted reflecting the values, beliefs, norms, rules, communicative behaviors, and social institutions of a group (Chen & Starosta, 1998). Based on the beliefs and values of our culture, we learn not only what are appropriate interaction scripts within our culture, but also the meanings that should be assigned to those interactions (Ting-Toomey, 1999). For example, we learn how to greet strangers, how older or ill individuals are (dis)valued, the relationship between our body and our self, and our own role within society.

Beliefs and values derived from a cultural group provide a guiding framework for social interaction and help shape expectations for those interactions. It is important to note, however, that cultures are not homogeneous (Gudykunst, 1998). For example, the United States is said to have an "American" culture that focuses on individualism, direct communication, and assumes a low power distance between individuals (Hofstede, 1991; Triandis, 1995). Not everyone living in the United States, however, adheres to this dominant style. Co-cultures (sometimes referred to as subcultures) are groups of individuals within a culture whose members share many values with the dominant culture, but also have some values that differ from the larger culture. Most of us belong to multiple co-cultural groups (e.g., age cohorts, health status, gender, and ethnicity; Al-Deen, 1997; Gudykunst, 1998; Orbe, 1998). The two primary co-cultural groups of interest in this chapter are age (Coupland, Coupland, & Giles, 1991; Coupland, Coupland, Giles, & Henwood, 1988; Gudykunst, 1998; Harwood, Giles, & Ryan, 1995) and health status (Charmaz, 1995, 2002; Frank, 1995; Hecht, Warren, Jung, & Krieger, 2005).

Membership in a co-cultural group shapes our attitudes toward people belonging to dissimilar groups (Allport, 1954; Ting-Toomey, 1999). Membership in a number of co-cultural groups necessitates the management of group boundaries (Ting-Toomey, 1999). For example, when we interact with a person outside of our co-cultural group we identify—usually subconsciously—our similarities and differences (see Tajfel & Turner, 1986). Interacting with others from our same group, then, is comfortable and safe because we know what to expect and do not have to explain or justify our behaviors (Gudykunst, 1995). Interacting with people from other groups, however, may lead to strong emotional reactions as our expectations, based on cultural norms, are violated (Burgoon, 1995; Mackie & Smith, 2002). Individuals tend to think that their own group behaviors are superior and that outgroup behaviors are inferior (i.e., ingroup bias; Brewer, 1979), resulting in a reaction of "it's just not right!"

As a consequence of these assumptions about group members, when individuals from different cultural groups communicate, they tend to operate on differing expectations for the interaction. Interactions between such individuals are labeled intercultural communication (Ting-Toomey, 1999). Because all cultures do not have the same underlying beliefs and values, we can compare the expectations of cultures—labeled cross-cultural communication (Ting-Toomey, 1999). An example helps to differentiate intercultural from cross-cultural communication. A physician from a large urban area in the United States may be seeing a patient who emigrated to the United States from a rural area in Colombia. Intercultural aspects of their interaction may include differences in language, social class, age, gender, and socioeconomic status. Cross-cultural aspects of their interaction may be revealed as they discover that each participant has different conceptions about the perceived causes and nature of illness and different definitions of and values for aging.

Age as a Co-Culture

A unique feature of age as a co-culture is that people move through a series of group memberships as opposed to other group categorizations that tend to be more stable, such as biological sex or national citizenship (Giles, Fox, Harwood, & Williams, 1994). As a result, age cohorts can be viewed as a separate culture—Generation X versus the Greatest Generation—or as a process that occurs within a culture (Coupland & Nussbaum, 1993; Giles et al., 1994). With regard to the former, an age cohort may be seen as having a culture itself that has distinctive experiences, values, norms, and use of language. Although none of us age and join successive age-group cultures in exactly the same manner, individuals often evaluate others to determine if the other is an age peer (Coupland, Coupland, & Giles, 1989; Coupland et al., 1991).

Williams and Nussbaum (2001) argued that communicative exchanges across the life span and into older adulthood become increasingly complex as older individuals have a greater range of experiences on which to draw while also needing to compensate for declining abilities. Intergenerational conversations, thus, are likely to require unique communicative approaches that account for distinctions between age segments of the population. However, even when age serves as a membership category, individuals are operating within a system of overlapping cultural systems (Hill, Long, & Cupach, 1997). The experience of being an older individual in the United States may be quite different for an urban Euro-American male compared with someone who is a rural First Nations female. The interpenetration and salience of an individual's cultures has implications for the aging process (Hill et al., 1997).

Health Status as a Co-Culture

Health status is another mechanism for group differentiation. In some cases, the boundaries of group membership based on health are clearly delineated. In other cases, the identity transformations that accompany long-term illness result in changes in group membership over time, similar to the aging process (Hecht, Warren et al., 2005). For example, people who have permanent physical or mental disabilities as a result of illness may experience feelings of isolation and alienation in our ableist society and begin to interact with similarly disabled others to gain a sense of belonging (Onken & Slaten, 2000).

Individuals with an illness might struggle with identity issues as they suffer physical losses and attempt to maintain a sense of identity integrity (Charmaz, 1995, 2002). They are still the same person, but they are a new person as well. Therefore, individuals with an illness such as cancer may attempt to maintain some continuity in their sense of self. As a consequence, they must re-evaluate and renegotiate their identities as they move from the "healthy" role to the "sick" role to, hopefully, the "cancer survivor" role (Frank, 1995).

Intergroup Interactions

When individuals interact with one another, they assess (consciously or subconsciously) which group memberships they have in common with one another, as well as which memberships they do not share. Which group memberships become the focus of this process depends on the context and situation. For example, an oncologist practicing medicine in the United States may see a variety of patients who are also U.S. citizens, but who may come from different ethnic backgrounds, have differing education levels, or be from different age groups, and, most obviously, are from a different health status role within their encounters. Which of these similarities and which of these differences will become salient during the interaction may affect the satisfaction each participant has with that interaction (see also Harwood & Sparks, Chapter 5, this volume). With this general discussion of the nature of age and health status as co-cultures, and definition of terms used in this chapter, we now turn more specifically to the literature that examines the role of culture in our social lives with regard to communication, aging, and cancer. Our treatment of the interconnections among culture, communication, aging, and cancer are somewhat uneven as there is limited research that examines all these factors in combination. However, what will become evident is that culture influences our attitudes and values regarding aging and health care, appropriate interactions within the health care setting, health-related decision making, and our communicative preferences regarding health.

CULTURAL INFLUENCES ON EXPERIENCES OF AGING

As discussed in the introduction to this chapter, culture plays an important role in defining the self, shaping the meaning of and attitudes toward aging, and defining the roles that are considered to be appropriate. To understand the influence culture has on the meanings assigned to the aging process, we provide a brief review of how cultural differences have been treated, particularly, in communication and related fields. Culture has garnered scholarly attention as a factor that mediates people's psychological, sociological, and communicative experiences (Gudykunst, 1983; U. Kim & Yamaguchi, 1995; Y. Kim & Gudykunst, 1988; P. Smith & Bond, 1999; Wiseman, 1995), which includes, of course, the aging process (Pecchioni, Ota, & Sparks, 2004). Most examinations of cultural differences focus on an East–West split of perspectives, bringing cultural variability in communication and aging into sharp relief. This perspective is adopted herein in order to highlight the differences in philosophical orientations across cultures and their impact on people's communication.

Eastern Cultures

Scholars have historically differentiated Eastern and Western cultures on the basis of societal tendencies toward collectivistic or individualistic norms. People in Eastern cultures tend to exhibit what are considered to be collectivistic tendencies. In essence, collectivism refers to a social norm that encourages individual behavior that corresponds with expectations of the larger group. One such expectation in many collectivistic societies is that group members will use an indirect communication style. Explicit verbal expressions of one's meanings are considered to be undesirable because of a high concern for the other's face (M.-S. Kim, 1995; Ting-Toomey, 1988; Ting-Toomey & Kurogi, 1998), and the high level of importance placed on maintaining harmony with others (Hofstede, 1991).

Groups that hold these norms are often referred to as "high context" because they rely heavily on contextual cues for deriving meaning (Hall, 1976; Holtgraves, 1997). In other words, people are expected to grasp the meanings others express in communication without explicit verbal expressions (Gudykunst, Matsumoto, Ting-Toomey, Nishida, & Heyman, 1996; Holtgraves, 1997). When there are foreseeable communication difficulties (e.g., conflict), group members are likely to turn to an intermediary for assistance to avoid negative consequences arising from direct communication (Ting-Toomey, 2004). This preference for indirect communication extends to the cancer realm. For example, Korean and Japanese patients often are not informed of their cancer diagnosis. Instead, the physician informs the family of the prognosis and allows family members to decide whether or not the patient should be told (Benowitz, 1999). Furthermore, medical decision making in many Eastern countries is customarily left to the physician, who is seen as the authority in these matters and is therefore given considerable latitude in decision making.

Western Cultures

Unlike Eastern cultures, Western cultures are considered to be individualistic in nature. Individualism is a social norm that cultivates behavior based on personal preference, rather than deference to the larger social group. People in individualistic cultures tend to use a more direct, or "low context," communication style (Hall, 1976; M.–S. Kim, 1993; Yum, 1988). Meaning is more commonly derived from explicit verbal messages (Cocroft & Ting-Toomey, 1994; Hall, 1976; M.–S. Kim, 1993, 1995) rather than contextual cues.

A preference for direct communication in Western cultures is consistent with expectations that patients have a right to know their personal health information. Thus, physicians are duty-bound to provide explicit health information to their patients, even when the prognosis is poor. In some countries, laws require that the patient be fully informed, and governments, health systems, and organizations support open access to health-related information. For example, in the United States, television stations are required to provide public service announcements for free to organizations promoting general public welfare and health. Thus, viewers are exposed to announcements related to smoking cessation, mammograms, diabetes treatments, and any number of other spots encouraging the adoption of healthy lifestyles and early intervention.

Culture, then, because it plays a role in defining all aspects of life, obviously plays a role in defining the aging experience and providing meaning for that experience. For example, individuals in Eastern cultures are more concerned with ingroup relationships, whereas individuals in Western cultures are more concerned with self-sufficiency (Keith, Fry, & Ikels, 1990). As a consequence, definitions of successful aging and quality of life vary across cultures (Fry, 2000; Torres, 1999). Individuals with similar life experiences and ages, but living in different cultures may report their satisfaction with their circumstances quite differently. An older person with cancer in a Western culture may wish to return to prior levels of self-sufficiency, such as living at home, driving a car, and doing his or her own shopping. On the other hand, an older person with cancer in an Eastern culture may desire demonstration of his or her place of honor within the family by having family members provide care, such as asking the older person to come live with an adult child and his or her family.

Culture in Cancer, Communication, and Aging

Definitions of health and illness, the causes of disease, and the appropriate roles of physicians, patients, and caregivers are culturally bound (Witte & Morrison, 1995). In many cultures, health involves the complex interaction of personal beliefs, cultural values, and physical, emotional, and spiritual factors (Ruiz-Beltran & Kamau, 2001). Through culturally bound communication, we learn definitions of health and illness, what causes disease, and what expectations are held for both formal and informal caregivers. Thus, when considering cancer and aging from a cultural perspective, several questions emerge: Is illness any condition that impairs one's ability to function fully? What does fully functional mean? Is disease caused by factors outside of one's control or by immoral behavior? Who steps in to provide individuals with assistance as they age or when they are diagnosed with cancer? How do the formal caregiving network and the informal caregiving network interact?

To date, many of these questions have yet to be addressed from a group perspective. We do know, however, that both physicians and patients often experience difficulties as they interact with a person from a different culture. Previous research has found that a patient's culture and cultural orientation influences his or her beliefs on issues on everything from the appropriateness of patient participation (M.S. Kim et al., 2000), to end-of-life beliefs such as the acceptability of physician-assisted suicide (Braun, Tanji, & Heck, 2001). Furthermore, different cultures define patient-provider roles in different ways. D. Smith and Smith (1999) found that individuals in mainland China rated their doctors' communication, asking for information, explaining, encouraging patient talk, and sharing decisions higher than individuals in either Hong Kong or the United States. The authors also found that doctors and patients in China and the United States need more communication about prescriptions and appropriate use of medicine than those in Hong Kong. Furthermore, communication with doctors may become more problematic when doctors use patronizing speech to older adults. Although data for this argument wait to be provided, extrapolating findings about nurse–older patient communication (Masataka, 2000) suggest the presence of problematic issues that need to be tackled across cultures. Differences in expectations for the patient–provider relationship are likely to be intensified by the process of medical decision making. Some patients with cancer prefer that their physician make all medical decisions (Benowitz, 1999), whereas others prefer involving friends and family members in cancer treatment decisions (Gorelick, Harris, Burnett, & Bonecutter, 1998).

Cultural differences often influence health care in ways that extend beyond the medical encounter. For some ethnic minority groups, attitudes toward the health care industry may lead to reluctance to use specific health services in the United States and elsewhere (Wykle & Ford, 1999; see also Jitapunkul et al., 1999, for older people in Thailand; Ushikubo, 1998, for older people in Japan). Even if trust in the medical establishment is not an issue, certain groups may hold health beliefs that are inconsistent with current medical recommendations. Despite a concerted effort in the United States to persuade older women to receive mammograms on a regular basis, some Korean Americans believe that once a woman has a mammogram, there is no need to repeat the procedure (Juon, Kim, Shankar, & Han, 2004). Group membership may also influence what types of health messages are preferred. A study of cancer patients in Hawaii found groups favored particular mediums for receiving cancer information (Kakai, Maskarinec, Shumay, Tatsumura, & Tasaki, 2003). Specifically, White patients preferred scientific and objective information sources (e.g., Internet, telephone cancer information services), patients of Japanese ancestry preferred commercial and mediated information sources (e.g., television, printed media materials), and non-Japanese Asian and Pacific Islanders preferred interpersonal sources (e.g., other cancer patients, family members, friends, co-workers, physicians).

Language can be an especially challenging facet of health care among older individuals who immigrated late in life or who interact primarily within linguistic minority co-cultural groups. An example of these challenges is exhibited by Jewish Russian émigrés who often moved to the United States with their children and grandchildren (Brod & Heurtin-Roberts, 1992). The Communist system of their homeland ensured that everyone received basic health services provided in an authoritarian manner. These émigrés find it difficult to get jobs in the United States and do not understand why they do not have greater access to services. Additionally, they are not accustomed to preventive care or the bureaucratic system of U.S. health care. Their physicians report feeling frustrated that they cannot meet all of their patients' needs and are expected to provide mental health and social services that are outside their area of expertise (Brod & Heurtin-Roberts, 1992). The issue of language difference is especially important to help older immigrants maintain satisfying communication and psychological health in hospitals and institutions (Ryan, Meredith, MacLean, & Orange, 1995).

Cultural variability is also reflected in the process of making decisions related to cancer treatment and, potentially, end-of-life care. Although not all cancer patients must deal with end-of-life decision making at the time of their illness, because of the nature of cancer, many patients engage in end-of-life ideation. Making cancer treatment decisions may be impacted by definitions of quality of life (Fry, 2000). Therefore, depending on the values of an individual and his or her family and culture, they may make decisions that medical professionals may not understand or support. For example, is it appropriate to make a morphine drip available so that the patient can control the level of pain endured, but is then unable to interact effectively with loved ones? Is the goal of treatment to sustain living, no matter the quality of life, or is the goal being able to spend time with loved ones and being aware enough to enjoy those interactions?

One of the most critical and difficult health-related decisions surrounding end-of-life care is the use of life-extending technology. Culture helps us to make coherent sense of our mortality, suffering, and death (Greenberg, Solomon, & Pyszczynski, 1997; Lynn, 2000). These issues are influenced not just by culture and co-cultural groups, but also by religious beliefs and personal experiences (Lynn, 2000). Ethnic minorities in the United States exhibit a range of preferences for varying reasons. African Americans are more likely to prefer life-sustaining treatments, but are reluctant to share their treatment preferences with health care professionals (Mouton, 2000). On the other hand, African Americans are less likely to use hospice care or agree to organ donation (Mouton, 2000). Hispanics are also less likely to agree to organ donation or autopsies (Talamantes, Gomez, & Braun, 2000). For both groups, the main reason for not selecting organ donation is the desire to present a whole body to God (Mouton, 2000; Talamantes et al., 2000). Hispanics, like African Americans, are likely to request life-prolonging treatments (Talamantes et al., 2000). Both groups express a desire to allow time for God to work miracles. Among Asian Americans and Pacific Islanders, considerable variability reflects the diversity of their countries of origin, their immigration histories, rural versus urban backgrounds, and education level (Yeo & Hikoyeda, 2000). However, as reflected in their more collectivistic approach to life, issues surrounding illness and death are managed primarily within their co-cultural groups where there is a preference for the family to be involved in all decision making (Yeo & Hikoyeda, 2000). In general, Asian Americans and Pacific Islanders are more likely to want life support because longevity is more important than quality of life. In order to provide a whole body to their ancestors, they prefer to avoid autopsy and organ donation (Yeo & Hikoyeda, 2000). Among Native Americans and Alaska Natives, who represent a diverse group with more than 300 federally registered tribes, death is seen as a natural part of the circular pattern of life, so they tend to have more positive attitudes toward dying than most other groups (Van Winkle, 2000).

Consequences of Culture for the Experience of Aging and Illness

Because culture plays a role in defining all aspects of life, it obviously plays a role in defining the aging experience and providing meaning for that experience. Indeed, definitions of successful aging and quality of life vary across cultures and social groups (Fry, 2000; Torres, 1999). Culture shapes our beliefs about role appropriateness, such as what is appropriate "for someone my age." For example, if older people are expected to serve as sources of wisdom, younger people may turn to them for advice. If the older person acts in wise ways, then he or she will be demonstrating appropriate role behavior. If, however, the older person does not seem to have any useful advice, then he or she will not be fulfilling role expectations. If older people are expected to stay out of sight and out of mind, an older person who speaks up about unjust treatment of older people may be in danger of a number of negative reactions and even retaliation.

In addition to conforming to role expectations about age, an older adult with cancer is also pressured to adhere to expectations for how a person in a given society should experience illness. If a person with cancer is expected to suffer silently and be noble, the person who complains about how he or she is feeling may end up being avoided by family, friends, and health care personnel. If the expectation is for a person with cancer to cry out against the injustice of being sick, a person who is silent may be assigned a diagnosis of depression. In some cases, cultural expectations will limit the number of options available to older adults to pursue treatment of their illness. To exemplify how cultural contexts and social expectations influence cancer treatment and management options, we offer the case of cancer clinical trials among older adults.

Cancer Clinical Trials

Cancer clinical trials are a prime example of how age bias can influence decisions as important as cancer treatment. Although older adults represent 63% of the U.S. population of patients with cancer, adults over the age of 65 make up only 25% of clinical trial participants (Hutchins et al., 1999). The reasons for this disparity lie in the clinical trial system, physicians, and older cancer patients.

For many years, older adults have been systematically excluded from participation in cancer clinical trials based on protocol requirements that exclude older adults because of comorbidities that might complicate or possibly confound their research design (Lewis et al., 2003). This exclusion occurs despite the fact that the majority of the population receiving treatment for cancer is older and that although they may have some normal age-related organ impairment or coexisting diseases, these conditions may not interact with the treatment under study (Hutchins et al., 1999).

To be enrolled in a clinical trial, a patient must be referred by his or her primary care physician. However, because physicians are often reluctant to refer older adult patients to clinical trials, many older patients are never even informed about this option (Comis, Miller, Aldigé, Krebs, & Stoval, 2003; Kenemy et al., 2003; Yee, Pater, Pho, Zee, & Siu, 2003). Many physicians cite concern for their older patients' physical ability, the possibility of increased toxicity of treatments, and comorbidities as reasons for not referring older cancer patients to clinical trials. They also question if older patients have the desire and resources (e.g., transportation, social support) to participate in medical research. These assumptions reflect physicians' ageist attitudes and personal judgments that ignore the scientific evidence that older adults fare just as well as their younger counterparts in clinical trials (Begg & Carbone, 1983; Chen et al., 2003; Hensing, Peterman, Schell, Lee, & Socinski, 2003; Sargent et al., 2001; Yancik, Ries, & Yates, 1989). Although physicians may point to concerns about their older patients, they also are sometimes reluctant to refer patients to clinical trials because of the additional time required of them to complete the relevant paperwork and follow-up with patients. Additionally, physicians may feel that conventional treatments are effective and their patients do not need to be subjected to less proven treatment regimens.

When physicians do suggest clinical trials as an option for older patients, patients themselves may decline involvement for a variety of reasons that reflect more on the physician's communicative abilities than on the patients' preferences. Patients who agree to participate in clinical trials are more likely to perceive their doctors as being friendly and having a better communicator image than patients who decline to participate (Grant, Cissna, & Rosenfeld, 2000). Therefore, the way the physician interacts with the patient impacts the patient's decision regarding enrollment. Moreover, the amount of information that the patient is provided also impacts the decision to enroll. Older patients have been found to ask their physicians fewer questions (Beisecker & Beisecker, 1990) and to receive less information from the physician than younger patients (Street, 1991). Thus, older cancer patients are less likely to have as much information on which to draw when making their decision on whether or not to enroll in a clinical trial than are younger adults. Additionally, older patients generally desire less autonomy in medical decision making than do younger patients (Arora & McHorney, 2000; Grant et al., 2000). Patients who agree to participate in clinical trials are significantly less autonomous with regard to decision making than are those who decline (Grant et al., 2000; Llewellyn-Thomas, McGreal, Theil, Fine, & Erlichman, 1991). This reliance on the physician as decision maker suggests that older patients should be more likely to agree to participate in clinical trails than younger patients, contrary to the current trend.

A few studies have examined differences in rates of agreeing or declining to participate in clinical trials based on age and ethnicity. One Australian study found that older women were significantly more likely to decline to participate in a clinical trial than younger women (Ellis, Butow, Tattersall, Dunn, & Houssami, 2001). However, a survey conducted in the United States found slightly different results. Although younger adults were more likely to have positive attitudes toward clinical trials than older adults, the *majority* of older adults (aged 65 and older) reported a positive attitude toward participating in a trial (Comis et al., 2003). Other studies have supported the idea that older adults are generally in favor of participating in clinical trials. Kenemy et al. (2003) found that although older and younger patients with Stage II breast cancer accepted participation in a clinical trial at similar rates, older patients were significantly less likely to be offered a chance to participate in a trial. Finally, Brown and Topcu (2003) reported that approximately 75% of both older White and Black Americans said they would participate in a clinical trial if diagnosed with cancer. Therefore, the empirical research supports the idea that older patients with cancer are willing to participate in clinical trials and receive greater health benefits than problems from such inclusion.

PRACTICAL APPLICATIONS AND CONCLUSION

Our coverage of the research related to culture, communication, aging, and cancer has been somewhat uneven because these factors have not all received the same amount of attention in past research, especially in combination. We do know that culture is pervasive, providing us with the values, beliefs, and attitudes that define appropriate definitions of self; of roles within the family, work place, and community; and even how to age or be sick. Thus, theoretical considerations of aging and health should place the individual within the context of his or her cultural place and time.

Acknowledging that all patients are not the same is an important first step. This acknowledgment should extend not just to the physical realm. Most health care professionals continue to operate based on the biomedical model of health and illness, in which the body is treated as a machine in isolation from its environment. The biopsychosocial model, however, provides us with a broader lens for examining patient responses to illness because it acknowledges that individuals operate within a web of individual and social roles. Conrad (1987) proposed the use of *disease* to refer to the physical ailment and *illness* to refer to the social elements of the disease. Thus, an individual is not his or her diagnosis, but makes sense of that diagnosis within a web of cultural expectations. In this perspective, then, health care personnel must identify each patient's attitudes toward the causes of illness and treatment options, definitions of quality of life, availability of social support, and the like. The body is no longer a machine, but a living organism in communication with its physical and cultural environments.

Another important issue to acknowledge is the ageism and racism that exists in the medical profession. When physicians do not provide older patients with information about clinical trials, even when they think they are acting in the patient's best interests, they are acting on assumptions that may be unfounded. In fact, the empirical evidence shows that older cancer patients fare well in clinical trials when compared to their younger counterparts. Older patients may well have physical differences from younger patients, but these differences should be established empirically rather than based on limited experience that may be filtered through negative attitudes toward aging. Think about how often you have heard a statement such as: "It's just so sad to see someone so young with such an awful disease." Such statements suggest that it is acceptable, even expected, for older people to suffer from disease. Co-cultural differences based on ethnicity, race, or nationality may be even more pervasive in health care than ageism as differences extend across the spectrum of care. Ethnic minorities have less access to health care, report lower levels of trust in health care professionals, delay going to doctors for tests, and are less likely to be offered high-quality care options with cutting-edge technology. This broad spectrum of differences in access make the cancer experience quite different depending on one's co-cultural group, at least in the United States.

Although scientists often have difficulty looking at an individual's life and identifying the factors that would predict a given outcome, individuals looking back over their own lives are quite adept at making sense out of what happened. Social gerontologists can advance knowledge about the aging process and the cancer experience, separately and in concert, by identifying the patterns that exist in the narratives of those individuals. What barriers do patients identify? How do patients and their families process information and make health-related decisions? How does a diagnosis of cancer within a family interact with other life events that may be unfolding in the family at the same time? How can health care professionals, in a medical system that focuses on efficiency, find the time to learn enough about patients to be able to tailor information and treatment? How does membership in multiple co-cultures (e.g., national, ethnic, socioeconomic status, age, gender, etc.) impact these processes? Such a theoretical undertaking leads to an ambitious research agenda to identify the key components and patterns that are available at any given time revealing underlying mechanisms of human nature.

REFERENCES

Al-Deen, H. S. N. (1997). Preface. In H. S. N. Al-Deen (Ed.), *Cross-cultural communication and aging in the United States* (pp. xi-xiii). Mahwah, NJ: Erlbaum.

Allport, G. W. (1954). *The nature of prejudice*. Reading, MA: Addison-Wesley.

Arora, N.K., & McHorney C.A. (2000). Patient preferences for medical decision making: Who really wants to participate? *Medical Care 38*(3), 335-341.

Begg, C., & Carbone, P. (1983). Clinical trials and drug toxicity in the elderly. The experience of the Eastern Cooperative Oncology Group. *Cancer, 52*(11), 1986-1992.

Beisecker, A., & Beisecker, T. (1990). Patient information-seeking behaviors when communicating with doctors. *Medical Care, 28*(1), 19-28.

Benowitz, S. (1999). To tell the truth: A cancer diagnosis in other cultures is often a family affair. *Journal of the National Cancer Institute, 91*(22), 1918-1919.

Braun, K., Tanji, V., & Heck, R. (2001). Support for physician-assisted suicide: Exploring the impact of ethnicity and attitudes toward planning for death. *Gerontologist, 41*(1), 51-60.

Brewer, M. (1979). In-group bias in the minimal intergroup situation: A cognitive-motivational analysis. *Psychological Bulletin, 86*, 307-334.

Brod, M., & Heurtin-Roberts, S. (1992). Older Russian émigrés and medical care. *The Western Journal of Medicine, 157*, 333-336.

Brown, D. R., & Topcu, M. (2003). Willingness to participate in clinical treatment research among older African Americans and Whites. *Gerontologist, 43*(1), 62-72.

Burgoon, J. K. (1995). Cross-cultural and intercultural applications of expectancy violations theory. In R. L. Wiseman (Ed.), *Intercultural communication theory* (pp. 194-214). Thousand Oaks, CA: Sage.

Charmaz, K. (1995). The body, identity, and self: Adapting to impairment. *The Sociological Quarterly, 36*, 657-680.

Charmaz, K. (2002). Stories and silences: Disclosures and self in chronic illness. *Qualitative Inquiry, 8*, 302-328.

Chen, G-M., & Starosta, W. J. (1998). *Foundations of intercultural communication.* Boston: Allyn & Bacon.

Chen, H., Cantor, A., Meyer J., Corcoran, M. B., Grendys, E., Cavanaugh, D., Antonek, S., Comarata, H., Haley, W., Balducci, L., & Extermann, M. (2003). Can older cancer patients tolerate chemotherapy? A prospective pilot study. *Cancer, 97*, 1107-1114.

Cocroft, B. A., & Ting-Toomey, S. (1994). Facework in Japan and the United States. *International Journal of Intercultural Relations, 18*, 469-506.

Comis, R., Miller, J., Aldigé, C., Krebs, L., & Stoval, E. (2003). Public attitudes toward participation in cancer clinical trials. *Journal of Clinical Oncology, 21(5)*, 830-835.

Conrad, P. (1987). The experience of illness: Recent and new directions. In J. Roth & P. Conrad (Eds.), *Research in the sociology of health care: A research manual* (Vol. 6, pp. 1-31). Greenwich, CT: JAI.

Coupland, N., Coupland, J., & Giles, H. (1989). Telling age in later life: Identity and face implications, *Text*, 9 129-151.

Coupland, N., Coupland, J., & Giles, H. (1991). *Language, society, and the elderly: Discourse, identity and ageing*. Oxford, England: Basil Blackwell.

Coupland, N., Coupland, J., Giles, H., & Henwood, K. (1988). Accommodating the elderly: Invoking and extending a theory. *Language and Society, 17*, 1-41.

Coupland, N., & Nussbaum, J. F. (1993). *Discourse and lifespan identity*. Newbury Park, CA: Sage.

Ellis, P., Butow, P., Tattersall, M., Dunn, S., & Houssami, N. (2001). Randomized clinical trials in oncology: Understanding and attitudes predict willingness to participate. *Journal of Clinical Oncology, 19*(15), 3554-3561.

Frank, A. W. (1995). *The wounded storyteller: Body, illness, and ethics.* Chicago: University of Chicago Press.

Fry, P. S. (2000). Guest editorial, Special issue: Aging and quality of life (QOL)—The continuing search for quality of life indicators. *International Journal of Aging and Human Development, 50*, 245-261.

Giles, H., Fox, S., Harwood, J., & Williams, A. (1994). Talking age and aging talk: Communicating through the life span. In M. L. Hummert, J. M. Wiemann, & J. F. Nussbaum (Eds.), *Interpersonal communication in older adulthood: Interdisciplinary theory and research* (pp. 130-161). Thousand Oaks, CA: Sage.

Gorelick, P. B., Harris, Y., Burnett, B., & Bonecutter, F. J. (1998). The recruitment triangle: Reasons why African Americans enroll, refuse to enroll, or voluntarily withdraw from a clinical trial: An interim report from the African-American Antiplatelet Stroke Prevention Study (AAASPS). *Journal of the National Medical Association, 90*, 141-145.

Grant, C. H., Cissna, K. N., & Rosenfeld, L. B. (2000). Patients' perceptions of physicians' communication and outcomes of the accrual to trial process. *Health Communication, 12*(1), 23-40.

Greenberg, J., Solomon, S., & Pyszczynski, T. (1997). Terror management theory of self-esteem and cultural worldviews: Empirical assessments and conceptual refinements. In M. Zanna (Ed.), *Advances in experimental social psychology* (Vol. 29, pp. 61–139). Orlando, FL: Academic Press.

Gudykunst, W. B. (1983). *Intercultural communication theory.* Beverly Hills, CA: Sage.

Gudykunst, W. B. (1995). Anxiety/uncertainty management (AUM) theory: Current status. In R. L. Wiseman (Ed.), *Intercultural communication theory* (pp. 8-59). Thousand Oaks, CA: Sage.
Gudykunst, W. B. (1998). *Bridging differences: Effective intergroup communication* (3rd ed.). Thousand Oaks, CA: Sage.
Gudykunst, W. B., Matsumoto, Y., Ting-Toomey, S., Nishida, T., & Heyman, S. (1996). The influence of cultural individualism-collectivism, self-construals, and individual values on communication styles across cultures. *Human Communication Research, 22,* 510-543.
Hall, E. T. (1976). *Beyond culture*. Garden City, NY: Doubleday.
Harwood, J., Giles, H., & Ryan, E. B. (1995). Aging, communication and intergroup theory: Social identity and intergenerational communication. In J. F. Nussbaum & J. Coupland (Eds.), *Handbook of communication and aging research* (pp. 133-159). Hillsdale, NJ: Erlbaum.
Hecht, M., Jackson, R. L., & Pitts, M. J. (2005). Culture: Intersections of intergroup and identity theories. In J. Harwood & H. Giles (Eds.). *Intergroup communication: Multiple perspectives* (pp. 21-42). New York: Peter Lang.
Hecht, M. L., Warren, J. R., Jung, E., & Krieger, J. L. (2005). The communication theory of identity: Development, theoretical perspective, and future directions. In W. Gudykunst (Ed.), *Theorizing about intercultural communication* (pp. 257-278). Thousand Oaks: Sage.
Hensing, T., Peterman, A., Schell, M., Lee, J., & Socinski, M. (2003). The impact of age on toxicity, response rate, quality of life, and survival in patients with advanced, Stage IIIB or IV nonsmall cell lung carcinoma treated with carboplatin and paclitaxel. *Cancer, 98*(4), 779-788.
Hill, L. B., Long, L. W., & Cupach, W. R. (1997). Aging and the elders from a cross-cultural perspective. In H. S. N. Al-Deen (Ed.), *Cross-cultural communication and aging in the United States* (pp. 5-22). Mahwah, NJ: Erlbaum.
Hofstede, G. (1984). *Culture's consequences.* Beverly Hills, CA: Sage.
Hofstede, G. (1991). *Culture and organizations: Software of the mind. New* York: McGraw Hill.
Holtgraves, T. (1997). Styles of language use: Individual and cultural variability in conversational indirectness. *Journal of Personality and Social Psychology, 73*, 624-636.
Hutchins, L., Unger, J., Crowley, J., Coltman, C., & Albain, K. (1999). Underrepresentation of patients 65 years of age or older in cancer-treatment trials. *New England Journal of Medicine, 341*(27), 2061-2067.
Jitapunkul, S., Songkhla, M. N., Chayovan, N., Chirawatkul, A., Choprapawon, C., Kachondahm, Y., & Buasai, S. (1999). A national survey of health service use in Thai elders. *Age and Aging, 28,* 67-71.
Juon, H., Kim, M., Shankar, S., & Han, W. (2004). Predictors of adherence to screening mammography among Korean American women. *Preventive Medicine, 39*(3), 474-481.
Kakai, H., Maskarinec, G., Shumay, D., Tatsumura, Y., & Tasaki, K. (2003). Ethnic differences in choices of health information by cancer patients using complementary and alternative medicine: An exploratory study with correspondence analysis. *Social Science and Medicine, 56*(4), 851-862.

Keith, J., Fry, C. L., & Ikels, C. (1990). Community as context for successful aging. In J. Sokolovsky (Ed.), *The cultural context of aging* (pp. 245-261). New York: Bergin & Garvey.

Kenemy, M. M., Peterson, B.L., Kornblith, A. B., Muss, H. B., Wheeler, J., Levine, E., Bartlett, N., Fleming, G., & Cohen, H. (2003). Barriers to clinical trial participation by older women with breast cancer. *Journal of Clinical Oncology, 21*, 2268-2275.

Kim, M.-S., Klingle, R. S., Sharkey, W. F., Park, H. S., Smith, D. H., & Cai, D. (2000). A test of a cultural model of patient's motivation for verbal communication in patient-doctor interactions. *Communication Monographs, 67*, 262-283.

Kim, M.-S. (1993). Cross-cultural comparisons of the perceived importance of the conversational constraints. *Human Communication Research, 21*, 128-151.

Kim, M.-S. (1995). Toward a theory of conversational constraints: Focusing on individual-level dimensions of culture. In R. L. Wiseman (Ed.), *Intercultural communication theory* (pp. 148-169). Thousand Oaks, CA: Sage.

Kim, U., & Yamaguchi, S. (1995). Cross-cultural research methodology and approach: Implications for the advancement of Japanese social psychology. *Research in Social Psychology, 10*, 168-179.

Kim, Y. Y., & Gudykunst, W. B. (1988). *Theories in intercultural communication.* Newbury Park, CA: Sage.

Lewis, J. H., Kilgore, M. L., Goldman, D. P., Trimble, E. L., Kaplan, R., Montello, M. J., Housman, M. G., & Escarce, J. J. (2003). Participation of patients 65 years of age or older in cancer clinical trials. *Journal of Clinical Oncology, 21(7)*, 1383-1389.

Llewellyn-Thomas, H. A., McGreal, M. J., Theil, E. C., Fine, S., & Erlichman, C. (1991). Patients' willingness to enter clinical trials: Measuring the association with perceived benefit and preference for decision participation. *Social Science and Medicine, 32*, 35-42.

Lynn, J. (2000). Preface. In K. L. Braun, J. H. Pietsch, & P. L. Blanchette (Eds.), *Cultural issues in end-of-life decision making* (pp. ix-xi). Thousand Oaks, CA: Sage.

Mackie, D. M., & Smith, E. R. (2002). From prejudice to intergroup emotions: Differentiated reactions to social groups. New York: Psychology Press.

Masataka, N. (2000). *Oiwakoushite tsukurareru: Kokorotokaradano kareihenka* [People age in this way: Psychological and physical aging]. Tokyo: Chukoshinsho.

Mouton, C. P. (2000). Cultural and religious issues for African Americans. In K. L. Braun, J. H. Pietsch, & P. L. Blanchette (Eds.), *Cultural issues in end-of-life decision making* (pp. 71-82). Thousand Oaks, CA: Sage.

Onken, S. J., & Slaten, E. (2000). Disability identity formation and affirmation: The experiences of persons with severe mental illness. *Sociological Practice: A Journal of Clinical and Applied Sociology, 2*(2), 99-111.

Orbe, M. P. (1998). From the standpoint(s) of traditionally muted groups: Explicating a co-cultural communication theoretical model. *Communication Theory, 8*, 1-26.

Pecchioni, L. L., Ota, H., & Sparks, L. (2004). Cultural issues in communication and aging. In J. F. Nussbaum & J. Coupland (Eds.), *Handbook of communication and aging research* (2nd ed., pp. 167-207). Mahwah, NJ: Erlbaum.

Pisani, P., Bray, F., & Parkin, D. M. (2002). Estimates of the world-wide prevalence of cancer for 25 sites in the adult population. *International Journal of Cancer, 97,* 72-81.

Ruiz-Beltran, M., & Kamau, J. (2001). The socio-economic and cultural impediments to well-being along the US–Mexico border. *Journal of Community Health, 26*(2), 123-132.

Ryan, E. B., Meredith, S. D., MacLean, M. J., & Orange, J. B. (1995). Changing the way we talk with elders: Promoting health using the communication enhancement model. *International Journal of Aging and Human Development, 41,* 89-107.

Sargent, D. J., Goldberg, R. M., Jacobson, S. D., Macdonald, J. S., Labianca, R., Haller, D. G., Shepherd, L. E., Seitz, J. F., & Francini, G. (2001). A pooled analysis of adjuvant chemotherapy for resected colon cancer in elderly patients. *New England Journal of Medicine, 345,* 1091-1097.

Schein, E. H. (1985). *Organizational culture and leadership.* San Francisco: Jossey-Bass.

Smith, D. H., & Smith, S. J. (1999). Chinese elders' communication about medicine. *Health Communication, 11,* 237-248.

Smith, P. B., & Bond, M. H. (1999). *Social psychology across cultures* (2nd ed.) Boston: Allyn & Bacon.

Street, R. L., Jr. (1991). Information-giving in medical consultations: The influence of patients' communicative styles and personal characteristics. *Social Science and Medicine, 32,* 541-548.

Stryker, S. (1987). Identity theory: Developments and extensions. In K. Hardley & T. Honess (Eds.), *Self and identity* (pp. 89-104). New York: Wiley.

Tajfel, H., & Turner, J. C. (1986). The social psychology of intergroup behavior. In S. Worchel & W. G. Austin (Eds.), *The psychology of intergroup relations* (pp. 7-24). Chicago: Nelson-Hall.

Talamantes, M. A., Gomez, C., & Braun, K. L. (2000). Advance directives and end-of-life care: The Hispanic perspective. In K. L. Braun, J. H. Pietsch, & P. L. Blanchette (Eds.), *Cultural issues in end-of-life decision making* (pp. 83-100). Thousand Oaks, CA: Sage.

Thois, P. A. (1991). On merging identity theory and stress research. *Social Psychological Quarterly, 54,* 101-112.

Ting-Toomey, S. (1988). Intercultural conflict styles: A face-negotiation theory. In Y. Y. Kim & W. B. Gudykunst (Eds.), *Theories in intercultural communication* (pp. 213-238). Newbury Park, CA: Sage.

Ting-Toomey, S. (1999). *Communicating across cultures.* New York: Guilford.

Ting-Toomey, S. (2004). The matrix of face: An updated face-negotiation theory. In W. B. Gudykunst (Ed.). *Theorizing about intercultural communication* (pp. 71-92). Thousand Oakes, CA: Sage.

Ting-Toomey, S., & Kurogi, A. (1998). Facework competence in intercultural conflict: An updated face-negotiation theory. *International Journal of Intercultural Relations, 22,* 197-225.

Torres, S. (1999). A culturally-relevant theoretical framework for the study of successful aging. *Ageing and Society, 19,* 33-51.

Triandis, H. C. (1995). *Individualism and collectivism.* Boulder, CO: Westview.

Ushikubo, M. (1998). A study of factors facilitating and inhibiting the willingness of the institutionalized disabled elderly for rehabilitation: A United States–Japanese comparison. *Journal of Cross-Cultural Gerontology, 13*, 127-157.

Van Winkle, N. W. (2000). End-of-life decision making in American Indian and Alaska Native cultures. In K. L. Braun, J. H. Pietsch, & P. L. Blanchette (Eds.), *Cultural issues in end-of-life decision making* (pp. 127-144). Thousand Oaks, CA: Sage.

Williams, A., & Nussbaum, J. F. (2001). *Intergenerational communication across the life span*. Mahwah, NJ: Erlbaum.

Wiseman, R. L. (1995). *Intercultural communication theory*. Thousand Oaks, CA: Sage.

Witte, K., & Morrison, K. (1995). Intercultural and cross-cultural health communication: Understanding people and motivating healthy behaviors. In R. L. Wiseman (Ed.), *Intercultural communication theory* (pp. 216-246). Thousand Oaks, CA: Sage.

Wykle, M. L., & Ford, A. B. (1999). *Serving minority elders in the 21st century.* New York: Springer.

Yancik, R. (1997). Cancer burden in the aged—an epidemiologic and demographic overview. *Cancer, 80,* 1273-1283.

Yancik, R., Ries, L., & Yates, J. (1989). Breast cancer in aging women: A population-based study of contrasts in stage, surgery, and survival. *Cancer, 63*(5), 976-981.

Yee, K., Pater, J., Pho, L., Zee, B., & Siu, L. (2003). Enrollment of older patients in cancer treatment trials in Canada: Why is age a barrier? *Journal of Clinical Oncology, 21*(8), 1618-1623.

Yeo, G., & Hikoyeda, N. (2000). Cultural issues in end-of-life decision making among Asians and Pacific Islanders in the United States. In K. L. Braun, J. H. Pietsch, & P. L. Blanchette (Eds.), *Cultural issues in end-of-life decision making* (pp. 101-125). Thousand Oaks, CA: Sage.

Yum, J. O. (1988). The impact of Confucianism on interpersonal relationships and communication patterns in east Asia. *Communication Monographs, 55,* 374-388.

13

An Organizational Communication Approach to Integrating Latino Cultural Values Into Cancer Care

Melinda M. Villagran

George Mason University

Mary F. Hoffman

Texas State University—San Marcos

A growing body of research demonstrates racial and ethnic disparities in health care for minorities including Latinos (Smedley, Stith, & Nelson, 2003). One potential source of these disparities is the lack of culturally and linguistically appropriate services provided by health care organizations (Office of Minority Health [OHH], 2003). Minority patients with cancer who enter into the health care system must overcome unique organizational barriers that arise based on cultural and linguistic differences between themselves and their providers. Organizational socialization of newly diagnosed patients with cancer into health organizations must include specific accommodations to make services more accessible to minority and Limited English Proficiency (LEP) patients (Hablamos Juntos, 2005).

After a brief review of literature related to Latino cultural issues and values specific to cancer care, we propose a culturally appropriate model of organizational communication to improve Latino patient socialization in the cancer context. Health organizations seeking to reduce health disparities among Latinos need to consider the role of cultural values in patients' information management and decision making. Values can then be used to create culture-specific strategies to increase support for intended health outcomes.

ETHNIC AND RACIAL DISPARITIES IN HEALTH CARE

The National Institutes of Health defines *health disparities* as "differences in the incidence, prevalence, mortality, and burden of diseases and other adverse health conditions that exist among specific population groups in the United States." Health care disparities among Latinos have been linked to patients' knowledge levels, attitudes, organizational factors in the health care system, and cultural and social values (Thomas, Fine, & Ibrahim, 2004). Research also suggests that health disparities are associated with higher mortality rates among lung cancer patients (Bach, Cramer, Warren, & Bragg, 1999). Moreover, minorities including Latinos have poorer health status and receive lower quality of health care than non-minorities (Solis, 2003). Comparing Latinos to non-Latino Whites, Latinos are 152% more likely to die from cervical cancer, 107% more likely to die from stomach cancer (63% higher for males and 150% for females), and 20% less likely to receive ongoing health care (CDC, 2003). Health organizations are less likely to provide clinically necessary and routine procedures for minorities, and are more likely to deliver low-quality health services to these patients (Smedley et al., 2003). Although some research links health disparities to sociodemographic characteristics of minority patients, other researchers demonstrate that racial and ethnic disparities exist even when patients' ages, income levels, insurance status, and severity of medical condition are consistent (OMH, 2003). At least 35.5 million people in the United States are Latino (U.S. Census, 2000), thus the need to eliminate racial and ethnic disparities in health is evident. Culturally competent communication by health care provider organizations could play a central role in helping to overcome health disparities among racially and ethnically diverse patients.

The relationships among communication, culture, and health disparities are especially salient for two major reasons. First, disparities may occur because of health organizations' ineffective dissemination of culturally sensitive messages regarding safety and prevention measures. If patients receive and manage prevention and treatment health information in culturally specific ways, it is important to clearly understand this process. For example, efforts to increase the number of mammograms performed on Latino women may be hindered by familial roles of women in Latino culture. For this reason, targeted health messages are essential to encourage cancer screening among this population (Villagran, Bains, Guajardo, Munoz, & Thomas, 2005).

Second, communication between patients and providers is the fundamental means through which high-quality medical care occurs. Health organizations wishing to reduce disparities must consider how variables such as culture affect provider–patient communication (Ashton et al., 2003). If there are organizational barriers that originate from culturally specific issues, then organizations interested in reducing health disparities for Latinos must identify those issues. Specific areas of concern are such issues as how to provide culturally and linguistically appropriate care for Latinos, and the role of family in cancer care.

Health organizations seeking to reduce potential racial and ethnic disparities occurring within their organization first need to understand the values of their patients, and then relate those values to effective patient decision making (McGorry, 1999). For older adult Latino patients with cancer, providers who are aware of socioeconomic characteristics and Latino cultural values can incorporate a sense of cultural competence into the way they construct and disseminate health messages.

INFORMATION MANAGEMENT AMONG LATINO PATIENTS WITH CANCER

Because information management plays such an important role in the health experience of patients with cancer, Brashers, Goldsmith, and Hsieh (2002) encourage researchers to examine how the cultural beliefs of patients affect their information-seeking and avoiding behaviors. Brashers et al. also suggest researchers examine how patient behaviors vary in terms of directness and indirectness, and whether patients or family members should be the primary recipients of health information. O'Hair et al. (2003) described information management as any behavior related to willingness to communicate by either seeking or avoiding information about health.

Despite an extensive body of research about information-management behaviors, most studies used culturally homogeneous populations (Butow et al., 1998; Degner et al., 1997; Johnson & Meishke, 1993; McCaughan & Thompson, 2000). These studies may lack generalizability for culturally heterogeneous groups such as Latino populations who tend to have different beliefs and values that may impact their information-management behaviors and other health outcomes. For this reason, it is important to consider an organizing framework from which to address the way Latinos manage health information upon organizational entry, and throughout their cancer care. Culturally and linguistically appropriate care services should integrate Latinos' cultural values in the form and content of health messages intended for Latino patients.

Derdiarian (1987) reported a hierarchy of patient information needs that breaks into the following distinct categories: concerns about the disease and treatment, and impact of the disease on personal life, family, and social relationships. Of these categories, disease information, like chances of cure and the spread of the disease, is rated most important (Adams, 1991; Degner et al., 1997; Derdiarian, 1987; Echlin & Rees, 2002; McCaughan & Thompson, 2000). Information needs can also be categorized by what patients desire at different stages of treatment (Adams, 1991; Echlin & Rees, 2002; Mills & Sullivan, 1999). Adams suggested five stages of disease: diagnostic, treatment, rehabilitation, survivorship, and recurrence/advanced. The stage of a patient's disease would impact his or her perceived importance of information. Each of these stages may be impacted by culture-specific values and characteristics.

LATINO CULTURAL VALUES AND CHARACTERISTICS AFFECTING CANCER CARE

Latino culture plays a role in some health care decision making for Latino patients with cancer and their families. Issues such as language barriers and cultural values including *fatalismo*, *familiasm*, *machismo*, *marianismo*, *respeto*, and *spiritualism* all have a potential impact on the way patients experience cancer care.

Language Barriers

Perhaps the most obvious barrier to quality health care for many Latinos is language. Language barriers impede access to health organizations, diminish the potential quality of health care services, and increase the risk of unintended health outcomes caused by miscommunication (Lu & Flores, 2005). Spanish-speaking patients face a multitude of obstacles in health organizations where English is the primary language for spoken and written communication. In addition to problems interacting with providers, language barriers for Spanish-speaking patients might include making appointments, locating appropriate health care facilities, reading signage in provider offices, completing patient intake forms, interacting with providers, and reading prescription and drug interaction information.

Although Title VI of the Civil Rights Act requires U.S. medical facilities to provide translators for LEP patients, translators are not typically involved in every aspect of patient care and decision making, and many are poorly trained or inexperienced with translating medical information (Lu & Flores, 2005). In some cases, family members who attend doctor visits with their parents act as translators (McGorry, 1999). Although their language skills allow them to speak in both English and Spanish, patient family members are not typically experienced with using specific medical jargon, or detailing treatment options and drug protocols. Moreover, using family members may lead to miscommunication between patients and providers if they need to translate sensitive or embarrassing information for the patient. For example, Latino men being screened for testicular cancer are less likely to share personal information about their symptoms if their child is asked to act as the translator.

Cultural Values

Fatalismo. Strong religious beliefs lead many Latinos to believe that illnesses such as cancer are predetermined by God, and should therefore be accepted or endured in accordance with God's will (Antshel, 2002). *Fatalismo* is the term for this type of cultural belief. Latinos who have a strong sense of fatalismo are more likely to feel anxiety and psychological distress about illness (Ross, Mirowski, & Cockerham, 1983). They are also less likely to comply with treatment recommendations by providers or seek treatment for themselves or their families (Baquet & Hunter, 1995).

Personalismo. An emphasis on personal relationships in Latino culture is referred to as *personalismo* (Antshel, 2002). Interactions with physicians may be influenced by respect, or *respeto*, and a high-context communication style. Personalismo explains the value that the Latino culture places on warm, sincere, and relational communication (Cora-Bramble & Williams, 2000). Underscoring this need for personalization of care, Trevino, Moyer, Valdez, and Stroup-Benham (1991) reported that when discussing health care, Latinos are more likely to refer to their medical care provider than they are the institution where they receive care. If a provider moves out of the area, Latinos families sometimes stop receiving health care services until they can receive an introduction to a new provider and build a relationship with him or her (Trevino et al., 1991).

A sense of respeto for persons in positions of power may lead to fewer questions asked in medical interviews because the patient is concerned about challenging the doctor's authority (Cora-Bramble & Williams, 2000; Kakai, Maskarinec, Shumay, Tatsumura, & Tasaki 2003). Personalismo as a cultural belief is antithetical to the current trends of short physician-patient interactions and fewer long-term relationships between providers and patients.

Familiasm. A strong emphasis on family, both nuclear and extended, is a central cultural value for many Latinos (Antshel, 2002). The collectivistic orientation of Latino culture leads to behaviors such as a sense of responsibility and sacrifice for the benefit of the family, generous assistance for family members, and expected obedience, loyalty, and respect toward senior members of the family (Martinez, 1988).

Anderson's (1995) behavioral model of access to health care includes a discussion of enabling factors that impact a patient's medical experience. Enabling factors that might be affected by Latino cultural values include a patient's social network and the patient's level of familiarity with the medical system, with various types of cancer, and with cancer treatment (Anderson, 1995; Czaja, Manfredi, & Price, 2003). Communication factors in a patient's social support system include frequency of communication, level of honesty, encouragement from relational partners, and the way unpleasant topics are handled. These variables positively impact a patient's adjustment to cancer with emotional support being the most important (Gotcher, 1993). Latino patients who possess a strong sense of familiasm may view their cancer diagnosis and care through that framework.

Machismo/Marianismo. Not only do many studies of information management related to health fail to account for variance among cultural groups, but some also fail to examine culture as a central variable in gender role orientation related to health information management (Czaja et al., 2003; Johnson, 1995; Johnson & Meiske, 1993). This results in a fragmented body of research that lacks explanatory power for patients' information management as a potential source of health disparities.

Gender roles within Latino families often highlight the patriarchal nature of Latino culture. *Machismo* is often treated as a negative value referring to "male domination" (Antshel, 2002, p. 439), and "aggressiveness, sexual domination, risky behavior" (Neff, 2001, p. 173) among Latino men. Machismo can, however, also refer to such positive masculine ideas as courage, honor, fearlessness, pride, and charisma (Neff, 2001; Stevens, 1973).

Marianismo refers to the corresponding female ideal of a nurturing, caretaker who takes the primary role in social support and care for immediate and extended family members (Antshel, 2002). Origins of marianismo as a behavioral pattern come from deep-rooted Catholic beliefs of the traditional Latin female as related to the Mary, the mother of Christ (Wood & Price, 1999). Implications of marianismo create an ideal of women who are morally superior and spiritually stronger than the man. In terms of health care, this may mean that Latino women choose not to undergo treatments that would take them away from family responsibilities, or fail to disclose negative health information to family or providers.

AN ORGANIZATIONAL MODEL OF VALUE-BASED SOCIALIZATION MESSAGES

Beginning from this understanding of health care disparities among Latinos, we propose a value-based approach to socializing Latinos into health care organizations in a culturally competent manner. Effective socialization messages must be grounded in shared values, and considered in the context of the process through which individuals are assimilated into organizations. Diagnosis and treatment of ethnic and racial minorities must include culturally and linguistically competent communication by health organizations. In the following, we provide a brief discussion of organizational socialization, then explain the importance and types of value-based messages appropriate for health organizations seeking to socialize racial and ethnic minority patients.

Organizational Socialization for Racial and Ethnic Minority Patients

Being socialized into a cancer care system is similar to being socialized into any other organization. Socialization is largely a process of information management, thus making the socialization process a useful tool for understanding how health organizations can positively influence decisions on the part of members. By creating effective, value-based socialization messages, health care and community-based organizations can influence the choices of Latinos, thus reducing health disparities. The following section explains the three-part socialization process with particular attention to values-based messages.

Organizational socialization is the process of adjusting the individual to the organization and the organization to the individual. In traditional research on socialization, the focus is more heavily on integration by conforming the individual to the organization (Jablin, 2001). In the case of health care organizations, however, the focus should be on adapting the organization or perceptions of the organization to the individual. Research on socialization in employment indicates that organizational newcomers experience a three-step process including an anticipatory phase, an entry phase, and an assimilation phase (Jablin, 2001).

Anticipatory Phase. Cancer patients who are in the *anticipatory phase* of socialization receive general information and form opinions about the larger health care system, and about specific health organizations. Jablin (2001) explained that before entering an organization, individuals already have expectations and beliefs about how organizations such as the health care system operate. That information has an impact on whether patients choose to interact with an organization. Most research on the anticipatory phase has focused on where people get anticipatory messages—educational institutions, the media, family and friends, and experiences with work. Despite the significant public relations efforts of many health organizations, very few messages are constructed to generate impressions of cultural sensitivity. Generally, these messages are more accidental or informal than they are strategic.

In socializing members into health organizations, the anticipatory stage must be much more strategically constructed to convey cultural sensitivity. This phase provides an opportunity for community organizations and specific health care organizations to begin to establish shared values with the larger Latino community. Demonstrating shared values between the organization and the individual serves a number of important functions at the anticipatory stage. First, it can help to create the underlying links so important to establishing a favorable decision-making climate. Second, it may create a more personal perception of the organization and enhance identification.

Messages in the anticipatory stage should also attempt to influence the decision-making climate. If members understand how making preferred health information management decisions helps them meet values shared by the organization, they are more likely to make those preferred choices. Messages in the anticipatory phase, for example, may link the shared value of family with decisions about cancer prevention and screening. By communicating in ways that identify shared values, community organizations and health care organizations alike can prepare patients for the entry and assimilation phase of socialization.

Miller and Jablin (1991) identified the entry phase as a key point for information-seeking on the part of newcomers. They argue that newcomers' choices of information-seeking strategies are related to perceived social costs of information seeking. This is particularly important in socializing newcomers in health organizations because of the impact that information-seeking behaviors has been shown to have on health outcomes (Czaja et al., 2003). In order for newcomers in health organizations to use more direct information-seeking strategies, organizations need to communicate in ways that lower the perceived social cost. One way of doing this is to create an environment where seeking information and taking action on health issues does not violate closely held cultural or personal values.

Entry Phase. During the *entry* and *assimilation* phases, organizations focus on creating the favorable decision-making environment just discussed. Part of being integrated into an organization is understanding how members are expected to make decisions, and sharing the values of the organization in making decisions. The entry phase begins when a member first interacts with the health care organization. In traditional work organizations, this phase often entails an orientation program. In health organizations, it may include an orientation with a representative of the organization, as well as printed materials or videotapes.

Louis (1980) recognized that organizational newcomers require two specific types of information—task or role information and cultural information. Likewise, in order to effectively socialize a newcomer into the system as a whole, organizational messages must address not only the specifics of a particular diagnosis, but also patient responsibilities related to long-term treatment and care. These messages will be most effective if they are based on shared values between the patient and the provider organization.

The personalization of the system suggested in the anticipatory stage must be reinforced at entry. Some specific strategies to increase personalization include identification of shared values, the use of collective pronouns like "we" and "our," and a consistent tone or unified voice across organizational documents (Cheney, 1983).

If Latino audiences can be encouraged to perceive a health care organization as a "person" of sorts, with a welcoming and friendly "voice" and a shared set of values, community organizations can help capitalize on the idea of personalismo by personalizing the health care institution and encouraging members to build a relationship not just with an individual provider, but with a system. Clearly, health care organizations can assist in this process after organizational entry by providing patient advocates, or "navigators" (Hablamos Juntos, 2005), who personalize interactions and maintain a consistent presence even as a patient moves from specialist to specialist.

Assimilation Phase. From entry, individuals move into a stage of organizational assimilation. Once newcomers have reached the assimilation stage, they feel like they are part of the organization. Assimilation is an ongoing process that is accomplished through a negotiation between individuals and organizations. For patients with cancer, this means gaining a clear understanding of patient and provider roles in cancer care, and a sense of agency on the part of patients in their ability to participate in health decision making (O'Hair et al., 2003). Fryer (1998) described this process as "striving for purposeful self-determination, attempting to make sense of, initiate, influence, and cope with events in line with personal values, goals, and expectations of the future in a context of cultural norms, traditions, and past experiences" (p. 12). Table 13.1 outlines a variety of other strategies for personalizing socialization into health care organizations for patients who are newly diagnosed with cancer.

TABLE 13.1
STRATEGIES TO PERSONALIZE PATIENT SOCIALIZATION IN HEALTH CARE ORGANIZATIONS

ORGANIZATIONAL ELEMENTS	PERSONALIZATION FOR LATINO PATIENTS WITH CANCER
Organizational structure	Inclusive governance with community advisory board
	Opportunities for informal interpersonal contact with providers such as provider-sponsored support groups
	Policies and procedures to require a balance between task and relational communication
Materials for patients and employees	Physical environment includes signage and graphics representing Latino culture
	All printed and audiovisual materials make use of shared values as well as inclusive ("we" and "our") language
	Distribution of staff bios to patients
Staff diversity	Representative staff for diverse patient populations on all work shifts
	Representation of multiple Spanish-language dialects
Staff training and development	Diversity training on Latino culture
	Spanish-language classes for staff
	Standardized curriculum and materials
	Evaluation of employee learning outcomes
Translation services	All printed materials available in Spanish
	Disease-specific materials in Spanish to aid in patient understanding
Interpreter services	All medical visits include qualified interpreter
	Interpreters trained in language and culture
	No family member interpreters
	Interpreters available for telephone consults
Tracking system for LEP patients	Patient satisfaction assessment throughout health care process
	Navigator/patient advocate program for LEP patients

Note: LEP, Limited English Proficiency (from OMH, 2003)

Value-Based Socialization Messages

For organizations, managing how members think about values is a key component to successful organizational socialization (Tompkins & Cheney, 1985). Anticipatory, entry, and assimilation messages that appeal to culturally specific values can be utilized by health organizations to socialize patients. When making a decision about how to manage health information, a cancer patient will weigh decisions against personal, cultural, and organizational values.

In order to encourage positive information management decisions by patients, organizations need to craft messages that demonstrate alignment between cultural and organizational values, and make use of shared values in advocating specific decisions. It is important that the values advanced by the organization are sensitive to those cultural values, or are framed in ways that integrate them. We call messages designed to accomplish this goal *value-building* and *value-aligning* messages. Table 13.2 outlines key message strategies to build, align, and target Latino values for patients with cancer.

Value-building messages establish what values are considered important by an organization. These messages will be most effective if they are in line with values already held by the target audience. Bostdorff and Vibbert (1994) suggested specific strategies for promoting shared values with an audience. They argued that organizations can identify shared values by praising them explicitly or by praising notable people who are models of the values. For example, health organizations may use notable cancer survivors such as Lance Armstrong to demonstrate the importance of values such as determination and courage in surviving cancer.

TABLE 13.2
KEY MESSAGE STRATEGIES FOR SUCCESSFUL SOCIALIZATION OF LATINO PATIENTS WITH CANCER

Key Message Type	Operational Definition	Stages of Socialization	Example Messages for Latino Cancer Patients	Representative Latino Cultural Value
Value-building	Messages that identify values held by the organization	Anticipatory	"Taking care of your family is important to us"	Familiasm
		Entry	"We take the time to get to know our patients as people"	Personalismo

TABLE 13.2
KEY MESSAGE STRATEGIES FOR SUCCESSFUL SOCIALIZATION OF LATINO PATIENTS WITH CANCER *(continued)*

Key Message Type	Operational Definition	Stages of Socialization	Example Messages for Latino Cancer Patients	Representative Latino Cultural Value
		Assimilation	"We take care of you so you can take care of your family"	Marianismo
Value-aligning	Messages that demonstrate compatibility between organizational and cultural values	Anticipatory	"We have faith in our ability to offer you the highest quality physical and spiritual care.	Fatalismo
		Entry	"We will always provide you with the highest quality Spanish-speaking providers"	Linguistic competence
		Assimilation	Through careful treatment and God's will, the path to survivorship is possible.	Fatalismo
Value-targeting	Use existing values to request particular decision	Anticipatory	"Getting screened for prostate cancer is the manly thing to do"	Machismo
		Entry	The best way to take care of your family is to take care of yourself	Familiasm
		Assimilation	"We are your partners during every step of your care"	Personalismo

Note: LEP, Limited English Proficiency (from OMH, 2003)

Cheney (1983) found that organizations create identification around shared values by explicitly appealing to those values, and by incorporating testimony from both insiders and outsiders. Additionally, narratives about the experiences of *patient-members* similar to the target audience can help demonstrate shared values and create identification (Pribble, 1990). *Familia* is an example of a shared, culturally sensitive value that might be built by a health organization.

Organizations seeking to communicate in a culturally sensitive way will also need to create value-aligning messages. These messages illustrate that apparently contradictory cultural and organizational values are, in fact, compatible. Rather than attempting to persuade people to let go of core cultural values, organizations should frame arguments in ways that take advantage of them. For example, the values underlying *machismo* and *marianismo* are currently believed to contribute to information management decisions that lead to disparities (Villagran et al., 2005). Value-aligning messages could demonstrate that the health organization also values strength and pride among men, and caretaking among women.

Once an organization has built shared values, or demonstrated that their values are in alignment with individual or cultural values, value-targeting messages come into play. Tompkins and Cheney (1985) established that individuals make specific decisions by measuring the consequences of the decision against values. If the health organization has successfully built or aligned values, then individuals should make decisions that promote the interests of the organization—in this case, wise information management or behavioral decisions. Value-targeting messages use existing shared values as a ground for requesting or suggesting particular information management decisions or health-related behaviors. For example, once an organization has built the value of "family," it can combat the belief that seeking treatment creates family hardship by using value-targeting messages to demonstrate how specific behaviors such as seeking treatment can uphold the value of "family." As illustrated previously, an organization might use value-alignment arguments to establish that its values and the cultural values of machismo and marianismo are compatible. The value-targeting message would focus on elements of machismo such as pride and honor, arguing that it is strong to ask questions about health and to see to the health of one's family. The value of marianismo could be used in the same way. Messages could demonstrate that women can best fulfill their role as caretakers by monitoring their own health in addition to the health of their families.

Value-building, value-aligning, or valuc-targeting messages might appear in newsletters, face-to-face presentations, video promotions, advertisements and events. Additionally, something as simple as a billing statement or an appointment reminder can also reinforce values that organizations want members to consider when making information management choices. Elsbach, Sutton, and Principe (1998) found that hospitals effectively used messages on bills to influence how patients felt about paying. It seems reasonable that messages designed to influence information management could be communicated in this way as well.

In addition to establishing a basis for decisions, value arguments can also enhance members' feelings of identification and belonging in the organization, and may create additional trust for later organizational messages (Cheney, 1983). This process is consistent with the Latino cultural value of personalismo.

CONCLUSION

Value-based arguments are key in the process of socializing individuals into the cancer-care system. By using value-building, value-aligning, and value-targeting messages to integrate individuals into the system, health care organizations can influence the information management choices of Latinos, thus reducing health disparities.

This is a preliminary model that attempts to create a framework for dealing with the role of culture in the cancer context. Patient choices about how to seek out or avoid information can be addressed by organizational concepts such as organizational socialization. Future work in this area should explicitly focus on measuring information management among Latino patients with cancer. Contextually, linguistically, and culturally appropriate messages can be constructed to reduce potential health disparities from differing information management strategies.

REFERENCES

Adams, M. (1991). Information and education across the phases of cancer care. *Seminars in Oncology Nursing, 7,* 105-111.

Anderson, R. M. (1995). Revisiting the behavioral model of access to medical care: Does it matter? *Health Services Research, 9,* 208-220.

Antshel, K. L. (2002). Integrating culture as a means of improving treatment adherence in the Latino population. *Psychology, Health and Medicine, 7,* 435-449.

Ashton, C. M., Haldet, P., Paterniti, D. A., Collins, T. C., Gordon, H. S., O'Malley, K., Petersen, L. A., Sharf, B., Suarez-Almazor, M. E., Wray, N., & Street, R. (2003). Racial and ethnic disparities in the use of health services. *Journal of General Internal Medicine, 18,* 148-152.

Bach, P. B.. Cramer, L., Warren, & Begg, C. B. (1999). Racial differences in the treatment of early stage lung cancer. *New England Journal of Medicine, 341,* 1198-1205.

Baquet, C. R., & Hunter, C. P. (1995). Patterns in minority and special populations. In P. Greenwald, B. Kramer, & D. L. Weed (Eds.), *Cancer prevention and control* (pp. 23-36). New York: Marcel Dekker.

Bostdorff, D.M., & Vibbert, S.L. (1994). Values advocacy: Enhancing organizational images, deflecting public criticism, and grounding future arguments. *Public Relations Review, 20,* 141-158.

Brashers, D. E., Goldsmith, D. J., & Hsieh, E. (2002). Information seeking and avoiding in health contexts. *Human Communication Research, 28,* 258-271.

Butow, P., Brindle, E., McConnell, D., Boakes, R., & Tattersall, M. (1998). Information booklets about cancer: Factors influencing patient satisfaction and utilisation. *Patient Education and Counseling, 33*, 129-141.

CDC. (2003). Health United States, table 68. Hyattsville, MD. Retrieved February 20, 2005, from http://www.cdc.gov/nchs/data/hus/tables/2003/03hus030.pdf.

Cheney, G. (1983). The rhetoric of identification and the study of organizational communication. *Quarterly Journal of Speech, 69,* 143-158.

Cora-Bramble, D., & Williams, L. (2000). Explaining illness to Latinos: Cultural foundations and messages. In B. B. Whaley (Ed.), *Explaining illness: Research, theory, and structure* (pp. 259-279). Mahwah, NJ: Erlbaum.

Czaja, R., Manfredi, C., & Price, J. (2003). The determinants and consequences of information seeking among cancer patients. *Journal of Health Communication, 8,* 529-562.

Degner, L. F., Kristjanson, L. J., Bowman, D., Sloan, J. A., Carriere, K. C., O'Neil, J., Bilodeau, B., Watson, P., & Mueller, B. (1997). Information needs and decisional preferences in women with breast cancer. *JAMA, 277*, 1485-1492.

Derdiarian, A. K. (1986). Information needs of recently diagnosed patients. *Nursing Research, 35,* 276-281.

Echlin, K. N., & Rees, C. E. (2002). Information needs and information seeking behaviors of men with prostate cancer and their partners: A review of the literature. *Cancer Nursing, 25,* 35-41.

Elsbach, K.D., Sutton, R.I., & Principe, K.E. (1998). Averting expected challenges through anticipatory impression management: A study of hospital billing. *Organizational Science, 9,* 68-86.

Fryer, D. (1998). Agency restriction. In N. Nicholson (Ed.), *The Blackwell encyclopedic dictionary of organizational behavior* (p. 12). Malden, MA: Blackwell Business.

Gotcher, J. M. (1993). The effects of family communication on psychosocial adjustment. *Journal of Applied Communication Research, 21,* 176-188.

Hablamos Juntos. (2005). A program of the Robert Wood Johnson Foundation. Retrieved August 9, 2005, from http://www.hablamosjuntos.org/default.asp.

Jablin, F.M. (2001). Organizational entry, assimilation, and disengagement/exit. In F.M. Jablin & L.L. Putnam (Eds.), *The new handbook of organizational communication: Advances in theory, research, and methods* (pp. 732-818). Thousand Oaks, CA: Sage.

Johnson, J. D., & Meischke, H. (1993). A comprehensive model of cancer-related information seeking applied to magazines. *Health Communication Research, 19,* 343-367.

Kakai, H., Maskarinec, G., Shumay, D. M., Tatsumura, Y., & Tasaki, K. (2003). Ethnic differences in choices of health information by cancer patients using complementary and alternative medicine: An exploratory study with correspondence analysis. *Social Science and Medicine, 56,* 851-862.

Lu, L., & Flores, G. (2005). Pay now or pay later: Providing interpreter services in health care. *Health Affairs, 24,* 435-444.

Lee, S. M., & Pope, C. R. (2001). *Patients who don't speak English: Improving language minorities' health care with professional interpreters.* Washington, DC: Office of Minority Health, U.S. Department of Health and Human Services.

Louis, M. R. (1980). Surprise and sensemaking: What newcomers experience in entering unfamiliar organizational settings. *Administrative Science Quarterly, 25,* 226-251.

Martinez, C. (1988). Mexican Americans. In L. Comas-Diaz & E. Griffith (Eds.), *Clinical guidelines in cross-cultural mental health* (pp. 182-203). New York: Wiley.

McCaughan, E. M., & Thompson, K. (2000). Information needs of cancer patients receiving chemotherapy at a day-case unit in Northern Ireland. *Journal of Clinical Nursing, 9,* 851-858.

McGorry, S. Y. (1999). An investigation of expectations and perceptions of healthcare services with a Latino population. *Journal of Health Care Quality Assurance, 12,* 190-197.

Miller, V. D., & Jablin, F. M. (1991). Information seeking during organizational entry: Influences, tactics, and a model of the process. *Academy of Management Review, 16,* 92-120.

Mills, M., & Sullivan, K. (1999) The importance of information giving for patients newly diagnosed with cancer: A review of the literature. *Journal of Clinical Nursing, 8,* 631-642.

National Institutes of Health. (n.d.). *Addressing health disparities: The NIH program of action.* Retrieved February 23, 2005, from http://healthdisparities.nih.gov/whatare.html.

Neff, J. A., (2001). A confirmatory factor analysis of a measure of "machismo" among Anglo, African American and Mexican American male drinkers. *Hispanic Journal of Behavioral Sciences, 23,* 171-188.

Office of Minority Health, US Department of Health and Human Services. (2003). *National study of culturally and linguistically appropriate services in managed care organizations.* Retrieved August 9, 2005, from http://www.omhrc.gov/cultural/MCOCLAS-1%20Final%20Report%20Main1.pdf.

O'Hair, D., Villagran, M. M., Wittenberg, E., Brown, K., Ferguson, M., Hall, H. T., & Doty, T. (2003). Cancer survivorship and agency model: Implications for patient choice, decision making, and influence. *Health Communication, 15,* 193-202

Pribble, P.T. (1990), Making an ethical commitment: A rhetorical case study of organizational socialization. *Communication Quarterly, 38,* 255-267.

Ross, C. E., Mirowski, J., & Cockerham, W. C. (1983). Social class, Mexican culture, and fatalism: Their effects on psychological distress. *American Journal of Community Psychology, 11,* 383-399.

Smedley, B. D., Stith, A. Y., & Nelson, A. R.. (2003). *Unequal treatment: Confronting racial and ethnic disparities in health care.* Washington, DC: National Academics Press.

Solis, H. L. (2003). Health disparities: A growing challenge in the Latino community. *Harvard Journal of Public Policy, 16,* 53-68.

Stevens, E. (1973). Machismo and marianismo. *Society, 10,* 57-63.

Thomas, S. B., Fine, M. J., & Ibrahim, S. A. (2004) Health disparities: The importance of culture and health. *American Journal of Public Health, 94,* 9-36.

Tompkins, P., & Cheney, G. (1985). Communication and unobtrusive control in contemporary organizations. In R. D. McPhee & P. K. Thompkins (Eds.), *Organizational communication: Traditional themes and new directions* (pp. 179-210). Beverly Hills, CA: Sage.

Trevino, F., Moyer, M., Valdez, R., & Stroup-Benham, C. (1991). Utilization of health services by Mexican-American, Mainland Puerto-Ricans and Cuban-Americans. *Journal of the American Medical Association, 265,* 233-237.

Villagran, M. M., Bains, Y. S., Guajardo, J., Munoz, O., & Thomas, C. R. (2005). *Preliminary investigation of preferred mediated and interpersonal sources of health information among low-income Hispanic program women receiving mammograms: The Laredo NCI U56 Health Care Disparities Navigator.* Paper presented at the American Society of Therapeutic Radiation and Oncology Conference, Denver, CO.

Wood, M. L., & Price, P. (1997). Machismo and marianismo: Implications for HIV/AIDS reduction and education. *American Journal of Health Studies, 13,* 44-53.

14

Finding Meaning in the Journey

Methods of Spiritual Coping for Aging Patients With Cancer

Nichole Egbert
Kent State University

Lisa Sparks
Chapman University

Gary L. Kreps
George Mason University

Athena du Pré
University of West Florida

> Cancer is a very frightening word, but it can also be a great teacher. . . . Stay strong, keep informed. Ask questions and most of all, stay faith-filled.

This advice, offered to *Newsday* columnist Saul Friedman (2005, p. B07), sums up many elements of a cancer experience—the fear, the learning, and the spirituality that are often involved. Few experiences change a person's sense of meaning and order more than a health crisis such as cancer. Patients diagnosed with cancer are likely to wonder "Why me?" and to feel, at times, hopeless and defeated (Fife, 2005). However, contrary to what might be expected, many cancer survivors report that—despite the pain, uncertainty, and stress—the experience actually enriches their lives. They find that life is more meaningful because they have changed their ideas about what is important. This perspective is not so hard to understand once we conceptualize a cancer experience (and life itself) as a quest for meaning.

As the stories in this chapter illustrate, a key component of coping with cancer is managing uncertainties and identifying meaning within the experience. In this respect, older adults may have an advantage over younger adults. Newman (2000) observed that diverse life experiences often engender a more sophisticated, and less egocentric, understanding of self and the world around us. This "expanded consciousness," as Newman called it, improves our ability to cope, to process novel information, and to find value and meaning within situations that seem, on the surface, meaningless or terrible.

As cancer survivor Regina Brett (2003) said, the challenge for people with cancer is to "get busy living or get busy dying" (p. B1). Faced with such an existential dilemma, cancer survivors young and old often seek spiritual understanding. In a study of an ethnically diverse sample of 248 cancer survivors, 40% reported wanting help with finding meaning in their experiences (Moadel et al., 1999).

Yet locating empirical communication studies that tackle issues of spirituality and/or religiosity is difficult (Egbert, Mickley, & Coeling, 2004). For whatever reason, these fundamental domains of human experience have been left largely unexplored by communication scholars until recently (see Parrott, 2004). When considering the impact of serious health issues such as cancer, understanding the processes of communicating and coping through spirituality is critical.

Our goal in this chapter is to discuss the role communication plays in facilitating coping with cancer through spirituality, a person's search for meaning in life's experiences. However, before the discussion can begin, we want to be clear about how we are conceptualizing *spirituality* and how this concept connects with related terms such as *religion* and *religiosity*.

DEFINITIONS OF RELIGION AND SPIRITUALITY

Although there is no general agreement regarding how the terms *religiosity* and *spirituality* should be defined, scholars largely agree that the terms represent separate, although overlapping, concepts (Koenig, McCullough, & Larson, 2001; Paloutzian & Kirkpatrick, 1995; Parrott, 2004; Thoresen & Harris, 2002). Historically, religiosity has received more scholarly attention than spirituality, especially in relation to health outcomes (Parrott, 2004). In 1967, a classic work by Allport and Ross differentiated between *intrinsic* (living according to one's religious beliefs because one truly believes in them) and *extrinsic* religiosity (using one's religion to meet needs such as social support, tradition, or status). This differentiation has been maintained by researchers for the past 40 years and has shaped our understanding of how religion and religiosity are defined. Thus, we rely on the related definition provided by Koenig et al. (2001):

> Religion is an organized system of beliefs, practices, rituals, and symbols designed (a) to facilitate closeness to the sacred or transcendent (God, higher power, or ultimate truth/reality) and (b) to foster an understanding of one's relationship and responsibility to others in living together in a community. (p. 18)

Spirituality, on the other hand, is a more expansive conceptualization of divinity. One may be a spiritual person, but not necessarily religious; likewise, being a member of a religion does not by definition make one spiritual. Whereas religion is associated with terms such as *formal*, *behavior-oriented*, and *doctrine-based*, spirituality is better characterized using words such as *individualistic*, *inward-directed*, and *not doctrine-oriented* (Koenig et al., 2001). Although both are concepts worthy of discussions related to cancer and aging, the central concept we highlight in this chapter is found in the term *spirituality*, meaning an individual's search for meaning in life (e.g., Dreyer, 1994; National Cancer Institute, 2005). Along these lines, we embrace Koenig et al.'s (2001) definition:

> Spirituality is the personal quest for understanding answers to ultimate questions about life, about meaning, and about relationships to the sacred or transcendent, which may (or may not) lead to or arise from the development of religious rituals and the formation of community. (p. 18)

Finding meaning after a diagnosis of cancer can be particularly difficult (Cole & Pargament, 1999). The diagnosis can challenge a person's core personal, vocational, and relational self-concepts. More to the point, how a person attributes meaning to these and other central beliefs can affect how he or she responds physically to medical interventions and therapies (Fife, 2005). Although experiencing a "loss of meaning and purpose" may be the result of clinical depression (a cause often overlooked by oncologists), feelings of meaninglessness may be the result of spiritual distress (Murray, Kendall, Boyd, Worth, & Benton, 2004).

In our effort to present a broad overview of spiritual coping mechanisms for people living with cancer, we chose to focus on the concept of *spirituality*, as opposed to religiosity, because spirituality is the more inclusive term. In the following analysis, we provide a context for individuals' search for meaning within cancer experiences.

MEANINGLESSNESS

The search for meaning within lived experiences is one of the most significant forces of human existence. To organize our discussion of this crucial journey, we draw on work in existential psychotherapy,[1] particularly that of Irvin Yalom, a contemporary scholar and therapist in the field. Yalom's (1980) model of the four "ultimate concerns of life" provides a revealing way to examine the quest by cancer survivors' for meaning and serves as the organizational structure on which our analysis is based.

In Yalom's model of meaning through struggle, he identified four struggles at the root of human experience: death, freedom, isolation, and meaninglessness. Yalom further proposed that there are six main strategies or mechanisms for spiritual coping: altruism, dedication to a cause, creativity, hedonism, self-actualization, and self-transcendence.

In the following sections, we discuss each of these strategies as it relates to coping with cancer. Additionally, we present stories and anecdotes of actual cancer survivors who have relied on these spiritual strategies in their own battles with cancer. Finally, we underline the communication processes that may help or hinder the search for meaning among those affected by cancer.

Spiritual Strategies for Creating Meaning

Although Yalom outlined six distinct strategies for combating meaninglessness, many of these strategies can overlap with one another; the strategies are not meant to be mutually exclusive. For example, one person may feel that appreciating life to the fullest (hedonism) means engaging in creative activities. Similarly, many cancer survivors find meaning in their circumstances by giving of themselves (altruism) to improve the situations of others struggling with cancer (dedication to a cause). Our goal in this discussion is to paint a broad picture of several different ways that people engage in a quest for meaning to relieve what Yalom (1980) called "existence pain," or the hurt that comes from common life experiences that are experienced differently by different individuals. The 12 examples presented here are stories from real cancer survivors who have found meaning through their own personal spir-

[1]Existential psychotherapy is based on the conviction that individuals should be treated as active, responsible agents in creating and understanding the circumstances of their lives. Existential therapists help clients make sense of their experiences, believing that the quest for meaning is the most profound of all human motivations and that each person's quest and understanding are unique. (This represents a divergent viewpoint from Freud's conviction that sex, not meaning, is human's most primary and powerful motivation.)

itual journeys. They share some common experiences as cancer survivors; however, many of their experiences of the illness are as unique as the people themselves.

> *The only ones among you who will be really happy are those who have sought and found how to serve.*
> —Albert Schweitzer

Altruism. Yalom explained altruism as the desire to leave the world a better place. History is filled with examples of people dedicated to improving the human situation; for example, Mother Teresa, Florence Nightingale, and Princess Diana were noted for their altruistic efforts on behalf of humanity. However, as laudable as their efforts were, how much more notable are the efforts of those who engage in selfless acts of altruism in the face of a serious illness such as cancer? In this section we describe the cases of Angie and Santiago.

Angie Alexander was 30 years old and 26 weeks pregnant when her husband noticed a lump in her breast that was quickly diagnosed as cancer. After delivering her baby early so that she could begin chemotherapy (which sent her into early menopause), she was fired from her job for not returning to work soon enough following her maternity leave (Strote, 2004). Yet even in these circumstances, Angie immediately began to give back to others. Following her treatments, Angie joined an organization called "ChemoAngels," a volunteer group that organizes support for people undergoing cancer therapies such as chemotherapy and radiation. She was paired with a 6-year-old boy in New Mexico so that she could send him hope through letters, cards, and gifts. "Being a ChemoAngel has helped tremendously with my own recovery" she says (Strote, para. 17).

Santiago was diagnosed with Stage IV bladder cancer at age 64. After enduring a 14-hour surgery during which his bladder, prostate, lymph nodes, and appendix were removed, and a new bladder created from part of his small intestine, he underwent chemotherapy ("Cancer Survivors' Network," 2002a). Since his recovery from cancer and from these invasive treatments, Santiago has dedicated his life to volunteering with organizations such as the American Association for Retired Persons and the Honor Guard at the National Cemetery in Riverside, California. He speaks very highly of the role of volunteering in cancer recovery:

> By doing volunteer work, this is something that I myself have decided to go forward to. I'm not being forced to do it; I'm doing it because I want to. And I think this is very important for a cancer survivor or any other survivor. You have to find a way to keep it going! We can't dwell

> on what we've been through, what we did, what could have been, whatever. You just got to keep going. ("Cancer Survivors' Network," 2002a)

In these instances, altruistic endeavors give life meaning even when cancer introduced uncertainty and hardship. The effect appears to be prevalent. In a study of older adults with cancer, Pentz (2005) found that the majority attribute their survival to spiritual faith, the support of others, and their commitment to work in the community. One participant in the study declared, "I don't have time to die" (p. 3).

Duty is never worthily performed until it is performed by one who would gladly do more if only he could.
—Harry Emerson Fosdick

Dedication to a Cause. Many cancer survivors find strength and meaning through dedication to worthy causes. Although not all worthy causes are cancer-related, many cancer survivors champion efforts to combat the disease that has affected their lives.

Lance Armstrong is perhaps the most visible cancer spokesperson of the last 10 years. His story of defeating testicular cancer and going on to win the Tour de France seven times made him a national hero; however, it was the creation of the Lance Armstrong Foundation in 1997 that made him one of the most influential celebrity spokespersons of his time. In 2004, the foundation began to sell the "Livestrong" yellow plastic bracelets for $1 each, donating the proceeds to youth cancer programs. To date, the foundation has sold more than 7 million bracelets and generated more attention for cancer research than any other communication campaign in recent memory.

Joseph Simone is another founder of an organization dedicated to discovering a cancer vaccine and to supporting cancer survivors and their families. Joseph, an entrepreneur who founded and runs Saratoga Food Group, a company that develops restaurants, has a great deal of personal experience with cancer. In addition to surviving cancer twice himself, he lost his wife, Merium Ann Simone, to liver cancer, and is watching his 3-year-old grandson fight leukemia (Landskroener, 2003). He and his wife founded the International Spirit of Life Foundation in 1999, an organization that partners with the Washington Cancer Institute to increase global awareness of cancer and share information about the disease. Joseph feels driven by his personal experiences to become a leader in the fight to cure cancer. "With genetic predispositions and environmental causes, we are seeing younger people with cancer. It's getting way out of control. Still I'm convinced the answer is out there, not in laboratories here in Washington but around the world" (Landskroener, 2003, paragraph 7).

Confusion is the welcome mat at the door of creativity.
—Michael J Gelb

Creativity. When Yalom (1980) described searching for meaning through creativity, he included any instance in which something new was generated. For some, creativity might lie in a scientific discovery, whereas for others, creativity means generating something artistic, engaging in storytelling, or creatively reframing an experience through humor or play.

When Calliope, a medical educator, learned at age 32 that she would lose her left eye in the process of removing a cancerous tumor on her optic nerve, she was immediately beset by uncertainty. First of all, could she function with sight in only one eye? To test herself, she drove home from the doctor's office with one eye closed. She recalls with a laugh: "I got home and I told my husband, 'I think I can do this. I tried it on the way home!'" Her optimism and coping ability were fueled by her creativity. Willing to experiment with new ways of performing everyday tasks, she felt less victimized and helpless than she might have.

Calliope also valued the role of humor and play. She says colleagues and physicians often used humor to reduce her uncertainty about what lay ahead.

> I was just so scared I would wake up [after surgery] and find they had made a mistake. I said, "If you take the wrong eye, just kill me, because I don't want to be completely blind." . . . I called up one of my doctor friends and shared my fear with him. He said, "I'll tell you what, just take yourself a big black marker and draw a ring around the eye they're supposed to take. Put a big arrow and write 'This one!' under it."

Calliope did not actually mark her eye before surgery, but the advice offered her humorous relief and perhaps a sense that she had more control over the situation than she imagined.

Calliope also enjoyed humorous rapport with the prosthetic specialist who crafted an artificial eye for her. He had lost an eye himself, and he shared humorous stories about clients and friends, including a football player who popped out his prosthetic eye on the field to unnerve his opponents. "I laughed until my stomach hurt," Calliope recalls.

In Calliope's case, coping with cancer involved creative behavioral adaptations, storytelling episodes, regular doses of humor, and a willingness to lay her fears on the table. She has been cancer-free since the surgery and follow-up therapy. The moral of her story, she says, is that you will have good days and bad days, but you can handle almost anything if you have the right attitude and keep on with your life.

> It was strange. Cancer of the eye is especially rare. You don't expect things like that to happen. But I just figured, I'm unique—this is unique. Let's take care of it and move on.

Likewise, Tonya Fowler Corbett's experience of creativity in the face of cancer is quite personal. She is one of only two women in the world who was able to give birth after surviving her type of ovarian cancer ("Cancer survivor story," n.d.). Doctors discovered this rare, and often fatal, form of cancer in Tonya in the form of a volleyball-sized tumor when she was only 17 years old. Her Stage III cancer had spread to her abdominal wall. She was treated with chemotherapy, and after a relapse and a few years had passed, she discovered that she was pregnant. Although the pregnancy was difficult, her baby was born healthy. "Oh Lord yes I feel lucky," she said. "All that time I was asking 'why me, why me.' Then you have him and it's all worth it" ("Cancer survivor story," n.d., paragraph 5).

B. Clare Goodwin is a therapist and survivor of cervical cancer from West Brookfield, Massachusetts. In 1997 she and 13 other women organized "Through the Eyes of Cancer," a multimedia show displaying creative works such as poetry, photography, weavings, and dance. She described the show as a sort of "show and tell" that got her and the others "in touch with our creativity" (Cahill, 1997, paragraph 7). Clare's creative expression of choice is her paintings known as "mandalas," or "bright circles filled with abstract or realistic shapes." She also displays her journal, filled with her writings and painted images. Clare and the other artists who participated in the show donated a portion of the proceeds to subsidize cancer survivors' enrollment in psychotherapy programs such as the one in which many of these women first met.

My cancer scare changed my life. I'm grateful for every new, healthy day I have. It has helped me prioritize my life.
—Olivia Newton-John

Hedonism. Although hedonism is often interpreted as self-centered pleasure-seeking, Yalom (1980) used the term to signify appreciating life to the fullest extent, not taking any moment or experience for granted. Many cancer survivors, such as the famous Australian pop singer and breast cancer survivor Olivia Newton-John, stress that surviving cancer has caused them to experience life on a different level: one at which every little blessing is cherished.

Nick Sullo has survived non-Hodgkin's lymphoma, chemotherapy, a bone marrow transplant, and a serious car accident. The 55-year-old husband and father leaned on his family and members of his cancer support group for strength ("Cancer Survivors' Network," 2002b). He now finds great reward in "little" things in life, such as planning vacations and his daughter's wedding. He stated:

> Many people waste their time because they think they're immortal! I try and utilize, as best I can, all the time that I can to do things that I enjoy doing in life with my family, with my friends, with people in my cancer support group. I'm living life. I'm part of life, and I want to continue doing that. ("Cancer Survivors' Network, 2002b)

Similarly, Carmen Mitchell relies on "living her life to the fullest" as a way to cope with Stage IV colon cancer. Although her condition was terminal (in 2002 she was told she had approximately 3 to 6 months to live), Carmen was still alive, fighting her cancer 2 years later in March 2005. She credits her longevity to a positive spirit.

> I live for today, I play for tomorrow, but I live for today to the fullest. I wake up in the morning and think, "What am I going to do today? And what am I going to do to contribute to someone else's happiness as well?" And live it that way. (Enersen, 2005, para. 4)

As a wife and the mother of three sons, Carmen also says her family and her faith contribute to her ability to remain positive. Soon after she found out about her terminal cancer diagnosis, she and her husband decided to renew their marriage vows as a celebration of their relationship.

Oh, my friend, it's not what they take away from you that counts. It's what you do with what you have left.
—Hubert Humphrey

Self-Actualization. Yalom's definition of self-actualization is not far removed from that of Maslow (1962). Both scholars described the quest for developing the self's fullest potential, although Yalom's focus is more on accepting one's own spiritual core, and therefore resolving inner conflicts and becoming more free. In any case, cancer survivors who exhibit the strategy of self-actualization demonstrate that they believe that even the experience of having cancer has contributed to their growth as human beings.

One example of self-actualization can be seen in Kaycee Hale, an African-American woman and self-proclaimed workaholic in her 50s, who was diagnosed with breast cancer in 2002. One of the most difficult and hidden struggles of Kaycee's cancer was the effect on her relationships. She found that many of the friends on whom she had counted in the past let her down, opening a void for new relationships that she calls "Survivor Sisters." These new friends, introduced through an extended network of Kaycee's friends and families, provided support by traveling to see her, participating in prayer circles, and even fasting on the day of Kaycee's chemotherapy. The new relationships have helped Kaycee feel at peace and conclude that although no one would purposely choose her path, she would not change anything, as her cancer was necessary for her to have the life she lives today. Says a writer familiar with Kaycee: "This disease gave her the opportunity to experience real support, real compassion, and real love" (Kaycee H., 2004, para. 8).

Dan Easterling also found opportunity for personal growth in his bout with germ cell cancer in 1991. Thinking that he was suffering from a cold, Dan's doctor ordered a lung X-ray only to find a football-sized tumor (Easterling, 1997). After three courses of chemotherapy and surgery, Dan began to reflect on his life, deciding that he needed a change that would provide more challenge and opportunity. He had been working as an auto mechanic, but decided to go back to school to earn his bachelor's degree in criminal justice. This choice was not without costs. Dan's wife divorced him and remarried soon after. This and the other difficulties in his life spurred him forward to achieve his goals. Dan finished a master's program in 1 year and enrolled in a PhD program in political economy at the University of Texas at Dallas in 1998. Although one might expect that Dan Easterling would be an unhappy, bitter person, he finds himself grateful for the cancer and his personal struggles, and is "profoundly happy. Cancer took many things from me, but what I have gained is so much greater I now say it was the best thing that ever happened to me" (Easterling, 1997, para. 16). Among the benefits that he attributes to his cancer experience are self-confidence, the desire to challenge himself, a sense of peace, deep relationships, a more loving spirit, and a greater self-awareness.

Let Go and Let God
—Author Unknown

Self-Transcendence. The last of Yalom's (1980) strategies to combat meaninglessness is self-transcendence, or the transfer of focus from oneself to something "higher," often God, religion, or another form of spiritual practice such as meditation or communing with nature. In this category we placed more traditional forms of spiritual coping, such as faith in God and prayer.

Dr. Carolyn Kinney is a therapist, nurse, and professor at the University of Texas Medical Branch at Galveston School of Nursing. Kinney, who lost her mother to breast cancer 30 years before she was diagnosed with it herself, believes that her cancer may have been an answer to her wish that she could have helped her mother more when her mother was battling the disease (Foote, 1999). She makes sense of her cancer as the impetus to "keep me on the path I should be on." Now Kinney leads a group of female cancer survivors in weekly meetings in her home. The 3-hour sessions consist of activities such as nutrition discussions, guided imagery exercises, and conversations about releasing control and expressing emotions. Every session ends in meditation, during which the women can listen to their inner voices and connect with a "higher spiritual language" (Foote, 1999, para. 9). She believes in meditation because "what healing is really about is being able to come to a place where you have a sense of understanding the meaning of your life and what has happened to you" (Foote, 1999, para. 9).

RuthAnn Lobo, mother of WNBA forward Rebecca Lobo, was a busy wife, mother, and school counselor when she noticed a lump in her breast while showering in 1993. At the time, her daughter Rebecca was playing for the University of Connecticut (UConn), and RuthAnn's life was a blur of activities (Lobo, n.d.). The days and weeks that followed, however, included a lumpectomy, mastectomy, as well as chemotherapy and participation in a clinical trial. Although she had the unfailing support of her husband, family, and the UConn women's basketball team, RuthAnn still struggled with dark, negative thoughts of death and dying. Then she made a commitment to herself to find new hope and positivity in her life through renewed spirituality. For RuthAnn, this spiritual nurturing came through seeking God in scripture, religious books and tapes, prayer, and church attendance. Her primary message: "Focus not on the disease, but on God" (Lobo, n.d., para. 17).

> I looked for God and He was there. I found Him in the faces of family, colleagues, friends, and teammates. I found Him in notes from strangers. I found Him in my local church on Sunday, but I also found Him in the healing services and prayer meetings of many denominations. (Lobo, n.d., para. 18)

CONCLUSION

Our cultural assumptions suggest that cancer is a dreadful diagnosis that leads to death. A closer look reveals that, along with the fear and uncertainty of cancer often comes unprecedented understanding, awareness, and appreciation for life. This chapter is part of an emerging field of research about the role of meaning, spirituality, and coping with health crises. A theme that arises with this and similar studies is that, no matter what their prognosis, cancer survivors are often grateful for cancer's role in redefining what their life is all about (see also, Charmaz, 1999; du Pré & Berlin Ray, Chapter 6, this volume).

As our understanding of spirituality, meaning, and health grows, we may change our ideas about what constitutes comforting communication. We may begin to acknowledge more fully people's unique quests for meaning. And we may rethink the popular notion that a health crisis is a purely organic phenomenon with nothing of value to add to a person's life experience.

Improved understanding may even challenge the assumption that illness and death are inherently bad. Casting illness and dying experiences in entirely negative terms masks the larger reality that almost nothing in life is entirely bad or entirely good. The work of Hospice of America is consistent with this viewpoint. Hospice volunteers and staff members treat illness as a natural part of life (McCormick & Conley, 1995). Hospice volunteers and staff members help others realize that avoiding talk about ill health often makes coping more difficult and may prevent people from attaining the new level of understanding such an experience can provide. Moreover, exposure to the narratives of cancer survivors may allow people to face their own misfortunes with greater confidence, knowing that others have managed similar crises and even gained something from them.

CancerCare, a national nonprofit organization that provides free support services to people affected by cancer, offers these five suggestions for nurturing one's spirit.

1. Take time regularly to meditate or pray. This can bring a sense of calm and stability during difficult times.
2. Read spiritual writings such as the Bible, the Koran, the Book of Psalms, Bhagavad Gita, or other faith-based texts. Delving into sacred texts can put you in touch with ancient traditions of wisdom and give you a sense of connection with a more divine reality. Recently published books on spirituality can also give new insights.
3. Seek the help of others. You might begin an ongoing dialogue with your clergy or counselor, or join a group for meditation, prayer, and support.
4. Retreat to spiritual spaces, natural settings, or concerts and museums to cultivate a spiritual sense of peace.
5. Keep a journal to express your feelings, thoughts, and memories. It can contribute to your process of self-discovery and spiritual development.
   http://www.cancercare.org/pdf/fact_sheets/fs_strength_spirit_en.pdf

We must not overlook the impact of cultural differences when studying (and ultimately trying to improve) the experiences of people living with cancer. Hispanic and African-American cancer survivors in Moadel and colleagues' (1999) study were particularly likely to describe unmet spiritual needs. Failing to address their spiritual concerns may not only leave an important life dimension unexplored, but may marginalize the experiences of underrepresented groups such as Hispanics and African Americans.

It is worth noting that health crises do not only affect the diagnosed individuals. Loved ones and caregivers also experience some of the losses and rewards involved in making sense of cancer experiences. When nurses were interviewed about their most rewarding experiences, it was surprising to find that nearly every one of them described caring for a terminally ill patient. As one nurse said, "People who are dying sometimes have an ability to see the world the way no one else can. You feel like you're in the presence of greatness sometimes." Another said:

> You don't expect the patients to offer you anything—I mean like wisdom or even a smiling "good morning" every day. Mostly we're there to offer them what they need and they're in hard times. But now and then a patient comes in and I think we should be paying him [or her] because we grow so much just knowing them. Those are the patients you never forget!

Perhaps the patients with the most to offer are the ones who cope effectively and even find something to marvel at within life's most trying times.

In a qualitative study investigating the spiritual dimensions of cancer survivors, Thomas and Retsas (1999) concluded that nurses and other professional health care providers can aid people with cancer in their quest for spiritual meaning. "The nurse may help clients during this process by engaging in behaviors that enhance the person's self-esteem and self-confidence and that help the person realize their wholeness through self-actualisation" (p. 200). The authors suggest that communication-related behaviors such as providing social support, encouragement, and a hopeful, positive attitude can facilitate the making of meaning through self-actualization.

Finding meaning within a cancer experience is no easy task. As Frankl (1959) and Yalom (1980) pointed out, the riches of self-transcendent or spiritual understanding are not easily won. The process typically involves letting go of previous assumptions and feelings and allowing the evolution of greater understanding. Whether this understanding is achieved through altruism, hedonism, self-transcendence, creativity, devotion to a cause, or self-actualization, it is not typically a passive or immediate process. However, the examples provided here remind us ultimately that health crises are not purely dreadful, that healing occurs in unexpected ways, and that adversity can be an opportunity for reflection and discovery. As Rachel Naomi Remen, a University of California-San Francisco medical professor, said, "Things that cannot be cured can still heal. Curing happens at the level of the body, healing happens to the whole person at the level of the heart and soul" (see http://www.givingvoice.org/learn/conference.html).

REFERENCES

Allport, G. W., & Ross, J. M. (1967). Personal religious orientation and prejudice. *Journal of Personality and Social Psychology, 5*, 432-443.

Brett, R. (2003, February 21). Life's great, say area survivors. *The Plain Dealer*, p. B1.

Cahill, P. (1997, December 15). Letters from eternity: Women who have been through cancer express their sorrows and triumphs in an Amherst exhibition. *Springfield (Massachusetts) Union News*. Retrieved online July 31, 2005, from http://www.abgoodwin.com/mandala/eyes.html

Cancercare. (n.d.). *Strengthening the spirit*. Retrieved November 13, 2005, from http://www.cancercare.org/pdf/reading/fs_stregtheningspirit.pdf

Cancer Survivors' Network. (2002a). *American Cancer Society*. Retrieved November 13, 2005, from http://www.acscsn.org/Talk_Shows_and_Stories/ Featured_Stories/901santiago.html

Cancer Survivors' Network. (2002b). *American Cancer Society*. Retrieved November 13, 2005, from http://www.acscsn.org/Talk_Shows_and_Stories/Featured_Stories/Nick_Sullo.html

Cancer survivor story: A local woman beats the odds and inspires others. (n.d.). New Hanover Health Network Online Cancer Center. Retrieved October 29, 2005, from http://www.nhhn.org/1140.cfm

Charmaz, K. (1999). "Discoveries" of self in illness. In K. Charmaz & D. A. Paternati (Eds.), *Health, illness, and healing: Society, social context, and self* (pp. 72-82). Los Angeles: Roxbury.

Cole, B., & Pargament, K. (1999). Re-creating your life: A spiritual/psychotherapeutic intervention for people diagnosed with cancer. *Psycho-Oncology, 8*, 395-407.

Dreyer, E. A. (1994). *Earth crammed with heaven: A spirituality of everyday life*. New York: Paulist Press.

Easterling, D. (1997, July). "I will not live in fear"—A story of cancer survivorship and hope. *THRIVEnet*. Retrieved August 4, 2005, from http://www.thrivenet.com/stories/stories97/stry9707.html

Egbert, N., Mickley, J., & Coeling, H. (2004). A review and application of social scientific measures of religiosity and spirituality: Assessing a missing component in health communication research. *Health Communication, 16*, 7-27.

Enersen, P. (2005, March 24). Living life to the fullest. *King5.com*. Retrieved July 31, 2005, from http://www.king5.com/health/specials/stories/NW_032305HEKcolonmitchellSW.144ba325f.html

Fife, B. L. (2005, November). The role of constructed meaning in adaptation to the onset of life-threatening illness. *Social Science & Medicine, 61*(10), 2132-2143.

Foote, K. (1999, Fall). Person, heal thyself. *University of Texas Medical Branch at Galveston Newsletter*. Retrieved from http://64.233.167.104/search?q=cache:0UP_hC88s_UJ:www.utmb.edu/utmbmagazine/archive/archive_pdfs/Fall99.pdf+%22UTMB+Quarterly+fall+99%22&hl=en (pp. 34-35).

Frankl, V. (1959). *Man's search for meaning* (I. Lasch, Trans.). Boston: Beacon Press.

Friedman, S. (2005, September 10). Gray matters: Some thoughts on cancer, which I'm beating, so far. *Newsday* (Nassau Ed.), p. B07.

Kaycee H. (2004, June). *Breastlink: Optimal cancer care*. Retrieved October 29, 2005, from www.breastlink.com/resources/survivor-kaycee_h.aspx)

Koenig, H. G., Mc Cullough, M. E., & Larson, D. B. (2001). *Handbook of religion and health*. New York: Oxford University Press.

Landskroener, M. (2003, Autumn). Forum: International spirit of life foundation. *International Network for Cancer Treatment and Research, 4*(2). Retrieved from http://www.inctr.org/publications/2003_v04_n02_a04.shtml

Lobo, R. (n.d.). About me: My story. *Loboline*. Retrieved August 3, 2005, from http://www.loboline.com/about_my_story.htm

Maslow, A. H. (1962). *Toward a psychology of being*. Princeton, NJ: Van Nostrand.

McCormick, T. R., & Conley, B. J. (1995). Patients' perspectives on dying and on the care of dying patients. *The Western Journal of Medicine, 163*(3), 236-243.

Moadel, A. L., Morgan, C., Fatone, A., Grennan, J., Carter, J., Laruffa, G., Skummy, A., & Dutcher, J. (1999). Seeking meaning and hope: Self-reported spiritual and existential needs among an ethnically-diverse cancer patient population. *Pyscho-Oncology, 8*, 378-385.

Murray, S. A., Kendall, M., Boyd, K., Worth, A., & Benton, T. F. (2004). Exploring the spiritual needs of people dying of lung cancer or heart failure: A prospective qualitative interview study of patients and their carers. *Palliative Medicine, 18*, 39-45.

National Cancer Institute. (2005, June 7). *Spirituality in cancer care*. Retrieved November 13, 2005, from http://www.cancer.gov/cancertopics/pdq/supportivecare/spirituality/healthprofessional/allpages#Section_4

Newman, M. A. (2000). *Health as expanding consciousness* (2nd ed.). Boston, MA: Jones & Bartlett.

Paloutzian, R. F., & Kirkpatrick, L. A. (1995). Introduction: The scope of religious influences on personal and societal well-being. *Journal of Social Issues, 51*(2), 1-11.

Parrott, R. (Ed.). (2004). Religious faith, spirituality, and health communication [Special Issue]. *Health Communication, 16*(1).

Pentz, M. (2005, January-February). Resilience among older adults with cancer and the importance of social support and spirituality-faith: "I don't have time to die". *Journal of Gerontological Social Work, 44*, 3-22.

Strote, M. E. (2004, October). Lessons in survival: Breast cancer changes everything. Here's what it taught three young women. *Shape*. Retrieved November 15, 2005 from, http://www.findarticles.com/p/articles/mi_m0846/is_2_24/ai_n6203847

Thomas, J., & Retsas, A. (1999). Transacting self-preservation: A grounded theory of the spiritual dimensions of people with terminal cancer. *International Journal of Nursing Studies, 36*, 191-201.

Thoresen, C. F., & Harris, A. H. (2002). Spirituality and health: What's the evidence and what's needed? *Annals of Behavioral Medicine, 24*, 3-13.

Yalom, I. D. (1980). *Existential psychotherapy*. New York: Basic Books.

15

Ending the End-of-Life Communication Impasse

A Dialogic Intervention

John W. Lannamann
University of New Hampshire

Linda M. Harris
U. S. Department of Health and Human Services

Alexis D. Bakos
National Institutes of Health

Kylene J. Baker
Texas A & M University

Gregory Bateson, famed anthropologist and communication scholar, died of cancer at his own funeral. Here is a portion of his daughter's, Mary Catherine Bateson, account of their extraordinary "Six Days of Dying":

> During those 6 days we were at San Francisco Zen Center, with most of the family and a few close friends sharing in the nursing and the Zen community providing practical help and a context of coherent tranquility. . . . Roger, a friend from Esalen, saw the pupils of his eyes dilate as his mind encountered the dark. So we gathered around the bed, some six of us who had been caring for him most closely, hardly breathing ourselves as we waited from breath to breath, the time stretching, the time

> stretching beyond the possible, and yet again and again followed by a gasping reflexive inhalation, and then again the lengthening pause. I kept praying that he would be free from each next compulsive effort, let go, rest, and when after a time no further breath followed, we still stood, slowly relaxing with the faintest sighs, barely able to return to a flow of time not shaped by that breathing. Lois reached forward, after her office, and gently closed his eyes.
>
> We did not at that time pause to mourn but slowly found our way into the expression of continuing care . . . in my turn, I reached out and began to straighten his arms, then folding his hands . . . we all worked together, removing soiled pads, cleaning away the final traces of excrement, lifting and turning and washing each limb. . . . Downstairs we drank sherry and ate the stilton cheese that Gregory loved . . . (Bateson, 1980, pp. 7-10)

Like many funerals, Gregory Bateson's was highly ritualized. Unlike most contemporary funerals, his was a continuation of the caregiving ritual, "so that the shadows of guilt and anger, which so often complicate grief . . . may be lightened by the experience of tending someone we love with our own hands, so that much that seems externally repellent and painful is transmuted by tenderness" (p. 4). What is striking about this description of the final days of Gregory Bateson's life is that the coherent tranquility afforded by his caregivers appears to have allowed him and those around him to preserve some of the qualities that had made his life meaningful. A persistent theme in Bateson's writing is that meaning, quality, and beauty are possible only in the context of a pattern of connections. In that sense, the meaning and quality of his end-of-life experience was a continuation of his pattern of living.

As life expectancies increase and the final effects of terminal illnesses are delayed, questions about the quality and meaning of the end-of-life become increasingly important. The medical advances that make new options possible for the terminally ill also present new burdens on the social support systems of patients and their families. In this chapter, we explore the communication implications of living longer with a terminal illness. Specifically, we explore what appears to be the paradox of end-of-life communication: Early family-led discussions regarding end-of-life decisions improve the quality of life for patients and their social support network, yet these discussions are often postponed until after many, if not all, of the options are closed off by death. We offer a therapeutic intervention of family-centered care-planning dialogues; a metaphor for interpersonal interactions in which patients and their significant others create their own communal meanings for what counts as postdiagnosis care and, in doing so, construct their own caring rituals, much like the Batesons did.

CONTEXT AND CONVERSATION MATTER

Context Matters

Context provides the social permissions and constraints for the kinds of things we can comfortably say and do together. And, in reciprocal fashion, the conversations that occur within these contexts help define their character as well (Pearce & Cronen, 1980). Hospitals, for example, to a large extent define and are defined by the conversations that are held and relationships that are sustained within them (Finnegan & Viswanath, 1990; Harris, Kobb, Ryan, Darkins, & Kreps, 2004). It should be expected, therefore, that certain kinds of hospital conversations are more easily held than others. Specifically, as we see in our overview of the evolution of hospital and hospice contexts, communication having to do with cure is quite a good fit within hospitals. Conversations about death and the end-of-life are permissible and even encouraged within a hospice context. However, the evidence of an impasse between patients and their providers regarding end-of-life communication, reviewed here, suggests there is no reliable way of initiating end-of-life conversations within the curative hospital context. Our review of recommendations for end-of-life conversations suggests they are helpful once the patient has shifted into a hospice context conducive to end-of-life communication but offer no reliable way to initiate the taboo subject of death within a curative hospital context. This chapter offers one way to manage this dilemma.

Rapid changes in U.S. medical care and technology have altered the communicative contexts in which patients and families make their decisions concerning end-of-life care. These contextual shifts have eroded traditional support systems that once guided patients and their families through the unfamiliar territories of death and dying. Although modern medical care has the potential to delay death, and in some cases even seems to offer some hope for avoiding it, ultimately death prevails.

We will ask: In what context can timely death preparations reliably occur?

Evolution of the Hospital Context in the United States. The success stories of modern medical care in the last 50 years make it difficult to recall a time when the hospital was not seen as a place to be healed but rather as a place signifying death. Our ancestors would find it surprising that the modern hospital is now a place where patients sometimes plead to extend their stays, contesting the limitations mandated by cost-conscious insurance programs. Yet, this is just part of an ongoing evolutionary drift involving hospitals and the larger culture context. In his history of hospitals, Risse (1999) traced the evolution of the cultural meanings of hospitalization. He observed that hospitals were originally thought of as houses of "mercy, refuge, and dying" (p. 676). But, as a rudimentary understanding of contagion emerged, hospitals became houses of segregation used to isolate contagious patients from the rest of society. During the Enlightenment, the hospital increasingly became a house of science and research. The contemporary hospital has now become a "house of high technology" (p. 677).

With the secularization of hospitals and the shift away from providing a place of mercy and refuge, the patient as a biological entity has benefited in many ways, but the patient as a social being has also lost access to some of the community resources that once provided comfort when facing death. Risse wrote:

> Historically, hospitals have dealt openly with death and dying, with patients assembled in large wards routinely witnessing such events with a mixture of fear and comfort. . . . Before the Enlightenment, dying in hospitals was considered a blessing for believers expecting salvation. Surrounded by prayerful care givers and provided with the last sacraments, their redemption was complete. (p. 678)

As hospitals became secularized, they were forced to compete for funding and this, Risse argued, meant that hospitals began "shunning the fatally ill, viewing their management as a waste of their limited resources and their ultimate death as detrimental to an image built on low mortality statistics" (p. 679). Risse suggested that a slightly more benevolent version of this attitude is still with us. He wrote that "dying is frequently equated with treatment failure, and heroic efforts are made to prolong life at all costs" (p. 679).

Cancer as Case in Point. Today, families facing a cancer diagnosis typically do so within the hospital's curative context. It is estimated that 570,280 cancer-related deaths are expected to occur in 2005 (Jemal et al., 2005). A majority of terminally ill cancer patients suffer with unrelieved pain, unwanted intrusive life-sustaining measures, and delayed hospice referrals (Field & Cassel, 1997; Fins et al., 1999; SUPPORT, 1995). This too often becomes a "chronic crisis for cancer patients and their families who find no relief for months or years." Caplan (1971) described a crisis situation as existing "when a person faces an obstacle which is, for a time, insurmountable through the utilization of customary methods of problem solving. A period of disorganization ensues, a period of upset, during which many different abortive attempts to a solution are made" (cited in Woolley, 1990, p. 1403). Unfortunately, many health care providers are constrained by their training and the curative model of care leaves them unprepared to help patients and their families reorganize themselves around the management of a life-threatening condition. Misunderstandings, missed opportunities and unnecessary suffering result, as the evidence presented here suggests.

Conversations Matter

Larson and Tobin (2000) wrote that "For patients and families facing advanced illness, the medical interventions and quality of life that lie ahead are largely determined through a series of conversations they have with their physicians and other health care providers" (p. 1573). This, we believe, is particularly the case for end-of-life conversations in which quality of life can be enhanced. However problematic, conversations can have a significant impact on the quality of life as well, as the evidence reviewed here reveals. There is little research documenting the actual provider–patient dynamics regarding end-of-life. But we do have access to findings that support Kelly et al.'s (1997) multisite ethnography demonstrating that families and health care providers hold competing interpretations and concerns related to end-of-life decisions. Our review of this literature takes each perspective in turn, followed by an analysis of the communication impasse these juxtaposed perspectives create.

From the Provider's Perspective. According to a 1979 survey 97% of doctors told their cancer patients about their diagnosis, compared to only 10% who did so 30 years earlier (Freedman, 1993; Okum, 1961). Physicians are not as forthcoming regarding prognosis. Miyaji (1993) found vagueness among physicians when it comes to informing patients about their prognosis. He found that 84% of physicians thought their dying patients were aware of their prognosis. Only 50% of physicians actually told their patients of their prognosis. In a national survey of internists, 90% believed that doctors should try to avoid prognostication. Seventy-five percent replied that they "sometimes find it helpful to shade prognoses to the positive." Of these internists, 92% were "reluctant to make predictions about a patient's illness when the clinical situation is uncertain" and believe that patients expect "too much certainty." Eighty-eight percent reported that their patients "might lose confidence in them" if they are mistaken (Christakis & Iwashyna, 1998). A study by S. Johnston, Pfeifer, and McNutt (1995) revealed several reasons, according to physicians, that they do not discuss advance directives, including their fear of depressing or upsetting the patient. Some physicians reported that advance directives were "perceived as the beginning, not the end of the discussion" (Pfeifer et al., 1994).

Providers may block end-of-life conversations to avoid their awkwardness (Morrison, 1998). Schneiderman Kaplan, Pearlman, and Teetzel (1993) found that physicians' projections of what they believed to be their patient's preferences correlated more closely to their own preferences for less cardiopulmonary resuscitation (CPR) and more artificial nutrition and hydration than their patients. Missed opportunities for communication were identified in 29% of the family conferences that took place surrounding end-of-life decision making in the intensive care unit. Missed opportunities were defined as opportunities to (a) listen and respond to family members, (b) acknowledge and address emotions, and (c) pursue key principles of medical ethics and palliative care (Curtis et al., 2005).

Professional training in communication skills has not yet met the perceived need of nurses and physicians (Samaroo, 1996). The landmark Study to Understand Prognoses and Preferences for Outcomes and Risks of Treatment (SUPPORT) project found that even when providing a nurse to facilitate end-of-life discussions, most patients had not discussed advance directives with their physicians (Teno et al., 1997).

Our assessment of the providers' perspective is that their options for managing end-of-life conversations are limited by the curative and technological context the medical setting has become. This context offers them multiple justifications to focus on and even intensify the curative tools that have currency in the hospital context. Introducing the topic of death in this curative context places them at perceived risk of awkwardness, for creating anxiety or depression in the patient, or undermining their own credibility.

From the Patient's Perspective. Passage of the Patient Determination Act (PSDA) in 1990 required health care institutions to inform patients regarding their rights about decision making and advance directives. However, survey research reveals that although many patients want to talk about end-of-life issues (Lo, McLeod, & Saika, 1986; Miles, Koepp, & Weber, 1996; Reilly et al., 1994; Smucker et al., 1993; Tulsky, Fischer, Rose, & Arnold, 1998), it rarely happens. Happ et al. (1999) found that end-of-life discussions with frail older adults and their families were delayed until the death was imminent if conducted at all. This delay is often accompanied by a knowledge deficit on the part of both caregivers and patients, denial by the patient, the caretaker's reluctance to disclose bad news, and an overreliance on high technology (C. Johnson & Slanika,1999; Morris & Branon Christie, 1995).

Most patients believed that it is their doctor's responsibility to initiate a conversation about advance directives, according to a study of primary care patients by S. Johnston et al. (1995). The great majority believed that doctors should discuss advance directives before their patients become seriously ill (91%), and most patients (61%) thought that discussion should include others, including spouse or significant others.

In a study of older, chronically ill patients, 66% expressed an interest in discussing end-of-life decisions, but less than 10% had actually spoken to their doctor in this regard (Lo et al., 1986). Gamble, McDonald, and Lichstein (1991) found similar results in a survey of older patients who had discussed terminal care with their doctors 1 year after the passage of the PSDA. Of these patients, 63% initiated end-of-life discussions themselves. In a study of the impact of the PSDA on doctor–patient communication,

Bradley, Peiris, and Wetle (1998) found of the 40% of alert residents, less than one-third had held a discussion with their doctor related to these rights. The SUPPORT project involved more than 9,000 patients in five hospitals. In a subset of seriously ill patients, only 23% had talked with their doctors regarding CPR (Hofmann et al., 1997). A study of cancer patients in London found that of 101 patients, 95 wanted "as much information as possible, good or bad" (Fallowfield, Ford, & Lewis, 1994). End-of-life conversations may occur more often among older, more educated patients (Walker, Schonwetter, Kramer, & Robinson, 1995).

Pfeifer et al. (1994) found that of the 30% of patients with a life expectancy of less than 18 months, most wanted to receive end-of-life information "in an honest and straightforward manner." Patients' conversations are not always in alignment with their medical condition. They may steer conversations away from their "pain, self-blame, anger, loss, fear and other difficult experiences that could be the content of end-of-life discussions" (Larson & Tobin, 2000, p. 1573). Weeks et al. (1998) found that patients often overestimated their chances of survival. Family members may avoid conversations that could move the patient from a curative to a comfort form of care (Lynn et al., 2000). Butow et al. (1996) studied the psychological adjustment of patients with cancer. Although 57% wanted to discuss life expectancy with their providers, this only occurred in 27% of the cases.

Often, patients are frustrated by the lack of end-of-life conversations, but are reluctant to initiate them. The physician usually initiates and sets the tone for end-of-life communication, which often relegates the patient to a passive role thereby impacting the flow of communication. Here it makes more sense to not ask difficult questions, placing the responsibility for initiating discussions about death on the professionals in charge of their care.

Evolution of the Hospice Context

The increasing emphasis on the curative and the technical aspects of a medical cure has created an opening for alternative contexts that offer palliative care. Hospice is one such alternative. Consistent with its roots in medieval times, hospice is primarily concerned with providing comfort rather than cure. Historically, hospices were located along routes popular with travelers, crusaders, and pilgrims. These early refuges were primarily places of care (Lundgren & Chen, 1986). Stoddard (1978) explained that the ancient hospice provided "hospitality in its original sense of protection, refreshment, 'cherysshing,' and fellowship, rather than the demand of a patient for a cure" (p. 7, cited in Lundgren & Chen, 1986, p. 137).

As modern medical advances made patient cure a realistic option and as the science of pain management developed in the controlled setting of the hospital, the societal appeal of the hospice declined for all but those for whom medical cures were no longer possible. As Morris and Branon Christie (1995) observed, "the hospice often is seen as the place one goes to die, the place that says to the patient 'your end is near'" (p. 21). This is one of the reasons that, even among the terminally ill, less than 50% receive hospice care (E. Emanuel & Emanuel, 1998). Approximately one in five Medicare beneficiaries used hospice care in 1998, but the average period of hospice use has declined over the years with half of Medicare hospice users receiving care for 19 days or less and average length of hospice care at 1 week or less (U.S. Government Accountability Office, 2000).

The "hospice-as-place-to-die" metaphor obscures the original sense of hospice as a place of refreshment, fellowship, and care. It is the recognition of these important elements of support that has contributed to the recent growth in hospice care, particularly among patients with cancer. It is precisely those characteristics along with the possibility of home-based palliative care that many find lacking in the more cure-oriented contexts of modern hospitals.

End-of-life Communication and the Hospice Context

Several researchers and practitioners have offered approaches to end-of-life communication which, we believe, are more reliably conducted in the palliative setting of hospice, given its nurturing context, than in the hospital context.

A recent Institute of Medicine (1997) report recommends that end-of-life communication should involve:

> not only the preparation of legal documents but also discussions with family members and physicians about what the future may hold for people with serious illnesses, how patients and families want their beliefs and preferences to guide decisions (including decisions should sudden and unexpected critical medical problems arise), and what steps could alleviate concerns related to finances, family matters, spiritual questions, and other issues that trouble seriously ill or dying patients and their families. (p. 199)

Lo, Quill, and Tulsky (1999) said that "as patients struggle to find closure in their lives, active listening and empathy have therapeutic value in and of themselves" (p. 744). This is consistent with recent calls for treating elderly patients as "active interpreters, managers, and creators of the meaning of their health and illness" (Vanderford, Jenks, & Sharf, 1997, p. 14; Ragan, Wittenberg, & Hall, 2003).

Curtis et al. (2001) recommended a "family conference" as a way to help patients and families hold on while letting go. Specifically, they suggested "moving from hoping for recovery to hoping for some quality time together or for a comfortable death without pain or dyspnea and with as much dignity and meaning as possible" (p. 30). von Guten, Ferris, and Emanuel (2000) in their seven step approach for structuring end-of-life communication, recommended a family meeting, joined by the physician, during which unresolved intrafamily issues can be addressed. Bowman's (2000) family systems approach to end-of-life communication offers a similar acknowledgment of the importance of exploring families' interpretations and unresolved conflicts. Fins and Soloman (2001), Quill (2000), and Chopra (2001) call attention to the value of fostering continual healing relationships, as does the Institute of Medicine's (2001) recent report on quality of care, *Crossing the Quality Chasm.*

Ragan et al. (2003) observed that "all patients, terminal or otherwise, want pain and other noxious symptom management, but patients and their families and caretakers also realize that there are other, equally important concerns at the end-of-life and that PC [palliative care], ideally, should address these meaning of life issues as well as pain control" (p. 221). Ragan et al. suggested that palliative care must engage "existential issues of meaning, relationships, autonomy, guilt, dignity, and communication."

Balaban (2000), in discussing the essential communication elements of palliative care, describes it as "fearless healing." Fearless healing means listening to and talking about the things that are painful, including patients' and family members' suffering and loss. Fearless healing can also mean helping patients and family members "hold on and let go." As Bowman claimed, the "tension between holding onto and letting go of a dying loved one is enormous for any family but can be overwhelming for a family with unreconciled conflict" (2000, p. S19).

Ironically, hospice is the one context in the health care system that offers permission and the expertise to implement the kinds of end-of-life conversations recommended here. Hospice care can be an important resource offering precisely the sort of "cherysshing" that may make it possible to experience a high quality of life all the days, even the final days, of our lives. Sadly, few patients with diagnoses of terminal conditions go through these doors.

In summary, hospitals and hospices are not the bricks and mortar that make up their structure. They are the conversations and relational contexts that reinforce each other in shaping what can and cannot be discussed without awkwardness or sanction. The hospital and hospice contexts have created a modern dichotomy between cure and death, and in the kinds of conversations that can comfortably be held about these topics.

There is significant ambivalence and avoidance on both sides, creating an impasse: Patients say they want to talk about issues related to the dying process and many indicate they want the bad news with the good, but when faced with the crisis, avoid the subject in practice. Physicians also want to engage in these conversations but have several motivations to avoid them as well. As a result, in the aggregate, many patients and providers are stuck in patterns of communication in which patients are likely to be both overly dependent upon professionals for defining their fate and overly optimistic regarding their prognosis. Providers often act as though their patients already know they are dying. Discussions about palliative care and hospice options are functionally blocked. As Bowman (2000) noted, there is no consensus on the ethical and/or legal approach to communicating about end-of-life. In fact, providers and patients are more likely than not to define the end-of-life period in radically different ways (Kelly et al., 1997). This communication gap "often causes an impasse that is perceived as an either/or choice, and the opportunity to find creative solutions is diminished" (Bowman, 2000, p. S19).

More of the Same is Not the Answer. Some have suggested that more accurate prognosis (Lamont & Christakis, 2001) can move beyond denial and avoidance. Gochman and Bonham (1990) pointed out that if information about hospice is not provided around the time of the terminal diagnosis, the probability that the patient will make use of hospice care is very small. But this moment is more profound than that. More information is not a reliable solution when patients and providers are determined to interpret each other in ways that avoid the topic of death.

There are times when the provider-centric knowledge transfer model of communication is extremely useful. It is efficient in its linear simplicity. It justifiably thrives in the curative medical context where providers' certainty regarding medical interventions are evidence based. However, a terminal diagnosis, which is a medically defined interpretation, is unique in all of medicine in that it offers nothing to cure in a curative context. At this point and beyond, no one has definitive knowledge regarding the best plan of care. The provider and the dying patient who continue in a dance of avoidance are unintentionally perpetuating a pattern of overdependence on the one hand, and substandard palliative care on the other. The patient is overdependent on a provider-defined plan loaded with potentially unnecessary curative services. The result is that attention and resources are shifted away from palliative care. Next, we explain how this is so.

UNDERSTANDING THE INTERPERSONAL DYNAMICS OF END-OF-LIFE COMMUNICATION

As the research reviewed here demonstrates, doctors often assume or hope that their patients are aware of their prognosis and so do not dwell on potentially discouraging news. But patients assume that the doctor knows, and take silence on the topic to mean that there is still hope for a medical cure. This creates an impasse despite the good intentions of providers and patients. Here, a focus on the intentions and interpretations of the individual provider or patient will do little to break the impasse because the problem is not with either party—it is between them in their jointly produced interaction.

Interpersonal Logics

One way out of the impasse is to shift the focus from an individual unit of analysis to an interactional unit of analysis. We find it useful to understand end-of-life communication by looking to the interpersonal dynamics as the source of the impasse. Specifically, we view the impasse as a problem in coordinating competing meanings that frame doctor–patient talk about death (Pearce & Cronen, 1980). This assessment requires an interactional unit of analysis in order to understand the way two or more participants are making sense of a conversation. Based on the Coordinated Management of Meaning (Pearce & Cronen, 1980), the concept of "interpersonal logics" fulfills this requirement.

Interpersonal logics are simply a way to account for the juxtaposition of participants' moment-to-moment answers to the question, "What should I do next?" Each act in a conversation is contingent on the emergent context and on the sorts of outcomes that each speaker hopes to create as a result of the conversation. The resulting actions have an interesting kind of logic in that they are always slightly out of control. No individual controls the way the other will interpret a given action and respond to it. But the resulting conversation is not a random collection of spontaneous acts either. The conversation is a function of the rhetorical obligations each speaker feels in response to the acts of the other.

For example, the initial greeting between two strangers has an interpersonal logic that is shared within our culture. It is made up of obligatory reciprocal salutes that guide the joint performance of this ritual. The obligations are so strong for greeting encounters that even the slightest variation (e.g., a greeting between friends is not returned) can lead to awkwardness and even insults if not repaired with a justification accepted by one's greeting partner. Yet, it is misleading to suggest that the meaning of the failed greeting was determined unilaterally by the actions of the single individual. For example, using an individual unit of analysis to understand this interaction, either greeting partner who breaks a normative greeting rule may be viewed as socially incompetent or uncooperative. But clearly, many friendly greeting patterns involve an unexpected and even superficially insulting response. In contrast, when we use an interpersonal unit of analysis, we can assess the responses as they fit into the *larger pattern* of conversation, perhaps even including the relationship or cultural pattern. In this case, it is the greeting ritual itself and its fit within the interpersonal system that determines the level of competence and willingness (Harris, 1979) of the participants.

A similar observation can be made about the end-of-life communication impasse. Although the research suggests that patients and providers as individuals are willing to discuss end-of-life options, these conversations are delayed and are often unsatisfying as a result of the interpersonal logic produced when each responds to the other based on competing interpretations and goals.

Because interpersonal logics often produce interactional knots that generate repetitive action, they have also been described in terms of loops. One type of loop is what Cronen, Pearce, and Snavely (1979) described as an "undesirable repetitive pattern" or URP. Their research suggests that people can become locked in undesired patterns of interaction when they feel a strong obligation to respond to a particular communicative act. The response is primarily motivated by the existing situation and what was just said or done. An interesting feature of the URP is that even as people feel compelled to react, they simultaneously disassociate their own responses from the emerging episode of communication. They feel compelled to respond in a particular way, but they do not experience their voluntary action as either a choice or as an intentional act that was selected to provoke the enactment of the undesirable episode.

Communication impasses concerning end-of-life decisions may exhibit this looped form of interpersonal logic. Doctors and patients may feel a strong obligation to say or do something, yet they may not be aware that in giving what seem to be appropriate responses, they play into a larger interpersonal pattern that neither individual would choose. For example, a doctor trained in medical interventions may feel a strong sense of obligation to offer options consistent with that training. Yet, even after a terminal diagnosis, merely mentioning a possibility for a cure, no matter how remote, can be heard by the patient and family members as an option that must be explored. For their part, the patient and family feel that they cannot walk away from what they interpret as a potential cure. Even when the provider does not provoke this chain of events with the mention of experimental medical interventions, the patient or family may initiate the pattern by asserting that some sort of treatment must be out there. The urge, or what Pearce and Cronen (1980) would call the "logical force," to look for a miraculous medical intervention is an understandable response when patients frame the context of their care as "healing requires curing." In this context, nearly all statements by the provider have the potential to trigger a sequence of increasingly intrusive medical interventions with little or no attention paid to palliative care and meaningful discussions about the social, psychological, and spiritual needs of the dying person.

A second type of looped interpersonal logic involves reflexivity between levels of meaning (Cronen, Johnson, & Lannamann, 1982). Unlike the URPs that subvert the good intentions of communicators, reflexive loops sometimes swallow the whole context in which actions are made meaningful. Cronen et al. (1982) use the term *strange loops* to refer to this form of reflexive loops. Strange loops confound the levels of context communicators use to make sense of their actions. A simple example of a strange loop is the command "be spontaneous." Here, the logic is looped because the relational context necessary to command another's action is contradicted by the content of the command. To be spontaneous requires that we not follow another's directions, yet the other has commanded we do precisely that. A strange loop puts people in a double bind where every action seems to change meaning and none of the options allow an escape from the loop. Trying harder within this logic only roots its participants more firmly in their competing justifications for repeating them as anyone who has told or been told "You never bring me flowers" can attest.

Not all reflexive loops are strange. We rely on contextual clues to understand the meaning of what is said. But, as the examples above illustrate, what is said and done is not just shaped by context—communicative action also shapes that context. When an action confirms or strengthens the expected context, it implies future actions that are consistent with that frame. In this situation, the loop is a self-confirming one and is referred to by Cronen et al. as *charmed*.

An example of a charmed loop in the curative context concerns the reflexivity between three levels: the context of cure, the relational context in which the doctor is seen as an expert, and the communicative episode of diagnosis. In this case, the curative context legitimates the doctor as having an expert opinion. The act of diagnosing a patient confirms this expertise and strengthens the contextual frame that gives shape to the entire enterprise as being about finding a cure. We can diagram this charmed loop as follows. The direction of the arrows can be read as a shorthand for "means that . . .".

Curative Context

↑ ↓

Doctor is the expert

↑ ↓

Give diagnosis

Each element in this charmed loop reinforces the other. In contrast, in a strange loop, one level paradoxically refutes the meaning of the other levels, producing shifts in meaning that can result in confusion, a sense of paralysis, or repetitive attempts to escape the paradox that ultimately continues the vicious cycle.

The end-of-life communication impasse offers one such example of a strange loop. One half of this strange loop looks like the charmed loop just described. In a context of seeking a cure, the doctor is considered an expert who is able to offer medical opinions to diagnose patients. However, offering a terminal diagnosis is a form of medical evaluation that then changes the context. The terminal diagnosis moves the patient from the frame of "seeking cure" to "facing death." This shifts the relational frame. Stripped of the possibility of offering a medical cure, the doctor is no longer the expert on how to proceed. Authority shifts to the patient who now must decide what to do. But here the loop continues. As we saw in the discussion of the undesirable pattern, the patient and family often feel compelled to seek options and their search for options can re-assert the "seek cure" context that then re-establishes the medical sequence. A temporary charmed loop may follow in which patients endure increasingly intrusive medical interventions, each of which confirms the expertise of the doctor in the medical context until, eventually, the terminal diagnosis is given. The loop becomes strange again until time or money runs out.

Strange Loop of Terminal Diagnosis:

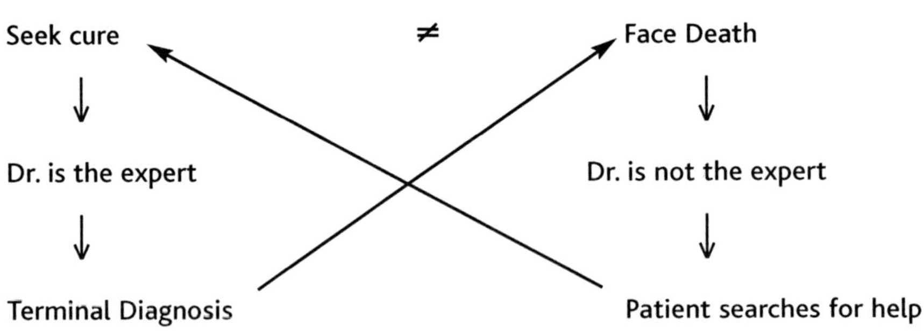

The result of this strangely looped interpersonal logic can be a desperate pattern of overdependence on medical technology with too little discussion of palliative care options.

A DIALOGIC INTERVENTION

Like many paradoxes, the end-of-life strange loop is held together by a cultural assumption that serves as the overarching context for the various intertwined levels of meaning. The organizing assumption of this loop is the commonsense premise that healing requires curing. Consistent with the historical evolution of hospitals and medical technology, the assumption that healing requires curing locates the physician at the center of decision-making discussions and marginalizes the voices of the patient and support givers. When a physician provides a terminal diagnosis, the patient is suddenly thrown into a new context with few signposts for guidance. The bleak choice of seeking a cure or facing death leaves little room for discussing new ways to construct the meaning of care at the end-of-life. A first step toward ending the end-of-life communication impasse would be to loosen the grip of the cure or death frame, not by doing more of the same, but by questioning the orienting assumption that healing requires curing. This necessitates a dialogue to open space for new voices and potentially, a new context of healing that is not limited to curing.

We propose an intervention in which dying patients and their significant others assume the lead in care planning conversations. This intervention has a broad interdisciplinary theoretical heritage spanning family systems theory, social construction, and complexity sciences that we review briefly here. These approaches feature an interpersonal unit of analysis and highlight dialogue as a central feature of knowledge creation and change. We then discuss the dialogical underpinnings of these approaches to set the stage for a family-centered care-planning scenario.

Theoretical Support

Watzlawick, Beavin, and Jackson (1967) and others (Selvini Palazzoli, Boscolo, Cecchin, & Prata, 1980; Watzlawick, Weakland, & Fisch, 1974) involved in family systems therapy and organizational change management would argue that to the extent that practitioners and patients are locked into a dysfunctional communication pattern there is little room for change. In fact, therapists often find that they are inducted into the dysfunctional pattern of the family by the compelling interpersonal logic that quickly incorporates attempts to change into a pattern of more of the same. Focusing on trying to change individual behaviors and meanings tends only to perpetuate the problem because the pattern is an interpersonal one. Therapists working in the systems tradition have long used an interpersonal unit of analysis for their understanding of communication, knowledge creation, and change. Social constructionists (Chumbler et al., in press; Harris et al., 2004;

McNamee & Gergen, 1999; Potter & Wetherell, 1987; Shotter, 1993) also call attention to the importance of relational processes as the source of meaning and action. Similarly, those working in the tradition of complexity sciences highlight the processual, interdependent nature of knowledge. Stacey (2001, 2003), in describing how people self-organize, argued that knowledge "is always a process, and a relational one at that. . . . Knowledge is the act of conversing, and learning occurs when ways of talking and therefore patterns of relationship change" (Stacey, 2001, p. 98). To change the patterns of relationships that characterize the end-of-life communication impasse, it is necessary to begin new conversations.

In the following sections, we review a dialogic model used in family therapy and organizational consulting. We then explore the implications of extending this model of communication to the end-of-life setting.

A dialogic approach to communication emphasizes the relational quality of understanding and the importance of joint action. It shifts attention away from the idea of knowledge as a commodity that is exchanged between two parties. A dialogic approach does not discount medical expertise and the value of specialized training. Rather, a dialogic approach suggests that to be useful, knowledge must be situated in a relational context. Knowledge becomes useful when it is addressed to someone who makes it relevant through a process of conversational give and take. This is consistent with recent calls by Vanderford et al. (1997) and Ragan et al. (2003) to tap into the meaning-making capabilities of patients.

The Russian literary critic Bakhtin, one of the pioneers of dialogic thinking, helps us to understand why dialogue is so important at times of crisis. He pointed out that "understanding is actively *responsive*" (Bakhtin, 1986, p. 69). Verbal information is not shared, as a book might be when passed from one friend to another. Rather, spoken words are shaped for the listener who understands them by answering to their call. Speakers, Bakhtin argued, expect "response, agreement, sympathy, objection, execution, and so forth" (p. 69) because these allow a mutual adjustment to and coordination of the emerging flow of conversation.

Dialogic understanding seems particularly important in end-of-life care because it opens a space for patients and their communities of support to actively shape the meaning of their lives together. Compared to models of communication that focus on transmission and information exchange, dialogic approaches are less likely to encounter the various barriers that inhibit initiating palliative care because a responsive dialogue requires that each person experience the multiple voices of the other, including both the hopes and fears of those facing a crisis. The dialogic approach is consistent with Balaban's (2000) notion of "fearless healing," which proposes that health professionals listen to and talk about the things that are painful, including patients' and family members' suffering and loss. A relationally situated, responsive encounter fosters a kind of understanding that is improvisational, going beyond the either/or interpretive frames of "cure or death" and "medical intervention or comfort." We expect that improvisational dialogue can help families reorganize around their crisis in ways that are not likely to be considered within the provider–patient dialogue alone. Additionally, a dialogic approach to end-of-life communication recognizes the multiple voices with which patients, doctors, family, and friends speak. Opening space for these multiple voices is the hallmark of a dialogic approach.

The Open Dialogue Model

Open dialogue is based on a dialogic model developed by Finnish psychiatrist Jaakko Seikkula and his colleagues (Seikkula, 2002; Seikkula et al., 1995). They have demonstrated the utility of social knowledge construction in their work with patients struggling with psychosis. Drawing on Bakhtin's (Bakhtin et al., 1986) observations about the dialogic basis of understanding, Seikkula shifted the traditional focus of medical intervention away from the isolated individual in order to treat the patient as a whole person who is sustained by a larger community. This commitment to understanding the patient as shaped by his or her community requires that Seikkula and his colleagues attempt to bring other voices into the therapeutic dialogue. These "other voices" may include the multiple aspects of the patient whose identity is a composite of many inner voices. The treatment discussion also engages the voices of those other significant people who respond to and define the patient. The result is what Seikkula called an "open dialogue," where the boundaries between the traditional "treatment team" are expanded to include all those who are invested in the patient's situation.

Seikkula et al. (1995) observe that when the treatment team is expanded and open dialogue encouraged, "the joint process itself started to determine the treatment, rather than the team itself or the treatment plan of the team" (p. 64). This observation suggests that a similar approach might interrupt the undesirable repetitive patterns characterizing the doctor–patient communication impasse at the end-of-life. Specifically, adding new voices to the discussion may provide unique resources for a patient in need of options when faced with a terminal diagnosis. Instead of continuing to search for new options only in the curative context of medical care, the patient can begin to explore healing options that are palliative, not just curative. This is an important shift because it diffuses the assumption that healing is limited to curing. When that context is changed, the interpersonal logic of the strange loop of cure or death loses some of its force.

Resource Inquiry. Resource inquiry (McNamee, 2004) aims to tap the potential creativity generated in open dialogue processes, particularly when the process involves envisioning possibilities that embrace the strengths of the dialogue participants. It involves asking questions that evoke participants' creative interpretations. Based on therapeutic and organizational change experiences we suspect that resource inquiry brings a comforting quality to the creative process. That is, people are comforted when their own meanings are given social life.

Resource inquiry is based on appreciative inquiry, which was originally developed for organizational consulting by Cooperrider (1990). This inquiry, based on a reframing of organizational problems, involves asking members of the organization to give voice to times when their commitment to the group was at its greatest, when they felt the organization was at its best. By engaging members in this discussion, Cooperrider is inviting the members to narrate what is possible and to imagine the specific steps that could be taken to construct that future. Although this approach has not yet been widely used to handle the organizational crises families face during end-of-life care, it is not unreasonable to assume that the same creative energies unleashed when organizations develop positive metaphors to imagine the future can also benefit families searching for ways to make sense of post-diagnosis decisions.

Through resource inquiry, end-of-life dialogues can become a context for exploring and appreciating the narrative and interpretive resources that members of the family and friends bring to the situation. It should lead to the collective constructing of future possibilities, some of which will diffuse the logic of the cure or death frame that fuels the patterns of avoidance and delay when it comes to planning for early palliative care.

Family-Centered Care-Planning Scenario

We have characterized the end-of-life communication impasse as caused by a paradoxical interpersonal logic, which is both guiding and justifying unintentional avoidance of talk about the implications of a terminal diagnosis. Our synthesis of this patterned discourse suggests a conflicting set of rhetorical obligations (Don't tell/Don't ask) constrains providers and patients to talk about curative care, while avoiding talk about palliative care.

Breaking Through. We envision an intervention scenario that would be triggered by a life-threatening diagnosis. This is in line with the recommendations of the World Health Organization, which has reconceptualized and redefined palliative care to begin at the time a diagnosis of illness is made. Likewise, Wenrich et al. (2001) suggested that the most appropriate time to consider all care options is at the time a terminal condition is diagnosed. Following Seikkula et al. (1995), we propose the doctor organize a family care-planning open dialogue in which the patient is asked to choose those family members, friends, and providers he or she would like to have included in the discussion. We expect that this will subtly shift the logic of the URP that constrains doctor–patient communication. The prescription by the doctor for an open dialogue plays into the "doctor is the expert" relational context, but the very structure of the open dialogue diffuses this authority and opens the possibility for creating novel responses to the crisis. Used this way, the open dialogue model is consistent with evidence that patients want to include others in their conversations at this time.

All dialogue participants would be invited to offer possibilities for diagnosis, prognosis, and future care options, and to respond to the possibilities offered by others. The knowledge regarding how to proceed reflects a dialogic understanding of the crisis; that is, a way of knowing what to do that is unique to each patient's support community.

This would differ from the current format of the conventional family conference in that we expect process, not the doctor to determine the agenda. In a fully responsive and open dialogue, no one leads the conversation. Instead, each participant responds to the emerging conversation in a way that gives voice to his or her concerns. This means that values will emerge as a function of the dialogue rather than being "discovered."

As Bateson and his family illustrated, family dialogue and palliative care can become one in the same when care becomes a ritual, even at the time of death.

A persistent theme in Bateson's writing is that meaning, quality, and beauty are possible only in the context of a pattern of connections. In that sense, the meaning and quality of his end-of-life experience was a continuation of his pattern of living.

For families who already have an open, dialogic form of patterned communication, the practice of planning care options will simply provide a platform for them to continue co-creating futures. For families who have not learned to perform meaning-creation rituals, the open dialogue at the time of diagnosis could usher in their first forms of therapeutic communication and may allow them to create comforting rituals before and after the end of a loved one's life. To the extent that the open dialogue model allows the construction of narratives that continue long after the initial meeting, there is, we believe, even a place for family conversational rituals among the survivors after a death because a life "carries on in a narrative sense, long after the physical body is dead" (Hedtke & Winslade, 2004, p. 199).

The barriers that inhibit an early discussion of the patient's prognosis and other end-of-life concerns are powerful in the context of cure or death, but when healing is expanded to include both the biomedical subject and the social subject, healing is no longer limited to cures. This suggests that dialogic interventions offer a way out of the paradox of end-of-life communication consistent with Cicely Saunders' declaration that "We don't have to cure to heal."

Based on the theoretical models, we propose that the dialogic intervention will have the following impact:

- By expanding the relational context to include significant others, each with a unique perspective on how to manage a crisis, the group is expected to self-organize around a future that is not constrained by the "Seek Cure or Face Death" dichotomy in which the doctor–patient dyad interaction had been stuck.
- By introducing new narratives through resource inquiry, members of the open dialogue sessions will generate alternatives to the "Healing = Curing" frame, thereby dismantling the context of the strange loop impasse at end-of-life.
- The self–organizing process will have its own therapeutic value for families that have become disorganized by this crisis, particularly as members see their own meaning come to life.
- By turning over the care planning to patients and their significant others, the overdependence on the doctor at a time when the doctor has limited solutions is diminished.
- Making family-centered care-planning dialogues a part of the standard of care at diagnosis normalizes a family framed plan of care, thereby granting it and its care options legitimacy.
- A family context will be a more reliable context for considering palliative and hospice care than the current medicalized context.
- Patients, as a result of continued care-planning dialogues, will participate in hospice care earlier than those locked in the end-of-life communication impasse.
- Patients who engage in continued care planning dialogues will experience a higher quality of life than those who receive standard post-diagnosis care.

CONCLUSION

We opened this chapter by asking: "In what context can timely death preparations reliably occur?" We have argued that within the curative context, doctor-led conversations about death are very difficult to bring about. We have also tried to make the case that in the unique instance in which the doctor believes the patient has a terminal condition, post-diagnosis planning conversations are best led by the patients and their self-selected support communities. We do not attempt to predict specific words that will be spoken to break through the end-of-life communication in this newly formed family context. We do expect that new ways of relating will yield new ways of knowing and doing that will become more precious to the participants than curative technologies.

REFERENCE

Bakhtin, M. M. (1986). The problem of speech genres. In C. Emerson & M. Holquist (Eds.), *Speech genres and other late essays*, (pp. 60-102). Austin: University of Texas Press.

Balaban, R. B. (2000). A physician's guide to talking about end-of-life care. *Journal of General Internal Medicine, 15*, 195-200.

Bateson, M. C. (1980, Winter). Six days of dying. *The CoEvolution Quarterly,* pp. 4-11.

Bowman, K. W. (2000). Communication, negotiation, and mediation: Dealing with conflict in end-of-life decisions. *Journal of Palliative Care, 16*(Suppl.), S17-S23.

Bradley, E. H., Peiris, V., & Wetle T. (1998). Discussions about end-of-life care in nursing homes. *Journal of American Geriatrics Society, 46*, 1235-1241.

Butow P. N., Kazemi, J. N., Beeney, L. J., Griffin, A. M., Dunn, S. M., & Tattersall, M. H. (1996). When the diagnosis is cancer: Patient communication experiences and preferences. *Cancer, 77*, 2630-2637.

Caplan, G. (1971). *An approach to community mental health.* New York: Grune & Stratton.

Chopra, A. (2001). Communicating effectively at the end-of-life. *Journal of the American Osteopathic Association, 101*, 594-598.

Christakis, N. A., & Iwashyna, T. J. (1998). Attitude and self-reported practice regarding prognostication in a national sample of internists. *Archives of Internal Medicine, 158*, 2389-2395.

Chumbler, N., Richardson, L., Harris, L., Ryan, P., Kobb, R., Darkins, A., & McCarthy, C. (in press). Cancer care dialogues: Empirical support for complex adaptive systems research and practice. In P. Whitten, G. Kreps, & M. Eastin (Eds.), *E-health: The advent of online cancer information systems.* Cresskill, NJ: Hampton Press.

Cooperrider, D. L. (1990). Positive image, positive action: The affirmative basis of organizing. In S. Srivastva & D. L. Cooperrider (Eds.), *Appreciative management and leadership: The power of positive thought and action in organizations.* San Francisco, CA: Jossey-Bass.

Cronen, V. E., Johnson, K. M., & Lannamann, J. W. (1982). Paradoxes, double binds and reflexive loops: A comparison of two theoretical perspectives and a suggested methodology. *Family Process, 21*, 91-112.

Cronen, V.E., Pearce, W.B., & Snavely, L.M. (1979). A theory of role-structure and types of episodes and study of perceived enmeshment in undesired repetitive patterns ("URPs"). In D. Nimmo (Ed.), *Communication yearbook* (Vol. 3, pp. 225-240). New Brunswick, NJ: Transaction Books.

Curtis, J.R., Engelberg, R.A., Wenrich, M.D., Shannon, S.E., Treece, P.D., & Rubenfeld, G.D. (2005). Missed opportunities during family conferences about end-of-life care in the intensive care unit. *American Journal of Respiratory and Critical Care Medicine, 171*, 844-849.

Curtis, J.R., Patrick, D.L., Shannon, S.E., Treece, P.D., Engelberg, R.A., & Rubenfeld, G.D. (2001). The family conference as a focus to improve communication about end-of-life care in the intensive care unit: Opportunities for improvement. *Critical Care Medicine, 29*(Suppl.), N26-N33.

Emanuel, E.J., & Emanuel, L.L. (1998). The promise of a good death. *Lancet, 351*(Suppl. 2), SII21-29.

Fallowfield, I.J., Ford, S., & Lewis, S. (1994). Information preferences of patients with cancer. *Lancet, 344*, 1576.

Field, M., & Cassel, C. (Ed.). (1997). *Approaching death: Improving care at the end of life.* Washington, DC: National Academy Press.

Finnegan, J.R., & Viswanth, K. (1990). Health and communication: Medical and public health influences on the research agenda. In J. Bryant (Ed.), *Communication and health: Systems and Applications* (pp. 9-24). Mahwah, NJ: Erlbaum

Fins, J.J., Miller, F.G., Acres, C.A., Bachatta, M.D., Huzzard, L.L., & Rapkin, B.D. (1999). End-of-life decision-making in the hospital: Current practice and future prospects. *Journal of Pain Symptom Management, 17*, 6-15.

Fins, J.J., & Soloman, M.Z. (2001). Communication in intensive care settings: The challenge of futility disputes. *Critical Care Medicine, 29*(Suppl.), 10-15.

Freedman, B. (1993). Offering truth: One ethical approach to the uninformed cancer patient. *Archives Internal Medicine, 153*, 572-576.

Gamble, E.R., McDonald, P.J., & Lichstein, P.R. (1991). Knowledge, attitudes, and behavior of elderly persons regarding living wills. *Archives of Internal Medicine, 151*, 277-280.

Gochman E. S., & Bonham, G. S. (1990) The social structure of the hospice decision. *Hospice Journal, 6*, 15-36.

Happ, M.B., Capezuti, E., Strumpf, N., & Wagner, L. (1999). Advance care planning and end-of-life care for nursing home residents. *The Gerontologist, 39* (Special Issue I), 60.

Harris, L. M., Kobb, R., Ryan, P., Darkins, A., & Kreps, G. L. (2004). Research as dialogue: Health communication and behavior change in patients' natural habitat. In P. Whitten & D. Cook (Eds.), *Understanding health communication technologies* (pp. 91-100). San Francisco: Jossey-Bass.

Harris, L. M. (1979). *Communication competence: Empirical tests of a systemic model.* Unpublished doctoral dissertation, University of Massachusetts, Cambridge.

Hedtke, L., & Winslade, J. (2005). The use of the subjunctive in re-membering conversations with those who are grieving. *Journal of Death & Dying, 50*, 197-215.

Hofmann, J. C., Wenger, N.S., Davis, R. B., Teno, J., Connors, A. F., Jr., Desbiens, N., Lynn, J., & Phillips, R. (1997). Patient preferences for communication with physicians about end-of-life decisions. *Annals of Internal Medicine, 127*, 1-12.

Institute of Medicine. (1997). *Approaching death: Improving care at the end-of-life.* Washington, DC: National Academy of Sciences.

Institute of Medicine. (2001). *Crossing the quality chasm: A new health system for the 21*st *century* (M. J. Field & C. K. Cassel, Eds.). Washington, DC: National Academy of Sciences.

Jemal, A., Murray, T., Ward, E., Samuels, A., Tiwari, R. C., Ghafoor, A., Feuer, E. J., & Thun, M. J. (2005). Cancer statistics, 2005. *CA: A Journal for Clinicians, 55*, 10-30.

Johnson, C. B., & Slaninka, S. C. (1999). Barriers to accessing hospice services before a late terminal stage. *Death Studies, 23*, 225-238.

Johnston, S. G, Pfeifer, M. P., & McNutt, R. (1995). The discussion about advance directives: Patient and physician opinions regarding when and how it should be conducted. End-of-life Study Group. *Archives of Internal Medicine, 155*, 1025-1030.

Kelly, S. E., Marshall, P. A., Sanders, L. M., Raffin, T. A., & Koeing, B. A. (1997). Understanding the practice of ethics consultation: Results of an ethnographic multi-site study. *Journal of Clinical Ethics, 8*, 136-149.

Lamont, E.B., & Christakis, N. (2001). Prognostic disclosure to patients with cancer near the end-of-life. *Annuals of Internal Medicine, 10*, 1096-1105.

Larson, D. G., & Tobin D. R. (2000). End-of-life conversations: Evolving practice and theory. *Journal of the American Medical Association, 284*, 1573-1578.

Lo, B., McLeod, G. A., & Saika, G. (1986). Patient attitudes to discussing life-sustaining treatment. *Archives of Internal Medicine, 146*, 1613-1615.

Lo, B., Quill, T., & Tulsky, J. (1999). Discussing palliative care with patients. *Annals of Internal Medicine, 130*, 744-749.

Lundgren, L.M., & Chen, S. (1986). Hospice: Concept and implementation in the black community. *Journal of Community Health Nursing, 3*, 137-144.

Lynn J., Arkes, H. R., Stevens M., Cohn, F., Koenig, B., Fox, E., Dawson, N. V., Phillips, R. S., Hamel, M. B., & Tsevat, J. (2000). Rethinking fundamental assumptions: SUPPORT's implications for future reform. *Journal of American Geriatrics Society, 48*(Suppl. 15), S214-S221.

McNamee, S. (2004). *Using conversational spaces to create communities of inquiry.* Seminar presented at Creating Communities of Inquiry: Using Conversational Spaces to Enhance Teaching and Learning, Fitchburg State College, MA.

McNamee, S., & Gergen, K. J. (1999). *Relational responsibility: Resources for sustainable dialogue*. Thousand Oaks, CA: Sage.

Miles, S. H., Koepp, R., & Weber, E. P. (1996). Advance end-of-life treatment planning: A research review. *Archives of Internal Medicine, 156*, 1062-1068.

Miyaji, N. T. (1993). The power of compassion: Truth-telling among American doctors in the care of dying patients. *Social Science & Medicine, 36*, 249-264.

Morris, R., & Branon Christie, K. M. (1995). Initiating hospice care: Why, when, and how. *Home Healthcare Nurse, 13*(5), 21-26.

Morrison, M. F. (1998). Obstacles to doctor-patient communication at the end-of-life. In M. D. Steinberg & S. J. Youngner (Eds.) *End-of-life decisions: A psychosocial perspective* (pp. 109-136). Washington DC: American Psychiatric Press.

Okum, D. (1961). What to tell cancer patients. *JAMA, 175*, 86-94.

Pearce, W. B, & Cronen, V. E. (1980). *Communication, action and meaning: The creation of social realities*. New York: Praeger

Pfeifer, M. P., Sidorov, J. E., Smith A.C., Boero, J. F., Evans, A. T., & Settle, M. B. (1994). The discussion of end-of-life medical care by primary care patients and physicians. *Journal of General Internal Medicine, 9*, 82-88.

Potter, J., & Wetherell, M. (1987). *Discourse and social psychology: Beyond attitudes and behaviour*. London & Newbury Park, CA: Sage.

Quill, T. E. (2000). Initiating end-of-life discussions with seriously ill patients: Addressing the "elephant in the room." *Journal of the American Medical Association, 284*, 2502-2507.

Ragan, S. L., Wittenberg, E., & Hall, H. T. (2003). The communication of palliative care for the elderly patient. *Health Communication, 15*, 219-226.

Reilly, B. M., Magnussen, C. R., Ross, J., Ash, J., Papa, L., & Wagner, M. (1994). Can we talk? Inpatient discussions about advance directives in a community hospital. *Archives of Internal Medicine, 154*, 2299-2308.

Risse, G. B. (1999). *Mending bodies, saving souls: A history of hospitals*. New York: Oxford University Press.

Samaroo, B. (1996). Assessing palliative care educational needs of physicians and nurses: Results of a survey. Greater Victoria Hospital Society Palliative Care Committee. *Journal of Palliative Care, 12*(2), 20-22.

Schneiderman, L. J., Kaplan, R. M., Pearlman, R. A., & Teetzel, H. (1993). Do physicians' own preferences for life-sustaining treatment influence their perceptions of patients' preferences? *Journal of Clinical Ethics, 4*, 28-32.

Seikkula, J. (2002). Open dialogues with good and poor outcomes for psychotic crises: Examples from families with violence. *Journal of Marital & Family Therapy, 28*, 263-274.

Seikkula, J., Alakara, B., Haarakangas, K., Keranen, J., & Sutela, M. (1995). Treating psychosis by means of open dialogue. In S. Friedman (Ed.), *The reflecting team in action* (pp. 62-80). New York: Guilford Press.

Selvini Palazzoli, M., Boscolo, L., Cecchin, G., & Prata, G. (1980). Hypothesizing-circularity-neutrality: Three guidelines for the conductor of the session. *Family Process, 19*, 3 .

Shotter, J. (1993). *Conversational realities: Constructing life through language*. London, Thousand Oaks, CA: Sage.

Smucker, W. D., Ditto, P. H., Moore, K. A., Druley, J. A., Danks, J. H., & Townsend, A. (1993). Elderly outpatients respond favorably to a physician-initiated advance directive discussion. *Journal of the American Board of Family Practice, 6*, 473-483.

Stacey, R. D. (2001). *Complex responsive processes in organizations: Learning and knowledge creation*. London & New York: Routledge.

Stacey, R. D. (2003). *Complexity and group processes: A radically social understanding of individuals*. Hove & New York: Brunner-Routledge.

Stoddard, S. (1978). *The hospice movement: A better way of caring for the dying*. New York: Stein & Day.

The SUPPORT Principal Investigators. (1995). A controlled trial to improve care for seriously ill hospitalized patients: The Study to Understand Prognoses and Preferences for Outcomes and Risks of Treatments (SUPPORT). *JAMA, 274*, 1591-1598.

Teno, J., Lynn, J., Wenger, N., Phillips, R. S., Murphy, D. P., Connors, A. F., Desbiens, N., Fulkerson, W., Bellamy, P., & Knaus, W. A. (1997). Advance directives for seriously ill hospitalized patients: Effectiveness with the patient self-determination act and the SUPPORT intervention. SUPPORT Investigators.

The Study to Understand Prognoses and Preferences for Outcomes and Risks of Treatment. *Journal of the American Geriatrics Society, 45*, 500-507.
Tulsky, J. A., Fischer, G. S., Rose, M. R., Arnold, R. M. (1998). Opening the black box: How do physicians communicate about advance directives? *Annals of Internal Medicine, 129*, 441-449.
U.S. Government Accountability Organization. (2000). *More beneficiaries use hospice but for fewer days of care* (GAO/HEHS-00-182). Washington, DC: Author.
Vanderford M. L., Jenks E. B., & Sharf B. F. (1997). Exploring patients' experiences as a primary source of meaning. *Health Communication, 9*, 13-26.
von Gunten, C. F., Ferris, F. D., & Emanuel, L. L. (2000). Ensuring competency in end-of-life care: Communication and relational skills. *JAMA, 284*, 3051-3057.
Walker, R. M., Schonwetter, R. S., Kramer, D. R., & Robinson, B. E. (1995). Living wills and resuscitation preferences in an elderly population. *Archives of Internal Medicine, 155*, 171-175.
Watzlawick, P., Beavin, J. B., & Jackson, D. D. (1967). *Pragmatics of human communication; a study of interactional patterns, pathologies, and paradoxes.* New York: Norton.
Watzlawick, P., Weakland, J. H., & Fisch, R. (1974). *Change; principles of problem formation and problem resolution.* New York: Norton.
Weeks, J.C., Cook, E. F., O'Day, S. J., Peterson, L. M., Wenger, N., Reading, D., Harrell, F. E., Kussin, P., Dawson, N. V., Connors, Jr., A. F., Lynn, J., & Phillips, R. S. (1998). Relationship between cancer patients' predictions of prognosis and their treatment preferences. *JAMA, 279*, 1709-1714.
Wenrich, M. D., Curtis, J. R., Shannon, S. E., Carline, J., Ambrozy, D., & Ramsey, P. (2001) Communicating with dying patients within the spectrum of medical care from terminal diagnosis to death. *Archives of Internal Medicine, 161*, 868-874.
Woolley N. (1990) Crisis theory: A paradigm of effective intervention with families of critically ill people. *Journal of Advanced Nursing, 15*, 1402-1408.

Author Index

B

D

K

L

N

Q

R

S

T

Y

Subject Index

Printed in the United States
136020LV00002B/14/P

9 781572 737549